PROGRESS IN OBSTETRICS AND GYNAECOLOGY

PROGRESS IN OBSTETRICS AND GYNAECOLOGY

Contents of Volume 11

ISBN 0443 05059 7

PROGRESS IN OBSTETRICS AND GYNAECOLOGY
Volume Twelve

EDITED BY

JOHN STUDD DSc MD FRCOG

Consultant Gynaecologist, Fertility and
Endocrinology Centre, The Lister Hospital and
Chelsea and Westminster Hospital,
London, UK

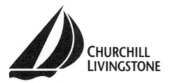
CHURCHILL
LIVINGSTONE

EDINBURGH LONDON NEW YORK PHILADELPHIA SAN FRANCISCO SYDNEY AND TORONTO 1998

CHURCHILL LIVINGSTONE
An imprint of Harcourt Brace and Company Limited

© Pearson Professional Ltd 1996
© Harcourt Brace and Company Limited 1998

⬗ is a registered trademark of Harcourt Brace and Company
Limited.

First published 1996
  Reprinted 1998

ISBN 0 443 05307 3
ISSN 0261 0140

British Library Cataloguing in Publication Data
A catalogue record for this book is available from the
British Library.

Library of Congress Cataloging-in-Publication Data
is available

Note
Medical knowledge is constantly changing. As new information
becomes available, changes in treatment, procedures, equipment
and the use of drugs become necessary. The editors/authors/contributors
and the publishers have, as far as it is possible, taken care to ensure that
the information given in this text is accurate and up to date. However,
readers are strongly advised to confirm that the information, especially
with regard to drug usage, complies with latest legislation and standards
of practice.

The
publisher's
policy is to use
**paper manufactured
from sustainable forests**

Produced by Addison Wesley Longman Singapore Pte Ltd
Printed in Singapore

Contents

PART ONE: OBSTETRICS

PART TWO: GYNAECOLOGY

Contributors

Julian W. Barrington MA MB BChir MRCOG
Senior Registrar, Department of Obstetrics and Gynaecology, Singleton Hospital, Swansea National Health Services Trust, Swansea, UK

Robin W. Burr MB ChB MRCOG
Research Fellow, Academic Department of Obstetrics and Gynaecology, Keele University and North Staffordshire Hospital, Stoke on Trent, UK

Tim Chard MD FRCOG
Professor, Department of Reproductive Physiology, St Bartholomew's Hospital, London, UK

F. A. Chervenak MD
Director of Maternal-Fetal Medicine, Department of Obstetrics and Gynecology, The New York Hospital-Cornell Medical Center, New York, USA

Ian D. Cooke FRCOG
Professor and Academic Head, Department of Obstetrics and Gynaecology, University of Sheffield, Jessop Hospital for Women, Sheffield, UK

Sean R. G. Duffy MD FRCS(G) MRCOG
Senior Lecturer in Obstetrics and Gynaecology, School of Medicine, Division of Obstetrics and Gynaecology, St James's University Hospital, Leeds, UK

Ailsa E. Gebbie MB ChB MRCOG
Senior Registrar in Community Gynaecology, Family Planning and Well Woman Services, Edinburgh Healthcare NHS Trust, Edinburgh, UK

Janesh K. Gupta MSc MRCOG
Senior Registrar in Obstetrics and Gynaecology, Department of Obstetrics and Gynaecology, Ninewells Hospital and Medical School, Dundee, UK

E. Hiadzi MRCOG
Senior Registrar, Ghana Police Hospital, Accra, Ghana

Laurie Montgomery Irvine MD MRCOG
Consultant Obstetrician and Gynaecologist, Department of Obstetrics and Gynaecology, Mount Vernon and Watford General Hospitals NHS Trust, Watford General Hospital, Watford, UK

Ian Jacobs MD MRCOG
CRC McElwain Fellow in Gynaecological Oncology, CRC Human Cancer Genetics Research Group, Department of Pathology, Cambridge University and Ovarian Cancer Screening Unit, The Royal London Hospital, The Royal London Trust, London, UK

Richard B. Johanson MB BChir MRCOG MD
Senior Lecturer in Perinatology/Consultant in Obstetrics and Gynaecology, Keele
University and North Staffordshire Hospital, Stoke on Trent, UK

Con Kelleher MB BS BSc
Research Fellow, Department of Obstetrics and Gynaecology, King's College
Hospital, London, UK

Frank Lawton MD MRCOG
Consultant Gynaecologist, Department of Obstetrics and Gynaecology, King's
College Hospital, London, UK

Christoph Lees MB BS
Research Fellow, Department of Obstetrics and Gynaecology, King's College
Hospital, London, UK

Rodney Ledward BSc(Pharmacy) DM FRCS FRCOG
Consultant Obstetrician Gynaecologist, Chairman Tutorial Systems International,
Ashford, Kent, UK

Richard J. Lilford MRCOG MRCP PhD
Chairman, Institute of Epidemiology and Health Services Research, Department of
Clinical Medicine, School of Medicine, University of Leeds, Leeds, UK

Allan B. MacLean BMedSc MD FRCOG
Professor and Head, University Department of Obstetrics and Gynaecology, Royal
Free Hospital School of Medicine, London, UK

Joan C. M. Macnab BSc PhD FRCPath
Senior Scientist, MRC Virology Unit, University of Glasgow, Glasgow, UK

Adam L. Magos BSc MD MRCOG
Consultant Obstetrician and Gynaecologist, Minimally Invasive Therapy Unit and
Endoscopic Training Centre, University Department of Obstetrics and
Gynaecology, The Royal Free Hospital, London, UK

Lawrence Mascarenhas MD MRCOG MFFP
Clinical Research Fellow/Senior Registrar, Academic Department of Obstetrics and
Gynaecology, Birmingham Maternity Hospital and Birmingham and Midland
Hospital for Women, Birmingham, UK

John J. Morrison BSc MD DCH MRCOG
Lecturer/Senior Registrar in Fetal Medicine, Department of Obstetrics and
Gynaecology, University College London Medical School, London, UK

Richard Neale FRCS(C) FRCOG
Consultant in Obstetrics and Gynaecology, Department of Gynaecology, Leicester
Royal Infirmary NHS Trust, Leicester, UK

John Newton LLM MD FRCOG MFFP
Professor, Academic Department of Obstetrics and Gynaecology, Birmingham
Maternity Hospital and Birmingham and Midland Hospital for Women,
Birmingham, UK

Patrick Neven MD
Consultant Obstetrician and Gynaecologist, Everberg (Kortenberg), Belgium

Rory A. O'Connor BSc FRCS(I) MRCOG
Consultant Obstetrician and Gynaecologist, Lister Hospital, North Herts NHS
Trust, Stevenage, UK

O. A. Odukoya MD MRCOG
Clinical Lecturer, Department of Obstetrics and Gynaecology, University of Sheffield, Jessop Hospital for Women, Sheffield, UK

Karl S. Oláh FRCS MRCOG
Lecturer, Department of Obstetrics and Gynaecology, The Royal Liverpool University Hospital, Liverpool, UK

David E. Parkin MD MRCOG
Consultant Gynaecologist, Aberdeen Royal Infirmary, Aberdeen Royal Hospitals NHS Trust, Aberdeen, UK

Rudigor Pittrof MRCOG
Lecturer in Maternal Health, London School of Hygiene and Tropical Medicine, University of London, London, UK

Martin J. Quinn MD MRCOG
Senior Registrar in Obstetrics and Gynaecology, Department of Obstetrics and Gynaecology, University Hospital of Wales, Cardiff, UK

Raj S. Rai BSc MB BS
Research Fellow, St Mary's Hospital, Recurrent Miscarriage Clinic, Samaritan Hospital for Women, London, UK

Lesley Regan MD MRCOG
Consultant/Senior Lecturer, St Mary's Hospital, Recurrent Miscarriage Clinic, Samaritan Hospital for Women, London, UK

Robert E. Richardson MB BS BSc MRCOG
Senior Registrar in Obstetrics and Gynaecology, Family Services Directorate, Department of Obstetrics and Gynaecology, Mount Vernon and Watford General Hospitals NHS Trust, Watford General Hospital, Watford, UK

Orla Sheil MD MRCOG
Senior Registrar, Department of Obstetrics and Gynaecology, National Maternity Hospital, Dublin, Eire

John Studd DSc MD FRCOG
Consultant Gynaecologist, Fertility and Endocrinology Centre, The Lister Hospital and Chelsea and Westminster Hospital, London, UK

Michael Turner MAO FRCP(I) MRCOG
Master, Coombe Women's Hospital, Dublin, Eire

Andrew D. Weeks MB ChB
Research Registrar, School of Medicine, Division of Obstetrics and Gynaecology, St James's University Hospital, Leeds, UK

Ann Yoong MD MRCOG
Lecturer, Department of Obstetrics and Gynaecology, St Mary's Hospital, Manchester, UK

PART ONE

Obstetrics

1 The effectiveness of current antenatal care

A. Yoong   T. Chard

The first book which specifically addressed the subject of antenatal care was 'Hints to Mothers for the Management of Health during the Period of Pregnancy and in the Lying-in Room with an Exposure of Common Errors in Connection with these Subjects'. This was written by Thomas Bull in 1837 at a time when pregnancy was regarded as a state of health.[1] A key event in the recognition that pregnancy could be a high-risk event was the paper by Ballantyne in 1901 entitled 'A plea for a Pro-Maternity Hospital'.[2] This secured an endowment for the Edinburgh Royal Maternity Hospital and the establishment of the first antenatal bed to be set apart specifically for the scientific investigation and treatment of disease in the expectant mother. However, it was only in 1915 than an antenatal clinic was opened in Edinburgh, following the establishment of such a clinic in Adelaide in 1910 by Wilson.

By 1950 there were around 2000 antenatal clinics in England and Wales. In 1948 a survey conducted by the Royal College of Obstetricians and Gynaecologists and the Population Investigation Committee established that 99.1% of expectant mothers in England and Wales had received some form of antenatal supervision.[3] With the advent of the National Health Service, antenatal clinics run by local authorities were closed and antenatal care was usually provided by general practitioners (GPs). The Cranbrook Committee[4] suggested that there should be a high level of co-operation between those responsible for care during pregnancy and delivery, and that the services of a doctor and a midwife should be available without charge.

Antenatal care as we know it today emerged in the 1960s with the development of new technologies and a redefined aim of preventing fetal death and congenital handicap. As a consequence, hospital antenatal care expanded and the role of the GP obstetrician was curtailed.

Probably, the greatest success of antenatal care in recent years has been the introduction of screening and early detection of fetal abnormalities using biochemistry and ultrasound. It has been clearly demonstrated in a prospective study that routine scanning of an unselected population at 19 weeks can reduce infant handicap and perinatal mortality: examination of 8849 fetuses led to the detection of 140 out of 166 fetal anomalies, with an overall sensitivity of detection of 85% and specificity of 99.9%.[5] Similar findings have been reported elsewhere in the UK.[6,7] In the past 20 years there has been a dramatic reduction in the frequency of neural tube defects at term as a result of alphafetoprotein measurement and ultrasound. It now seems likely that similar reduction will be seen in other common anomalies including Down's syndrome and cystic fibrosis.

AIMS OF ANTENATAL CARE

Commonsense suggests that it is better to prevent disease than to cure it, and antenatal care has been described as the perfect example of preventive medicine. The aim of antenatal care, which is to ensure the well-being of mother and child, is self evident. This objective can be subdivided into the screening and prevention of maternal or fetal problems, management of maternal or fetal problems, and the preparation of the couple for childbirth and childrearing.

The purpose of this chapter is to review current customs in antenatal care and their effectiveness.

UTILIZATION OF ANTENATAL CARE

The quality and effectiveness of antenatal care is often judged by the number of antenatal visits, and perinatal outcome is related to this number. The shortcoming of this approach is that the duration of the pregnancy will significantly alter the number of visits: a longer pregnancy will, by definition, result in more attendances. Similarly, women from better social circumstances who have a better perinatal prognosis, irrespective of antenatal care, will attend earlier and will have a greater number of attendances. By contrast, mothers whose pregnancies are curtailed by preterm labour, whether spontaneous or induced, will have made fewer visits and suffer higher perinatal loss. Therefore, an apparent relationship between a greater number of antenatal visits and outcome is created.

The Kessner scoring system has been used to assess the amount of antenatal care, taking into account late attendance and/or early delivery.[8] Care is divided into adequate, intermediate or inadequate according to the gestational age at which the first visit takes place and the number of visits before particular gestations (Table 1.1). Antenatal care is deemed 'adequate' if the first visit occurs at or before 13 weeks, with nine or more subsequent antenatal visits, and 'inadequate' if women start their antenatal care at or after 28 weeks or if they have made less than five visits at, or after, 34 weeks. Anything in between is deemed as 'intermediate'. Using this score, the Alan Guttmacher Institute reported in 1989 that 16% of pregnant women (585 000 women) in North America received inadequate antenatal care and that another 18% (661 000 women) had received intermediate care.[9] This type of scoring has not been used in the UK.

What stops pregnant women from taking advantage of antenatal care? In

Table 1.1 Kessner index of adequacy of antenatal care (modified from Kessner et al, 1973)[8]

Antenatal care	Gestational age (weeks)		Number of antenatal visits	Notes
Adequate	13 or less	and	1 or more or not stated	In addition the 1st visit
	14–17	and	2 or more	has to be at 13 weeks or
	18–21	and	3 or more	less
	22–25	and	4 or more	
	26–29	and	5 or more	
	30–31	and	6 or more	
	32–33	and	7 or more	
	34–35	and	8 or more	
	36 or more	and	9 or more	
Inadequate	14–21	and	0 or not stated	All women who start
	22–29	and	1 or less or not stated	their antenatal care at
	30–31	and	2 or less or not stated	28 weeks or later are
	32–33	and	3 or less or not stated	considered to have had
	34 or more	and	4 or less or not stated	inadequate care
Intermediate	All combinations other than those specified above			

the USA lack of medical insurance is a major barrier, and in some areas antenatal care for low income women is completely absent. Clinic waiting time has the greatest effect on patient satisfaction for antenatal care.[10] Long distances to the clinic and the absence of good public transport are also obstacles. Women who have no one to care for their other children are twice as likely to have incomplete antenatal care. Cultural barriers also exist. These include language incompatibility, preference to be seen by a female, or a belief that pressure will be imposed to alter certain behaviours such as substance abuse or heavy smoking. Unplanned pregnancy, fear of medical procedures and parental response, and negative feelings towards the pregnancy can all result in poor participation.[11] There is good if not surprising evidence that patient satisfaction can be raised by improving continuity of care, increasing the sympathy of health care workers and providing more social support and financial assistance.[12–16]

'Outreach' or home visiting exists in certain countries and is usually intended to support high-risk women. Although domiciliary care does not necessarily reduce hospital admission there is a very positive response from the women themselves.[17,18] However, outreach services are expensive. They should be only one component of a well-designed maternity care system and should not supplant other means of improving access.[14]

ANTENATAL CARE IN THE UK

In this country the routine antenatal care offered to symptom-free pregnant women includes a visit to the hospital clinic or GP early in pregnancy followed by monthly visits until 30 weeks gestation, fortnightly until 36 weeks and then weekly until delivery. This basic structure was defined in a Ministry of Health memorandum in 1929.[19] It was not scientifically validated but derived from a survey of what most clinics were doing at that time. This traditional approach was further propagated in a paper in the British Medical Journal by Coope & Scott in 1982.[20] In contrast to this received wisdom, Hall suggested in 1980[21] that for most pregnant women only five full antenatal checks were necessary, with more frequent measurement of blood pressure alone in the third trimester in primigravidae. Antenatal care could thus be redirected at women presenting with problems.

The present system of 'shared' antenatal care commonly used in the UK involves a division of labour between hospital obstetrician, family practitioner and community midwife. This should be effective and convenient for mothers, but relies heavily on good communication. The main method of communication is usually the 'co-operation card' which can be supplemented by letters, telephone calls and personal contact. In 1983 Thomas & colleagues[22] demonstrated that better co-operation and co-ordination between health care personnel involved in shared antenatal care was required and suggested increased use of community midwives, alternative antenatal care systems, with the hospital specialist travelling to community clinics, and the use of a more comprehensive co-operation card or patient-held case records. Patient-held records are becoming increasingly popular. They remove the need for the duplication which occurs with 'co-operation cards' and allow the GP and midwife ready access to results of investigations. In the Newbury Maternity Care study[23] women carrying their full case notes rather than a co-operation card felt more in control of their antenatal care and found it easier to talk to doctors and midwives. The policy led to savings on clerical time. The disadvantages feared before the trial, that women would lose their notes or would be made to feel unnecessarily anxious, did not materialize. These benefits have been substantiated by a similar study at St Thomas' Hospital.[24]

The uptake of new forms of information technology in obstetric care has been slower than anticipated. At one time it was envisaged that computerised multi-terminal systems would obviate the need for any paper records allowing almost simultaneous data access by community and hospital, as well as emphasizing risk factors and providing instructions on appropriate actions.[25–30] But the paperless record system imposes a heavy financial burden on health districts already under severe budgetary constraints. At present there are only 100 obstetric computer systems in England and Wales; 97 of these collect data on labour and delivery and only 36 collect data on antenatal visits. Their commonest applications were replies to ad hoc enquiries and the preparation of perinatal statistics; the least common was preparation of care plans. Links between obstetric computer systems and patient administration systems (PAS) were infrequent and connections to other relevant services such as radiology and haematology were uncommon.[31]

THE RISK APPROACH

In an attempt to improve the effectiveness of antenatal care Boddy[32] devised a scheme using risk cards whereby each pregnant woman was formally assessed against a check list of risk factors. Each risk factor initiated appropriate action. A continuing plan of management using specialist and community services and based on locally agreed protocols was then organized and delays in communication between members of the antenatal care team were avoided. The 'Sighthill' scheme has subsequently been adopted by many centres in the UK. Some schemes allow use by illiterate traditional birth attendants.[33]

Identification of high and low-risk pregnancies begins at the first (booking) antenatal visit. Determinants of obstetric risk include: maternal characteristics such as age, height and weight and social circumstances; factors indicating that gestational age may be uncertain; items in the past obstetric, previous medical history and family history which relate to adverse fetal or maternal outcome; and irregularities noted at the first antenatal examination (Table 1.2).

Subsequent antenatal surveillance will detect factors such as anaemia, poor maternal weight gain, reduced fetal movement, vaginal bleeding or infection, proteinuria or glycosuria, raised blood pressure, abnormal uterine size for gestation, excessive or diminished liquor volume and malpresentation (Table 1.3). The system should be flexible so that low-risk mothers can be transferred into the high-risk group. On the other hand, if it is clear that the risk is not confirmed (for example mothers with transient hypertension), then they should be referred back to primary care.

The aim of the risk approach is to predict problems before they arise so that women designated as high-risk can receive special attention and further care in a hospital setting. The risk approach provides a rationale for resource allocation; low-risk pregnant women can receive antenatal care locally without specialized personnel and equipment and the overall costs for antenatal health care are thereby reduced. The risk approach attempts to quantify risk in a coherent and logical manner rather than relying on the rather nebulous process of human intuition.

Unfortunately the risk approach has many weaknesses. The data on which risk estimates are based is taken from large groups of women, to determine relationships between antenatal problems and problems at birth, and analysed by probabilistic methods such as Bayes theorem or logistic regression. The derived statistical weightings, that is to say 'risks', are then applied to each pregnant woman to determine her 'risk score'. But applying population data to individuals is fraught with difficulty. For this reason, the efficacy of risk scores in the prevention of perinatal morbidity and mortality has never been conclusively proved. All studies on obstetric-risk scoring systems have demonstrated a correlation between increasing risk and poor outcomes.[34-40] However, most scoring systems have positive predictive values of less than 0.3,

Table 1.2 Identification of obstetric risk at the booking visit

Maternal characteristics	Age <18 y, age >35 y Height of less than 152 cm Weight of < 45 kg or > 100 kg Smoking > 10/day Alcohol > 4 units/day Substance abuse Lack of social support
LMP details	LMP uncertain +/- 2 weeks Pill stopped up to 2 periods before LMP Cycle length prior to LMP greater than 30 days IUCD in situ/on OCP after conception Vaginal bleeding since LMP
Past obstetric history	Parity ≥ 5 Congenital abnormality Perinatal death IUGR or macrosomy Preterm labour Previous cervical suture Antibodies in previous pregnancy Hypertension/eclampsia Caesarean section 3rd stage complications
Past medical history	Surgery to the female genital tract Chronic disorders such as diabetes, cardiac, thromboembolism, renal disease and medication
Family history	Fetal abnormality Diabetes mellitus Multiple pregnancy
Booking examination	Blood pressure ≥ 140/90 mm Hg Maternal weight ≥ 85 kg Maternal weight ≤ 45 kg Maternal height ≤ 152 cm Cardiac murmur detected/referred Uterus large/small for dates Other pelvic mass detected Blood group Rhesus negative

LMP = last menstrual period; OCP = oral contraceptive pill; IUCD = intrauterine contraceptive device; IUGR = intrauterine growth retardation.

implying that 70% or more of adverse perinatal outcomes cannot be predicted by existing assessment methods. The predictive accuracy of risk scores can be improved by separate prediction for multiparous and primiparous women, separate prediction of specific poor perinatal outcomes and the inclusion of late antenatal and intrapartum risk factors in the scores.[41,42] As events in a previous pregnancy make an important contribution to risk status it is obvious that risk scoring is more effective in multiparae than primiparae. Separation of the various components of poor perinatal outcome allows for more precise analysis; the predictive accuracy for preterm delivery and low birth weight is higher than that for perinatal mortality in most studies. The use of late

Table 1.3 Identification of obstetric risk at subsequent antenatal visits

Factors arising in pregnancy	Haemoglobin < 10g/dl
	Poor weight gain
	Fetal movement not felt
	Vaginal bleeding
	Vaginal infection
	Rh negative/Antibodies
	Proteinuria
	Glycosuria
	Raised blood pressure
	Uterus large for dates
	Uterus small for dates
	Excess liquor
	Reduced liquor
	Malpresentation
	Head not engaged
	Preterm labour

antenatal and intrapartum risk factors also increase the predictive accuracy but at this stage the opportunity to influence the level of risk is at its lowest.

As with all screening tests, the clinical accuracy of risk scores will depend on the prevalence of the condition in the population and on the cutoff point used. Because of the low prevalence of adverse perinatal outcome, identification of such mothers requires a very low cutoff point for 'high risk'; conseqently it will include large numbers of normals. Possibly the most difficult question raised by studies of risk factors is the determination of a cutoff point between 'normal' and 'abnormal', recognizing that there will be a massive overlap between the two. It has been suggested accordingly that the cutoff point should be chosen in line with financial constraints so that a fixed proportion of the obstetric population becomes the target of increased antenatal surveillance.[40]

Another problem in assessing risk is the benefit of an action initiated when a risk is identified, especially when the action turns an unsatisfactory outcome into a satisfactory one. This is the 'treatment paradox'. If the intervention is 100% successful then the risk factor will apparently have no predictive value.

The risk approach emphasizes the dangers of pregnancy, focusing on the negative rather than the positive, and perpetuates an ever increasing demand for technology. The belief of the clinician is passed on to the pregnant woman. Consequently, any woman who is labelled as high-risk may be under considerable stress.[43]

THE EFFECTIVENESS OF ANTENATAL CARE

It is generally accepted that routine antenatal care has an overall beneficial effect on the health of the woman and fetus but the exact elements of antenatal care which are responsible for this remain unknown.[44] Evidence can be sought by examining the history of antenatal care, using international comparisons, by looking at enhanced antenatal care and at audit performed on antenatal care.

Historical evidence

Initially, antenatal care was uncritically viewed as conferring an unspecified benefit, and the extent of this benefit was considered to be directly related to the amount of care delivered. Indeed, it was confidently suggested that proper antenatal care would reduce fetal death by 20%.[45] In his last address, delivered 3 weeks before his death in 1923, Ballantyne outlined expected benefits from antenatal care, including an immediate decline in stillbirths, and a fall in the maternal death rate as a result of obstetric complications such as sepsis and haemorrhage, and to the resulting interventions. In a classic study of maternal mortality in the Glasgow Royal Maternity Hospital from 1926 to 1930, the primary cause of death in 35% of patients was stated to be inadequate or absent antenatal care.[46] However, disillusionment with antenatal care followed. A series of papers[47,48] suggested that antenatal care had made no impression on the national maternal mortality rate and that the incidence of and death rate from eclampsia were still far too high. Indeed, overzealous practice of antenatal care might have actually increased mortality: while there were fewer deaths from obstructed labour there were many more deaths attributable to induction of preterm labour and to Caesarean section. Therefore, more antenatal care did not necessarily lead to less perinatal or maternal mortality. The cynic might attribute the remarkable reduction in maternal and perinatal mortality in the last 50 years to coincidental factors such as improved economic conditions, less unemployment, smaller family size, improved nutrition, the advent of antibiotics, better anaesthesia and the availability of blood for transfusion.

European comparisons

One way to investigate the effects of antenatal care is to compare the various systems of antenatal care in different countries. In the European Community, antenatal practice differs widely in the member states yet all have remarkably low perinatal and maternal mortality rates. A feature of these comparisons is that the quality of available information varies widely. In most European countries, including the UK, data on antenatal care are incomplete or based on samples of the population. Many countries do not have systems for collecting data on perinatal events. National perinatal surveillance systems are feasible in any industrialized country with an existing health care structure; solutions for developing countries include periodic surveys, exemplified by that conducted in Greece by Tzoumaka-Bakoula.[49] Another approach is the recruitment of motivated local lay people to collect data on pregnancy and birth, a method which has provided data more accurate than the official statistics in Turkey.[50]

Table 1.4 Number of antenatal visits (modified from Blondel[50,51])

| Country | Number of visits | | Women who receive no antenatal care (%) | Policy for non-attenders | |
	Legal or recommended number	Average actual number		Home visits	Financial incentive
UK: England and Wales	12–13	No data	< 2	×	
UK: Scotland	12	10–12	0.1	×	
France	7	5.9	0.6		×
Denmark	10	8	< 1	×	
Sweden	12–13	14	–		
Norway	14	#	–		
Finland	14	14	–		
Netherlands	12	12–14	–		
Federal Republic of Germany (FRG)	10	8.5	1.1		×
Switzerland	3–4	5	–		
Belgium	7	No data	4.3		
Luxembourg	5	5	–		×
German Democratic Republic (GDR)	10	No data	–		

39% of women have more than 10 visits

International comparisons allow comments on specific aspects of antenatal care. Blondel's work compares the organization of antenatal care in 13 European countries which have a fetal and infant mortality rate lower than 20 per 1000:[51]

Number of antenatal visits

The number of antenatal visits varies widely in Europe (Table 1.4). The number recommended by the state or medical profession ranges from 3 to 14 visits. The actual number of visits is smaller (Table 1.4). Between 0.1 and 4.3% of women receive no antenatal care. To reduce non-attendance, some countries offer home visits and others offer financial inducements: the minimum number of visits necessary for a pregnant woman to be eligible for antenatal allowances were four in France (increased to seven in 1992), five in Luxembourg and eight in the Federal Republic of Germany (FRG). In Switzerland the cost of only three visits is refunded by insurance unless there is a medical complication.

Qualification of person in charge of antenatal care for normal pregnancies

In the UK and France, obstetricians work alongside midwives and general practitioners: the most common pattern is the 'shared care' system (Table 1.5). In Denmark it is recommended that a woman should attend her

Table 1.5 Qualification of people in charge of antenatal care for normal pregnancies (modified from Blondel[50,51])

Country	Midwife	GP	Obstetrician
UK: England and Wales	Y	Y	Y
UK: Scotland	Y	Y	Y
France	Y	Y	Y
Denmark	5	3	2
Sweden	10	Y	Y
Norway	11	3	N
Finland	10	3	N
Netherlands	Y	Y	N
FRG	Rare	Y	Y
Switzerland	Rare	Y	Y
Belgium	Rare	Y	Y
Luxembourg	Rare	1	4

midwife five times, the general practitioner three times and the obstetrician twice. In other Scandinavian countries and the Netherlands midwives are pre-eminent; general practitioners are less involved and visits to an obstetrician are only reimbursed if there is a specific complication. By contrast, in Germany, Switzerland, Belgium and Luxembourg obstetricians assume an essential role.

In most countries in which midwives are responsible for antenatal care they also perform most normal deliveries. Only in France and particularly in the UK are midwives more involved in care during delivery than during pregnancy.

Home visiting systems

Blondel also examined home visiting and found that some countries provide health workers to visit pregnant women at home and others do not.[51,52] In Finland, France, the Netherlands and Sweden a planned home visiting system is provided for individual cases, especially non-attenders. Home visiting systems for women at low-risk are in place in the UK, Denmark and Belgium, although the availability of this service is patchy.

Therefore, there is no single model of antenatal care among countries having similar low rates of fetal and infant deaths. The number of intended or actual antenatal visits, the qualification of the 'carer' and the presence or absence of home visiting are not necessarily related to better outcome. These different patterns of antenatal care reflect contrasting development of health care systems in each country.

Kaminski[53] and Mascarenhas[54] compared obstetric care in England and Wales to obstetric care in France. They confirmed that there were no major differences in perinatal outcome with respect to crude perinatal mortality, low birth weight and preterm birth from the national statistics of these two countries. Important differences in obstetric practice were noted. In England

Table 1.6 Published studies on the benefit associated with enhanced antenatal care

Authors	Findings
Sokol (1980)[55]	Mothers within the Maternity and Infant Care project experienced 60% less perinatal mortality than mothers not within the project
Olds (1986)[56]	Nurse home visits in socially deprived mothers led to higher birth weight (395 g) and longer gestation (75% reduction of preterm delivery) but only for the offspring of smokers and adolescents aged less than 17 years
Spencer (1989)[57]	Controlled study demonstrated no benefit of antenatal social support
Heins (1990)[58]	Intensive education and surveillance by nurse-midwives had no effect on incidence of low birth weight
Goldenberg (1990)[59]	Controlled study indicated no benefit of intensive antenatal surveillance on the incidence or consequences of preterm delivery
Oakley (1990)[17]	Controlled study showing that social support did not influence the rate of low birth weight babies but did improve mothers' emotional well-being
Pagel (1990)[60]	Controlled study showing that measures of anxiety, life events and family social supports can predict a statistically significant proportion of variance in pregnancy outcome after controlling for simultaneous influences of demographic, biomedical and lifestyle variables, but their contributions to variance were not always large
Hobel (1991)[61]	Intervention program led to 18.7% reduction in preterm labour (P not significant)
McLaughlin (1992)[62]	Comprehensive antenatal care led to a significant increase in mean birth weight of 144 g among first born but not subsequent infants
Graham (1992)[63]	No reduction in low birth weight rate in low-income black mothers who received home visits, focusing on smoking, drug abuse, nutrition and emphasizing links with community services, as compared with those receiving no visits. Increasing the number of prenatal visits did not reduce the rate of low birth weight deliveries.
Clarke (1993)[64]	Participants in a public prenatal care program had lower neonatal mortality than those of a matched comparison group.

and Wales there were more antenatal visits, especially to GPs and midwives, and more inductions of labour. In France there was more acceleration of labour with oxytocin, more instrumental and Caesarean section, more specialist care in labour and longer postpartum stay.

Enhanced antenatal care

Ethical considerations prohibit randomized prospective studies which compare the use of antenatal care with no antenatal care. An alternative is to compare standard forms of care with enhanced intervention. In general, the effects of 'enhanced' antenatal care on perinatal outcome seems very slight. Table 1.6 summarizes published controlled studies on the benefits of enhanced antenatal care.

Audit of antenatal care

Another approach to determining the effectiveness of antenatal care is to examine the ability of the process to identify women with important non-symptomatic disease. This approach is equivalent to an 'audit of process' and is concerned with whether or not the task has been carried out correctly and efficiently.

Hall[21] analysed 19 451 return antenatal visits to hospital or general practice. Only 83 of 189 (44%) cases of intrauterine growth retardation (IUGR) were correctly diagnosed, while the condition was suspected in 289 but confirmed in only 83 (29%) women. Fifty-one of 58 (88%) cases of breech presentation were detected antenatally. Seventy-six of the 259 (30%) women developing pre-eclampsia presented for the first time in labour or the puerperium, thus preventing antenatal diagnosis. On the other hand, 256 women with transient hypertension were falsely diagnosed as having pre-eclampsia; their blood pressure settled after hospital admission without the need for treatment. Despite the process of antenatal care elective admissions were still outnumbered by emergency admissions to hospital.

Backe's study of 1908 Norwegian women found a 94% detection rate for twins, 69% for breech presentation, 57% for placenta praevia, 57% and 75% for pre-eclampsia.[65] Only 14% of small for gestational age (SGA) fetuses were identified before delivery. It was recommended that stricter standards be set: for example, all twin pregnancies should be diagnosed before 20 weeks, and no pregnant woman should have raised blood pressure for more than 7 days before diagnosis and referral to specialist care.

In our own study, retrospective audit of the case notes of 2000 pregnant women demonstrated that only one-quarter of action protocols dictated by identified antenatal risk factors were actually implemented.[66] It was suggested that good compliance with protocols reflected routine rather than selective obstetric practice, while low compliance was associated with disagreement or simple ignorance of guidelines.

THE FUTURE OF ANTENATAL CARE

The effectiveness of the current 'rituals' of antenatal care have never been scientifically proven. For example, there has been no significant change in the incidence of preterm labour in most obstetric populations during the last two decades, despite much increased awareness of risk factors and the availability of sophisticated diagnostic procedures. There are now moves to discard outdated procedures and, rather than the haphazard implementation of untested regimens, to focus on prospective trials of more promising antenatal interventions.

Although most countries emphasize biological interventions in pregnancy, social and psychological support is equally important.[50] The social model of pregnancy uses a health education and counselling approach and emphasizes reduction of smoking, improvement of diet, alleviation of stress and providing financial benefits, better housing and support before, during and after birth. Women require protection against potential hazards in the workplace and at home. Legislation on the employment rights of the pregnant woman may compensate for disadvantaged social circumstances.[11,17,68]

Antenatal services should be conveniently sited in the community, with creche facilities, and have access to relevant services such as the dentist, drug rehabilitation, social workers and HIV counsellors. The approach should be multidisciplinary and comprehensive but flexible enough to take into account maternal wishes. Only if the mother perceives the service as being in her own interest and actually meeting her needs, will she actually use it.[69]

An alternative scenario to the interaction of the pregnant woman and the health care professional is the development of self-help groups whereby small groups are taught by a midwife to take each other's blood pressure, test each other's urine and measure uterine growth. Such an approach demystifies the antenatal process and strengthens the role of the mother.[50]

In-patient antenatal care has now been substantially replaced by day care facilities. Most tests of maternal or fetal well-being, for example cardiotocography and Doppler studies, can be carried out on an outpatient basis. Results appear to indicate that day care is as effective as in-patient care but with genuine reduction in hospital admissions and cost savings.[70]

CONCLUSIONS

Antenatal care began in the UK in 1901 and was hailed as the panacea for all perinatal problems. Unfortunately this has not proven to be the case. Very little is known about the true nature of the care any pregnant woman receives. Routine antenatal visits vary in content, care provider, timing, frequency, setting and duration and the usual record for the visit does not adequately document the full nature of this supervision. The components of antenatal care which actually work are still unknown and antenatal interventions, whether biological or social, require appropriate evaluation.

REFERENCES

1 Browne F J, McClure Brown J C. Antenatal and postnatal care. London: Churchill Livingstone, 1955
2 Ballantyne J W. A plea for a pro-maternity hospital. Br Med J 1901; i: 813–814
3 Royal College of Obstetricians and Gynaecologists and the Population Investigation Committee. Maternity in Great Britain. Oxford: Oxford University Press, 1948
4 Cranbrook Committee. Report of the Maternity Services Committee. London: HMSO, 1959
5 Luck C A. Value of routine ultrasound scanning at 19 weeks: a four year study of 8849 deliveries. Br Med J 1992; 1474–1478
6 Chitty L S, Hunt G H, Moore J, Lobb M O. Effectiveness of routine ultrasonography in detecting fetal structural abnormalities in a low risk population. Br Med J 1991; 303: 1165–1169
7 Shirley I M, Bottomley F, Robinson V P. Routine radiographer screening for fetal abnormalities by ultrasound in an unselected low risk population. Br J Radiol 1992; 65: 564–569
8 Kessner D M, Singer J, Kalk C E, Schlesinger E R. Infant death: An analysis by maternal risk and health care. Washington DC: National Academy of Sciences, 1973

9 Singh S, Forrest J D, Torres A. Prenatal care in the United States: A state and county inventory. New York: The Alan Guttmacher Institute, 1989

10 Flynn S P. Continuity of care during pregnancy: the effect of provider continuity on outcome. J Fam Pract 1985; 21: 375–380

11 Brown S. Prenatal Care. Reaching mothers, reaching infants; Committee to study outreach for prenatal care. Washington DC: National Academy Press, 1988

12 O'Brien M, Smith C. Women's views and experiences of antenatal care. Practitioner 1981; 225: 123–125

13 Oakley A. The relevance of the history of medicine to an understanding of current change: some comments from the domain of antenatal care. Soc Sci Med 1982; 16: 667–674

14 Brown S. Drawing women into prenatal care. Fam Plann Perspect 1989; 21: 73–80

15 Witwer M B. Prenatal care in the United States: reports call for improvements in quality and accessibility. Fam Plann Perspect 1990; 22: 31–35

16 Hansell M J. Sociodemographic factors and the quality of prenatal care. Am J Public Health 1991; 81: 1023–1028

17 Oakley A, Rajan L, Grant A. Social support and pregnancy outcome. Br J Obstet Gynaecol 1990; 97: 155–162

18 Blondel B, Bréart G. Home visits for pregnancy complications and management of antenatal care: an overview of three randomised controlled trials. Br J Obstet Gynaecol 1992; 99: 283–286

19 Ministry of Health: Memorandum 145/MCW: Maternal mortality in childbirth in antenatal clinics: Their conduct and scope. London: HMSO, 1929

20 Coope J K, Scott A V. A programme for shared maternity and child care. Br Med J 1982; 284: 1936–1937

21 Hall M H, Chng P K, MacGillvray I. Is routine antenatal care worth while? Lancet 1980; July 12: 78–80

22 Thomas H, Draper J, Field S. An evaluation of the practice of shared antenatal care. J Obstet Gynaecol 1983; 3: 157–160

23 Elbourne D, Richardson M, Chalmers I, Waterhouse I, Holt E. The Newbury Maternity Care Study: a randomized controlled trial to assess the policy of women holding their own obstetric records. Br J Obstet Gynaecol 1987; 94: 612–619

24 Lovell A, Zander L I, James C E, Foot S, Swan A V, Reynolds A. The St Thomas' Hospital Maternity case notes study: a randomised controlled trial to assess the effects of giving expectant mothers their own maternity case-notes. Ped Perinat Epidemiol 1987; 1: 57–66

25 Rosen M G, Sokol R J, Chik L. Use of computers in the labor and delivery suite: an overview. Am J Obstet Gynecol 1978; 132: 589–594

26 Morgan M, Studney D R, Barnett G O, Winickoff R N. Computerized concurrent review of prenatal care. Qual Rev Bull 1978; 4: 33–36

27 Lilford R J, Chard T. Microcomputers in antenatal care: a feasibility study on the booking interview. Br Med J 1981; 283: 533

28 Maresh M, Beard R W, Combe D, Gillmer M D G, Smith G, Steer P J. Computerization of obstetric information using a microcomputer. Acta Obstet Gynecol Scand (suppl) 1982; 109: 42–44

29 Lilford R J, Bingham P, Fawdry R, Setchell M, Chard T. The development of on-line history-taking systems in antenatal care. Meth Inform Med 1983; 22: 189–197

30 Gonzalez F A, Fox H E. The development and implementation of a computerized on-line obstetric record. Br J Obstet Gynaecol 1989; 96: 1323–1327

31 Yoong A, Das S, Carroll S, Chard T. A national survey to assess current use of computerised information systems in obstetrics. Br J Obstet Gynaecol 1993; 100: 205–208

32 Boddy K, Parboosingh I J T, Shepherd W C. Schematic approach to prenatal care. In: Report of the Royal College of Obstetricians and Gynaecologists working party on antenatal and intrapartum care. London: RCOG, 1982: pp 40–46

33 Chabot H T, Rutten A M. Use of antenatal cards for literate health personnel and illiterate traditional birth attendants: an overview. Trop Doct 1990; 20: 21–24

34 Goodwin J W, Dunne J T, Thomas B W. Antepartum identification of the fetus at risk. Can Med Assoc J 1969; 101: 57–67

35 Wilson E W, Sill H K. Identification of the high risk pregnancy by a scoring system. NZ Med J 1973; 78: 437–440

36 Haeri A D, South J, Naldrett J. A scoring system for identifying pregnant patients with a high risk of perinatal mortality. J Obstet Gynecol Br Commonwlth 1974; 81: 535–538

37 Morrison I, Olsen J. Perinatal mortality and antepartum risk scoring. Obstet Gynaecol 1978; 53: 362–366
38 Wall E M. Assessing obstetric risk. J Fam Prac 1988; 27: 153–163
39 Pattison N S, Sadler L, Mullins P. Obstetric risk factors: can they predict fetal mortality and morbidity? NZ Med J 1990; 103: 257–259
40 Chard T, Yoong A, Macintosh M. Obstetric risk scores. In: Van Geijn H P, Copray F J A, eds. A critical appraisal of fetal surveillance. Amsterdam: Elsevier, 1994
41 Herman A A B, Irwig L M, Groenveld H T. Evaluating obstetric risk scores by receiver operating characteristic curves. Am J Epidemiol 1988; 127: 831–842
42 de Caunes F, Alexander G R, Berchel C, Guengant J P, Papiernik E. The Guadeloupean perinatal mortality audit: process, results, and implications. Am J Prev Med 1990; 6: 339–345
43 Chalmers B. Stressful life events and pregnancy complications: a summary of research findings. Humanitas 1982; 8: 49–57
44 Banta D, Houd S, Ojeda E S. Prenatal care – An introduction. Int J Technol Assess Health Care 1985; 4: 783–788
45 Holland E. Report on the causation of fetal death. Report on public health and medical subjects No 7. London: HMSO, 1922
46 Kerr J M M. Maternal mortality and morbidity. Edinburgh: E&S Livingstone, 1933
47 Browne F J. Antenatal care and maternal mortality. Lancet 1932; ii: 1–4
48 Wrigley A J. A criticism of antenatal care. Br Med J 1934; 1: 891–894
49 Tzoumaka-Bakoula C. The Greek national perinatal survey: design, methodology, case ascertainment. Ped Perinat Epidemiol 1987; 1: 43–51
50 Wagner M. Pursuing the birth machine. Australia: ACE Graphics, 1994
51 Blondel B, Pusch D, Schmidt E. Some characteristics of antenatal care in 13 European countries. Br J Obstet Gynaecol 1985; 92: 565–568
52 Blondel B. Antenatal care in the European Community countries over the last 20 years. In: Kaminski M, Bréart G, Buekens P, Huisjes J, Mcllwaine G, Selbmann H, eds. Perinatal care delivery systems: Description and evaluation in EC countries. Oxford: Oxford University Press, 1986: pp 3–15
53 Kaminski M, Blondel B, Bréart G. Management of pregnancy and childbirth in England and Wales and in France. Ped Perinat Epidemiol 1988; 2: 13–24
54 Mascarenhas L, Eliot B W, Mackenzie I Z. A comparison of perinatal outcome, antenatal and intrapartum care between England and Wales, and France. Br J Obstet Gynaecol 1992; 99: 955–958
55 Sokol R J, Woolf R B, Rosen M G, Weingarden K. Risk, antepartum care, and outcome: impact of a maternity and infant care project. Obstet Gynecol 1980; 56: 150–156
56 Olds D L, Henderson C R Jr, Tatelbaum R, Chamberlin R. Improving the delivery of prenatal care and outcomes of pregnancy: a randomised trial of nurse home visitation. Pediatrics 1986; 77: 16–27
57 Spencer B, Thomas H, Morris J. A randomised controlled trial of the provision of a social support service during pregnancy: South Manchester Family Worker Project. Br J Obstet Gynaecol 1989; 96: 281–288
58 Heins H C, Webster N W, McCarthy B J, Efird C M. A randomised trial of nurse-midwifery prenatal care to reduce low birth weight. Obstet Gynecol 1990; 75: 341–350
59 Goldenberg R L, Davis R O, Copper R L, Corliss D K, Andrews J B, Carpenter A H. The Alabama preterm birth prevention project. Obstet Gynecol 1990; 75: 933–939
60 Pagel M D, Smilkstein G, Regen H, Montano D. Psychosocial influences on new born outcomes: a controlled prospective study. Soc Sci Med 1990; 30: 597–604
61 Hobel C J, Ross M, Bemis R, Bragonier J, Bear M, Mori B. Abstract of Phase I report Los Angeles area prematurity prevention project. J Perinat Med 1991; 19: 15–18
62 McLaughlin J J, Altemeier W A, Christensen M J, Sherrod K B, Dietrich M S, Stern D T. Randomised trial of comprehensive prenatal care for low income women: effect on infant birth weight. Pediatrics 1992; 89: 128
63 Graham A V, Frank S H, Zyzanski S J, Kitson G C, Reeb K G. A clinical trial to reduce the rate of low birth weight in an inner-city black population. Fam Med 1992; 24: 439–446
64 Clarke L L, Miller M K, Vogel W B, Davis K E, Mahan C S. The effectiveness of Florida's 'Improved Pregnancy Outcome' program. J Health Care Poor Underserved 1993; 4: 117–132
65 Backe B, Nackling J. Effectiveness of antenatal care: a population based study. Br J Obstet Gynaecol 1993; 100: 727–732

66 Yoong A, Lim J, Hudson C, Chard T. An audit of antenatal protocols. Br Med J 1992; 305: 1184–1186
67 Steer P. Rituals in antenatal care – do we need them? Br Med J 1993; 307: 697–698
68 Wagner M. Health services for pregnancy in Europe. Int J Technol Assess Health Care 1985; 1: 789–798
69 Hepburn M. Social problems. Baillières Clin Obstet Gynaecol 1990; 4: 149–168
70 Twaddle S, Harper V. An economic evaluation of daycare in the management of hypertension in pregnancy. Br J Obstet Gynaecol 1992; 99: 459–463

2 Drugs in pregnancy

R. S. Ledward

When prescribing for the pregnant woman, the practitioner should use a small armamentarium of drugs that have a well proven value with known and recorded minimal side effects. Many drugs have been used with enthusiasm in the past, only later to be withdrawn or discontinued because of side effects, and examples include thalidomide and betasympathiomimetics. Continued pharmacovigilance by all practitioners, indicating that continuous observation and reporting of any side effects is ongoing, will help reduce the potential for iatrogenic disease in the mother, her fetus and the newborn.

In an overview of the 15 months of therapy for the potentially pregnant and pregnant patient and her fetus, the general principles and obstetric rules include:

1. Consider that all drugs have the potential for affecting the fetus except heparin, which is a large molecule and does not cross the placenta.
2. Remember the patient may be exposed to 'over-the-counter medicines' with potential risks arising from, for example, excessive vitamins D or A. Approximately 6% of women take drugs during the first trimester of pregnancy, especially 'over-the-counter' drugs including narcotics or antacids, but this figure is generally falling from a high of 64% in 1960 to 6% at the present time. These figures relate to the UK and may be higher in other countries.
3. Consider that all patients are at risk of pregnancy during their reproductive years.
4. Remember there is a balance of the risk of therapy against the potential for not treating the primary medical disorder.

The general principles of therapeutics apply to the pregnant woman as much as to any other patient, although some of the conditions which are treated are peculiar to pregnancy.

There are two additional features of prescribing for the pregnant woman which must be considered by the practitioner in relation to medicinal and all other forms of therapy. First, the physiological adaptions of pregnancy may alter the effects of the therapeutic agent – for example, by affecting drug absorption; and second, that the therapeutic agent may affect the fetus detrimentally, or occasionally beneficially, as well as the mother.

The physiological changes during pregnancy affect the distribution and elimination of the drug and this may lead to ineffective therapy owing to inadequate drug concentration. Examples include anticonvulsants, theophylline derivatives or antidepressants, including lithium, and blood levels should be monitored during therapy; a knowledge of the absorption, distribution, metabolism and excretion of the drug in the mother and fetus can be of value for active fetal therapy.

MATERNAL PHARMACOKINETICS

Drug absorption

The pharmacokinetic variables of drug absorption, distribution, metabolism and excretion can all be influenced by physiological changes that occur during pregnancy. Almost all drugs can cross the placental barrier and affect the fetus (in clinical doses, heparin is the exception). A physiological adaptation to pregnancy may alter the therapeutic agent by absorption and a therapeutic agent can harm the fetus or may prove beneficial. Gastrointestinal transit is prolonged owing to slow emptying of the stomach and reduced gut motility, but this is only of clinical importance during late pregnancy and labour when parenteral administration of drugs is indicated. Mendelson's syndrome remains a potential hazard, especially if general anaesthesia is required, and a 'nil by mouth' regimen has its advocates once labour is established. Control of the acid content of the stomach can be achieved with magnesium trisilicate or sodium citrate, metoclopramide or an H_2 receptor antagonist such as ranitidine or cimetidine.

Drug distribution

Lipid solubility and protein binding affect the molecular distribution of drugs. Total body water and plasma volume increase during pregnancy, and the concentration of plasma albumin falls from 15 g/l to 10 g/l. Plasma drug concentration is greatest for drugs with low lipid solubility that are highly bound to plasma protein. The therapeutic dose for drugs monitored by total plasma concentration must be reduced if their binding changes during pregnancy, e.g. phenytoin.

Drug metabolism

Water-soluble drugs are eliminated unchanged. Lipid-soluble drugs are metabolized by oxidation, or conjugated in the placenta and fetal liver before being excreted in bile or urine.

Drug excretion

Renal plasma flow, glomerular filtration rate and creatinine clearance are all increased in pregnancy; drugs excreted unchanged are excreted more quickly.

FETAL PHARMACOKINETICS

Distribution, metabolism and fetal excretions occur in the fetus and placenta. The fetal liver or adrenal gland metabolizes drugs by oxidation, oxidative dealkylation, reduction hydroxylation, hydrolysis and conjugation. Metabolism is mainly an inactivating process but metabolites and intermediate compounds may be harmful to the fetus.

Low-molecular-weight compounds diffuse easily across the placenta. Amino acids may be transported across the placenta by active transfer, with lipid solubility and plasma protein binding contributory factors.

SPECIFIC HAZARDS

Prescriptions in pregnancy are intended to contribute to maternal health with minimal risk to the baby. The best estimate of the fetal hazards of medication given for maternal disease should be presented to the patient who may elect a termination of pregnancy if the hazards are unacceptable to her. The basic rules of prescribing in pregnancy are:

1. Encourage preconceptual counselling and review all patients with a medical disorder. Advise all patients about potential hazards of tobacco, alcohol and over-the-counter medicines.
2. Question the need for any drug in pregnancy; 'first do no harm' is the basic rule.
3. Review all drug regimens in pregnancy, e.g. the epileptic patient may be able to manage on a single drug rather than be exposed to polypharmacy.
4. Use those drugs where experience has shown minimal side effects rather than new drugs.

PRINCIPLES OF PRESCRIBING IN HUMAN PREGNANCY

The first principle is to evaluate every drug prescribed for a pregnant (or possibly pregnant) woman with respect to whether it is really necessary and whether equivalent results can be obtained by alternative therapeutic measures.

The second principle of prescribing for pregnant women is to use drugs which have been widely used in pregnancy for many years in preference to recently introduced agents with ill-established or merely theoretical advantages.

The third principle is medicolegal. In the UK, under the Congenital Disabilities (Civil Liability) Act of 1977, a doctor is immune from civil liability

Table 2.1 Basic rules of prescribing in pregnancy

Remember the obstetric rules
1. First do no harm
2. Never be the first to use the new, nor the last to use the old
3. Remember that all women are pregnant until proved otherwise

Prescribing in pregnancy
1. Preconception phase; the patient may be taking drugs or require drugs prior to conception
2. The patient may be taking drugs and find she is pregnant
3. The patient who is pregnant may require drug treatment

---

for the ill effects on the fetus of a drug he has prescribed if (a) he has informed the mother of any known potential hazard, or (b) the drug is currently prescribed in pregnancy as established medical practice. In cases where the doctor considers it desirable to be vague, or to withhold from the patient the knowledge of a small established risk, it is clear that if this decision is taken in good faith and in the best interests of the patient, then this provides an adequate defence in law.

'Data sheets' and commercial literature are not good sources of information on whether a drug may be used safely in pregnancy. In the majority of cases where a drug is stated in these documents to be contraindicated in pregnancy the warning is given for the medicolegal protection of the pharmaceutical company and there is no concrete evidence that the drug is harmful. If in doubt, the doctor should consult with the pharmaceutical company.

Prescribing for the pregnant or potentially pregnant patient will be required in the preconception phase for any associated medical condition. The patient may be taking drugs when she finds she is pregnant, or she may require drug treatment for conditions specific to pregnancy. Therapy is, however, not without risk and trial by media and medicolegal hazards have led to therapeutic nihilism. It is only in recent years that positive fetal therapy for specific conditions has become more acceptable. Obstetric rules for prescribing are listed in Table 2.1.

The practitioner will recognize that there is more to therapy than drugs alone and as well as treating the mother, her uterine activity and her fetus, the importance of psychotherapy, including an explanation of any associated condition, is paramount. This alone may be a factor in reducing drug intake. Total therapy includes:

1. consideration of the place of therapy; hospital versus home
2. provision of appropriate nursing care
3. dietary advice
4. psychotherapy
5. physiotherapy
6. investigations
7. surgery
8. and only then the potential for drug therapy including therapy for minor ailments should be considered.

Placental transfer of drugs

The great majority of drugs cross the placenta by simple diffusion from a high to a low concentration, and the rate of transfer is related to the concentration gradient and to the thickness and surface area of the membrane as well as to the diffusion constant for the substance being transferred. The rate of diffusion is described by Fick's diffusion equation:

$$Q/t = \frac{K.A. (Cm - Cf)}{L}$$

Q/t = rate of diffusion (quantity per unit of time); Cm = maternal blood concentration; Cf = fetal blood concentration; A = placental surface area; L = transplacental distance; K = diffusion constant.

Only those molecules of the drug not bound to protein are available for transfer. The diffusion constant K depends on the molecular weight of the drug and the spatial configuration of the molecule and only molecules with a molecular weight of less than 1500 can normally pass the placenta by simple diffusion. Highly fat-soluble molecules that are uncharged reach the fetus more rapidly than drugs with a low fat solubility which are ionized.

PRECONCEPTUAL COUNSELLING

The 15 months of potential and definitive cyesis are prone with difficulties for the mother, her fetus and her adviser (Fig 2.1). The preconception phase is of paramount importance, especially for those who have demonstrated a poor obstetric performance in the past. However, many others – the very young, the socially deprived or the more senior potential mother may need advice, and practitioners should be alert to potential problems in the general practice clinic (not specifically in the preconception clinic).

Preconception clinics provide a forum for counselling and indications for referral are wide ranging and tailored to specific individuals (Table 2.2). Subjects for discussion can include:

1. Age – the potential for chromosomal abnormality with elderly mothers needs discussion.
2. Drugs of abuse: cigarettes, alcohol, heroin. This may be the most appropriate time for discontinuing these toxins.
3. Drugs needed by the mother for any medical condition. The patient may request therapy including antibiotics without realising she is pregnant, and be prone to teratogenesis.

Whilst the preconception clinic provides an excellent forum for discussion, realism shows that most patients (especially those that need the actual

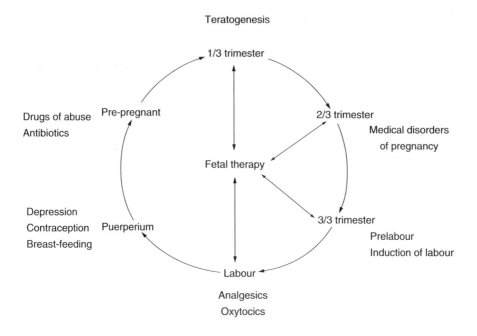

Fig. 2.1 Potential and definitive months of pregnancy.

counselling) present during pregnancy and may already be on medication. Patients who receive medication may:

1. be already taking drugs or require drugs prior to conception
2. be taking drugs and find herself pregnant
3. require drug therapy during the present pregnancy.

DIETARY ADVICE

Dietary deficiencies in proteins, vitamins, minerals or trace elements can all affect fetal growth and development.[1] Fetal malnutrition has been implicated in adult cardiovascular disease and diabetic mellitus.[2] The total energy requirement of pregnancy is 80 000 KCal, and a steady rate of 400 KCal/day manifests as a 400–500 g weekly weight gain. Approximately 3 kg of fat will be stored by 30 weeks, providing energy, and 10 g of protein is required daily. The well-nourished woman will show a slight increase in appetite and this will provide all her protein and energy requirements. The optimal weight gain for thin women in pregnancy is 12.5 kg or more; the optimum weight gain for obese women in pregnancy is 5–10 kg and this is associated with

Table 2.2 Indications for referral to the preconception clinic

---

Age
Screening tests; chromosomal analysis; a full discussion on testing for chromosomal abnormalities by detailed scan for nuchal oedema; chorionic villus biopsy or amniocentesis for other abnormalities. Referral to a tertiary centre may be indicated for genetic counselling

General advice including nutrition

Past obstetric history
Including ovulation-inducing drugs; recurrent miscarriages

Social history
Drugs of abuse including cigarettes, alcohol; sexually transmitted disease; travelling; vaccinations; malaria

Medical history
Epilepsy; psychiatric disorder; transplantation; hypertension; diabetes mellitus

Industrial history
Video computer; farming

Family history
Gender choice

Teratogenesis

---

optimal perinatal mortality; these figures relate to UK patients and may differ for patients from the Indian subcontinent and elsewhere.

Food preparation and general advice

To prevent listeriosis all fruit and vegetables should be washed and soft cheeses avoided.[3] Meat products should be stored and carefully prepared. To prevent infection with *Chlamydia psittaci*, which can cause miscarriage, the patient should not provide help when lambing or milking ewes and should avoid contact with aborted or newborn lambs.

To prevent toxoplasmosis, contact with cat litter trays should be avoided and gloves should be used for gardening. Screening for toxoplasmosis is routine in France and Austria but not routinely performed in the UK,[4] and allows parents the opportunity to make an informed decision about the future management of the pregnancy, be it either termination or medical therapy with pyrimethamine, sulphadiazine and folic acid.

Dietary supplementation will be required for:

1. strict vegans
2. those suffering from malabsorption
3. a proportion of malnourished individuals.

One aim of supplementation, amongst other factors, is to reduce congenital malformations and should include the following:

Table 2.3 Levels of folate/folic acid in various foods

Food	Folate/folic acid per typical serving (µg)	Food	Folate/folic acid per typical serving (µg)
Vegetables (boiled unless stated)		*Fruit*	
Broccoli	30	Banana	15
Brussels sprouts	100	Grapefruit	20
Cabbage	25	Orange	50
Carrots	10	Orange juice	40
Cauliflower	45		
Green beans	50	*Cereals and cereal products*	
Peas	30	White rice, boiled	5
Potatoes old	45	Brown rice, boiled	15
Potatoes new	40		
Spinach	80	Spaghetti, boiled	9
Sweet corn	10	White bread, average (2 slices)	25
Cucumber, raw	2	Wholemeal bread, average (2 silces)	40
Lettuce, raw	15	Soft grain bread (fortified with folic acid)	105
Tomatoes, raw	15	Cornflakes (unfortified)	3
		Comflakes (fortified with folic acid)	100
		Branflakes (unfortified)	40
		Branflakes (fortified with folic acid)	100
		*Other foods**	
		Bovril (per cup)	95
		Yeast extract (on bread)	40
		Milk, whole/semi-skimmed (one pint)	35

Note. To ensure vegetables do not lose folate: eat fresh vegetables; boil only lightly.

Vitamins

Vitamin D. Supplementation with a daily dose of 400 U vitamin D will lower the risk of neonatal rickets, dental enamel displacer and neonatal calcium derangement.

Vitamin A. It should be noted that excessive use (e.g. 40 000 I U) of vitamin A, either as capsules or food including liver pate or liver sausage, can be hazardous and the recommended maximum dose is 2500 I U (750 µg) rising to 2700–3300 µg/day (800–10 000 I U). Eating normal quantities of liver in pregnancy, however, does not do any harm but additional vitamin A preparations or analogues are not indicated.

Folic acid. Defects of the neural tube are amongst the most common neonatal congenital deformations with a prevalence of between 24 and 38 per 10 000 in the UK and Ireland: spina bifida comprises an important part of these defects in 44% of cases.[5] Folic acid deficiency was first diagnosed in India in

1930[6] and in 1980, Smithells et al[7] suggested the possible prevention of neural tube defects by a periconceptual vitamin supplement, and as a consequence of this folic acid is now present in fortified foods (see Table 2.3). Neural tube closure occurs between day 21 and day 27 postconception. Therefore, to prevent neural tube defects, folic acid (0.4 mg daily) should be given prior to conception and continued for at least 3 months. For those who have a history of neural tube defect, and patients with low folate levels or who are receiving antiepileptic therapy, 5 mg daily is required to reduce the risk by 70%. However, folic acid can reduce serum phenytoin levels and therefore extra phenytoin will be required.[8]

Haematinics

Opinions differ with regard to the need to provide iron supplements for healthy women starting pregnancy with a normal haemoglobin level (> 11 g/dl). Iron preparations are not without their problems of nausea, constipation and diarrhoea – and they may not be needed. Anaemia in pregnancy can have a number of causes including haemodilution, iron deficiency, folate deficiency, infection, haemorrhage or pre-existing haematological disorders.

High-risk groups such as deprived populations, vegetarians or those with a history of anaemia may be treated prophylactically, but all anaemic patients should be investigated fully – haemoglobin, full blood count, blood film, serum or red cell folate, haemoglobin electrophoresis, serum iron-binding capacity, plasma transferrin, serum ferritin, stool examination for hookworms, and possibly bone marrow examination if the haemoglobin level fails to improve after the patient has been put on oral ferrous salts.

Iron preparations can be given orally or parenterally.

Oral preparations. Ferrous salts: sulphate, gluconate and fumarate are commonly used. They are also available as delayed-release preparations and combination preparations with folic acid and vitamin supplements. Many commercially available haematinics contain multivitamins but there is no need to give them to healthy pregnant women on a normal diet. Similarly, added minerals such as zinc and calcium are not required.

Prophylaxis involves a daily dose of 50 mg elemental ferrous iron plus 300 µg folic acid. The treatment regimen is 100–300 mg elemental ferrous iron plus 5–15 µg folic acid daily.

Parenteral preparations. These may be used if the serum iron or bone marrow iron stores are depleted. However, if the pregnancy has not progressed beyond 36 weeks, oral preparations are recommended. Intramuscular injections of iron sorbitol citric acid complex at weekly intervals should suffice. Total dose iron infusions given by the intravenous route are reserved for patients where there are social reasons for completing treatment rapidly. They may provoke a hypersensitivity reaction and so a test dose is mandatory.

PAST OBSTETRIC HISTORY

Ovulation-inducing drugs

Ovulation-inducing drugs are being evaluated for possible teratogenic effects – a two to threefold increase of risk of neural tube defects has been suggested following clomiphene therapy;[9] ovarian malignancy has also been mentioned after excessive use, i.e. large doses after 12 months' therapy.

Hormones

Diethylstilboestrol

Prenatal exposure of this hormone given for threatened abortion has been associated with adenocarcinoma of the vagina.[10,10a]

Progestogens

These have been used for patients who have a poor obstetric history as evident by recurrent miscarriages and poor luteal phase.

There is little or no place for this therapy except for the patient who has previously had a successful pregnancy after progesterone therapy following many miscarriages.

Oral contraceptives

Oral contraceptives suppress folate and pyridoxine levels. Patients who conceive whilst taking the oral contraceptive pill and who are happy to continue with the pregnancy should, however, be reassured that there is no additional teratogenic risk. Oral contraceptives reduce folate and pyridoxine levels.

Anticoagulants

Aspirin and heparin (75 mg die) are recommended where systemic lupus erythematosus is diagnosed as being associated with recurrent miscarriages. It should be prescribed from conception to 14 weeks gestation in a dose of 10 000 U twice daily.[10b,10c]

Miscellaneous

Aspirin and nitric oxide have also been advocated to improve uterine perfusion in patients suffering from recurrent miscarriages.[11]

SOCIAL HISTORY

Drugs of abuse

Patients experienced in drugs of abuse are also subject to sexually transmitted diseases including hepatitis B or human immunodeficiency virus (HIV). Social deprivation is also a common associated feature.[11a]

Cigarettes

The vasoconstrictor in nicotine and the associated elevated carbon monoxide levels leads to growth retardation of the fetus.[12] Many patients will try to reduce their cigarette intake in pregnancy but others will confirm 'they only want a small baby!' and advice should be generally supportive.

Alcohol

Alcohol intake should be restricted to zero; however, many patients will participate in a minimal intake and no harm will be evident. Alcohol intake should be restricted to:

1. two glasses of wine per day
2. one pint of beer or two mixed drinks per day. But even these low levels can lead to a slow reaction, a low IQ and hyperactivity. Excessive alcohol intake leads to the fetal alcohol syndrome.[13]

Narcotics

Narcotics cause:

1. reduced fetal growth
2. increased stillbirth rates
3. neonatal abstinence syndrome
4. sudden infant death syndrome.

Benzodiazepines

These lead to withdrawal effects on the baby.

Cocaine

This is the only drug of abuse that is truly teratogenic and results in a lower birth weight, preterm delivery, increased placental abruptus, increased fetus death and structural anomalies.[14]

Marijuana

There is reported to be an absence of major adverse affects.

Caffeine

Caffeine is found in social drinks of coffee, tea, chocolate, dietary aids and 'over-the-counter' preparations. However, it has been associated with an increased miscarriage and stillbirth rate.

Drug management

In pregnancy, drug management is aimed at:

1. withdrawal from the drugs, and
2. a maintenance of total abstinence.

Social deprivation and associated factors need to be reviewed and sexually transmitted disease treated, including HIV infection. Zidovidine has been used in doses of 300–1200 mg/day. The drug is well tolerated and not associated with malformations. Anaemia and growth retardation occurring in a minority of patients may have resulted from zidovidine therapy.

Sexually transmitted disease

Sexually transmitted diseases are now the commonest group of communicable diseases in the world. The greatly increased incidence has occurred despite improvements in diagnosis and effective treatment (Table 2.4).

Contact tracing is important in preventing the spread of infection. Whilst serology for syphilis may still be routinely performed in antenatal clinics, investigations for other diseases such as AIDS should only be undertaken when informed consent is given. Women who are seropositive for HIV should be checked for other sexually transmitted diseases.[15, 16] They should also be screened for toxoplasmosis, tuberculosis and urinary tract infection. About 30% of their babies will be HIV positive and of these the great majority will develop AIDS. Breast-feeding should be avoided in these women.

Vaccination and travel

Cholera

Cholera is best prevented by paying close attention to personal hygiene.

Typhoid

Systemic reactions can follow repeated doses of vaccine when given subcutaneously or intramuscularly; however, these reactions are less common when

Table 2.4 Sexually transmitted diseases

Organism	Disease	Treatment
Bacteria	Gonorrhoea	Penicillin
	Chancroid	Sulphadimidine
	Granuloma inguinale	Erythromycin
Viruses	Non-specific genital infection	Erythromycin
	Chlamydial infection	Erythromycin
	Herpes genitalis	Caesarean section
	Genital warts	Cautery
	Lymphogranuloma venereum	Erythromycin
	Molluscum contagiosum	Phenol
	Hepatitis B	Specific immunoglobulin to neonate
	Acquired immune deficiency syndrome (AIDS)	Zidovidine
Spirochaetes	Syphilis	Penicillin
	Balanitis	Penicillin
Protozoa	Trichomoniasis	Metronidazole
Fungi	Candidiasis	Tropical imidazoles
Parasites	Scabies/Pediculosis pubis	Benzyl benzoate

vaccines are given intradermally and this is an acceptable alternative for booster doses (0.1 ml).

Vaccines

Vaccines for yellow fever, cholera, poliomyelitis and influenza may be given in the antenatal phase. Rubella vaccination is allowed only in the preconception or postpartum phase.

GENERAL MEDICAL DISORDERS

Patients should be reviewed in the combined medical obstetric clinic by the physician and obstetrician.

Epilepsy

The child born to a woman with epilepsy has an increased risk of malformation and this risk is further increased by taking an antiepileptic drug.[17, 18]. Abnormalities fall into two categories:

1. Minor abnormalities defined as structural deviations from the norm not constituting a threat to health.
2. Major abnormalities of medical, surgical or cosmetic importance, i.e. cleft lip, spina bifida and congenital heart disease.

Antiepileptic drugs are not without side effects including:

1. Valproate, which is associated with spina bifida and cranial and facial anomalies.
2. Carbamazepine, which is associated with spina bifida.
3. Phenobarbitone, which is associated with congenital heart disease and cleft palate.
4. Phenytoin or trimethadione can cause the hydantoin syndrome.

Management

In the preconception clinic, counselling and screening are indicated to advise the epileptic patient of the potential risks should they wish to conceive:

1. In the interim they should be advised to take higher doses of oral contraception.
2. They should be advised of the risk of neural tube defects and a daily dose of 4–5 mg folic acid recommended before conception and up to 12 weeks after conception.
3. The practitioner should aim to control their symptoms using a single-dose drug therapy in the lowest possible dose. Carbamezepine is thought to be the drug of choice.
4. Blood levels of the drug should be monitored during pregnancy; serum phenytoin levels can be lowered by folate therapy.
5. Additional vitamin K should be given at birth to protect the infant.

Psychiatric illness

Non-psychotic depression

Meprobamate or benzodiazepines can cause serious symptoms in the neonate, but there is no evidence of a teratogenic effect.[19]

Monoamine-oxidase inhibitors, including tranylcypromine, phenelzine and isocarboxazid are contraindicated in pregnancy in view of the potentially fatal interaction between these and the drugs normally used in anaesthesia.[19] In an emergency the anaesthetist should be informed if the patient has been taking these drugs.

Tricyclic antidepressants such as amitriptyline, butiptyline, clomipramine, imipramine and nortriptyline should be used with care during pregnancy and lactation.[19] Babies born to mothers who have continued therapy have been jittery and refused to feed.

Lithium salts. Whilst lithium clearance increases in pregnancy, infants may occasionally be born with cyanosis, lethargy, hypotonia, poor suckling, poor respiratory effort or congenital heart disease; serum lithium values should be monitored.

Phenothiazines can cause Parkinsonism when given in large doses for schizophrenia or to control vomiting of pregnancy.

Transplantation

Many patients have been subjected to transplant procedures including renal, lung, liver, bone marrow and heart.[20] Subsequently, their general health has improved and they have ovulated, conceived and delivered. The preconception clinic offers a unique opportunity for general discussion on their general worries including the therapy that will be required. Experience with liver transplantation is limited but figures from 84 centres in the USA and 30 centres from other countries show an 80% survival rate of heart transplant and 70% for a heart and lung transplant. The management of the pregnancy is complex and drug therapy is just one aspect; drugs that are used include immunosuppressive agents such as adrenal steroids, azathioprine and cyclosporin.

Adrenal steroids

The side effects of adrenal steroids are well listed and include peptic ulceration, osteoporosis, hypertension, increased maternal infection and poor tissue healing.

Azathioprine

This is associated with hepatic toxicity, bone marrow depression, an increased risk of infection and an increased risk of neoplasia. There may be chromosomal gaps in the lymphocytes of the fetus which revert to normal at 32 weeks. There is thought to be a 3% malformation rate.

Cyclosporin

Nephrotoxicity is dose related, and because it is associated with an elevated serum uric acid is not a good marker for pre-eclampsia. There is an increased risk of lymphomas and viral infections in patients receiving cyclosporin therapy, and this affects the management of their pregnancy, which is complex anyway, requiring team care including: the transplant team; the obstetrician, who should provide a resume of the drugs used and their potential for side effects; the neonatologist; and the social services.

Hypertension

A number of agents have a favourable benefit – risk profile for use of women with pregnancy-induced hypertension, methyldopa, beta blockers, hydralazine, prazosin and calcium channel antagonists.[21, 22] Angiotensin-converting enzyme inhibitors are contraindicated. Low-dose aspirin may have a major preventative role in high-risk categories.[23]

Diabetes mellitus

Oral agents are contraindicated and soluble insulin should be used for monitoring during pregnancy.[24, 25]

INDUSTRIAL HISTORY

Operating theatres

The volatile gases present in operating theatres may theoretically be associated with spontaneous abortion and congenital abnormality; there is no definite proof but on general principles scavenger systems should be installed.

Laundries

Organic solvents used in cleaning processes can cause anencephaly or fetal dysmorphology.

Computers

Pregnant women who work at computer terminals do not have a higher risk of suffering miscarriage, or having babies with congenital deformities, than pregnant women with no exposure to computers.

Saunas

Maternal hyperthermia has been associated with malformations in the fetus of some animals but has not yet been elucidated in humans; hot sauna baths are not associated with malformation.[26]

FAMILY HISTORY

Gender choice

It is fashionable for many patients to ask for appropriate dietary advice to ensure that they acquire a fetus of their chosen sex (Tables 2.5 & 2.6).[27] Diets high in sodium and potassium and low in calcium and magnesium are reported to give an 80% chance of a male fetus.

TERATOGENESIS

A teratogen is an agent that causes physical and/or developmental abnormalities in the embryo or the fetus. The timing of embryonic and fetal

Table 2.5 Boy diet

General points	Specific Foods	
Lots of salt (in foods such as ham, bacon, smoked salmon)	Artichokes	Aubergines
	Mushrooms	Avocado pears
	Sweetcorn	Figs
Salty mineral water	Tomatoes	Dates
Very limited dairy products	Celery	Prunes
No shellfish	Broad beans	Raisins
No nuts	Baked beans	Apricots
	Brussel sprouts	Cherries
	Leeks	Bananas
	Beetroot	Melons
	Lentils	Peaches
	Dried beans	Raspberries
		Oranges

Note. This diet is unsuitable for anyone with high blood pressure.

Table 2.6 Girl diet

General points	Specific foods
No salt or salty foods	Lettuce
Lots of dairy products	Watercress
Reduced fat and fibre	Radishes
Avoid a few other food constituents, such as the fizz in fizzy drinks, which prevent the absorption of calcium	Cucumber
	Broccoli
	Green pepper
	Asparagus
	Runner beans
	Peas
	Cabbage
	Carrots
	Cauliflower
	Onions
	Turnips
	Apples
	Pears
	Kiwi fruit
	Clementines
	Nuts

Note. This diet is unsuitable for anyone prone to kidney stones.

development is important (Fig. 2.2). The pre-embryonic phase lasts from day 1 until 17 days postconception; the embryonic phase is from 18–55 days postconception and this is followed by the period of organogenesis and postorganogenesis. Drugs can still affect the fetus, e.g. danazol, causing virilization of the female and warfarin or non steroidal anti-inflammatory drugs.

In 1961 thalidomide,[28] originally thought to be a benign sedative, affected 40% of humans – it caused phocomelia (reduction defects of limbs, and visceral, eye and auricle malformations) but it had no effect on animals, other than monkeys. There are two stereoisomers of thalidomide – one responsible

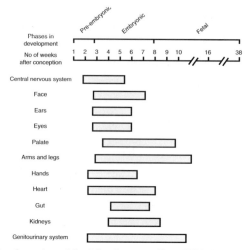

Fig. 2.2 Timing of embryonic and fetal development (from Whittle M. and Hanretty K. P., Br Med J 1986; 293: 1485)

Table 2.7 First reports on exogenous factors as causes of human birth defects

Year	Type of factor causing birth defects
1929	Malformations caused by X-rays
1939/1942	Malformations caused by infections (toxoplasmosis and rubella)
1952	Malformations presumably caused by a drug (aminopterin)
1959	Malformations caused by exposure to a chemical agent (methyl mercury)
1961	Thalidomide tragedy

for teratogenesis; one for the hypnotic effect. Other teratogens include: methylmercury (1959); aminopterin (1952); rubella and toxoplasmosis (1939); X-rays (1925) (see Table 2.7). In 1940 Gregg[29] showed the affect of rubella on fetal development and in 1961 McBride[28] showed the relationship between thalidomide and phocomelia.

Recent correspondence has followed the re-emergence of thalidomide on a named patient basis for Behcets syndrome as to whether thalidomide is a human mutagen as well as a potent teratogen;[30] the classic malformation resulting from thalidomide is caused by interference with the way in which genetically normal embryos develop, and not by mutations.[31]

Major malformations in the general population range from 2–5% and up to 6% with epileptic patients. Drugs cause anything from 1–5% of severe congenital abnormalities. Drug metabolites can also cause adverse reactions; examples include metabolites of paracetamol, sedatives, tranquilizers and anticonvulsants.

Media reports that birth defects including missing hands and arms, in babies born in UK seaside towns, is only thought to be, at the present time, due to chance.

Table 2.8 Drugs with a potential for fetal damage

Contraindicated in pregnancy
Antimitotics*
Alkylating antimitotic drugs – chlorambucil, busulfan
Actinomycin D
Antimetabolites – mercaptopurine, methotrexate
Vitamin A derivatives used for acne or psoriasis – tretinoin, isotretinoin
Radiochemicals
Radioactive iodine (^{131}I) associated with fetal goitre
Sedatives
Thalidomide associated with phocomelia, neurological abnormalities
Antibiotics
Tetracycline associated with discolouration and enamel hypoplasia in deciduous teeth;
maternal liver failure in late pregnancy

Known or suspected to carry a teratogenic risk
Narcotics
Reduce intrauterine activity and depress respiration in the newborn infant
Some antibiotics
See above
Some anticoagulants
Antidepressants
Lithium; infants may be born with cyanosis, lethargy, hypotonia, poor suckling, congenital
heart disease. The action of lithium is unknown
Antiepileptics
Some hypotensive drugs
Sex hormones
Stilboestrol treatment is associated with adenosis or adenocarcinoma of the vagina in the
mother and female offspring; progestogens: 19-norethisterone or its derivatives (components of
many oral contraceptives) may cause masculinization of a female fetus, with clitoral
enlargement or labial fusion; oral contraceptives
Antivirals
Idoxuridine

Drugs subject to an anecdotal adverse report
The prescriber must select an alternative drug or balance the reported risks of the drug with the
stated advantages and discuss the situation with the patient before use

* All cause an increased abortion rate or increased fetal abnormality rate.

Teratogenic drugs (Table 2.8)

Teratogenic drugs act by three main mechanisms:

1. Direct embryo toxicity.
2. Indirect toxicity by alteration of the metabolic endocrine or physicochemical factors.
3. Genetic factors determining the susceptibility to teratogenesis, e.g. warfarin.

Teratogenic drugs can be classified into two categories:

1. Major teratogens. Drugs with a proven and considerable risk of causing a congenital abnormality, e.g. thalidomide, cytotoxics and radiochemicals.

Table 2.9 Effect of low risk drugs on the fetus during pregnancy

Drug	Effect	Reason for Effect
Antithyroid drugs		
Carbimazole	Increase fetal thyroid-	Inhibit thyroxine
Propylthiouracil	stimulating hormone (TSH) with resultant goitre	secretions by fetus
Antidepressants		
Lithium	Hypotonia Bradycardia Cyanosis Neonatal goitre	Unknown
Sedatives/narcotics		
Opiates and barbiturates	Respiratory depression at birth	Smaller proportion of myelin allows greater penetration into cerebral tissue
Phenothiazines	Cerebral depression Neonatal temperature regulation disturbance Extrapyramidal signs	As above
Benzodiazepines Chlordiazepoxide Diazepam Nitrazepam	Depressed respiration in the neonate	Placental transfer
Anticoagulants Warfarin Coumarin	Fetal and neonatal haemorrhage	Low level of vitamin K-dependent clotting factor
Salicylates Aspirin	Haemorrhage (near term)	Hypothrombinaemia caused by Factor XII platelet dysfunction
Prostaglandin Synthetase Inhibitors Indomethacin	Premature closure of ductus arteriosus and pulmonary hypertension	Smooth muscle in ductus arteriosus is mediated by prostaglandin

2. Drugs with a known but small risk (Table 2.9). Such drugs are usually necessary for the health of the woman. Any potential problems should be discussed with the patient.

Drugs which are known or suspected to carry a teratogenic risk include the following.

Antineoplastic drugs

Antimetabolites or alkalizing agents, i.e. methotrexate, azauridine, cyclophosphamide, chlorambucil.

Folic acid antagonists. Aminopterin can cause central nervous system (CNS), limb and renal malformations and spontaneous abortion.

Anticonvulsants

Epilepsy, with or without therapy, has a three times higher risk of congenital abnormality.

Phenytoin or trimethadione can give the hydantoin syndrome (cranial or facial defects, digital hyperplasia, microcephalin, mental deficiency and growth retardation).

Carbamazepine causes fetal and head growth retardation and spina bifida.

Sodium valpamates are indicated in spina bifida.

Coumerol anticoagulants

In the first trimester, warfarin causes nasal hyperplasia and chondrodysplasia puntaton.

PREGNANCY

Vomiting in pregnancy

Nausea and vomiting are common complaints during the first trimester of pregnancy and may be severe enough to merit hospital admission for intravenous fluid replacement. Clinically, there appears to be less demand for antiemetics possibly owing to improved psychotherapy and/or fears of teratogenesis from anecdotal reports, and many patients will put up with bland measures such as biscuits or milk. However, if the symptoms do not improve then an antiemetic, chosen in confidence from the list in Table 2.10, should be given.

It remains mandatory to exclude non-obstetric causes of vomiting, which can include: gastroenteritis, cholecystitis, pancreatitis, peptic ulceration, intestinal obstruction, diaphragmatic hernia, pyelonephritis, uraemia, diabetes mellitus, appendicitis, jaundice, twisted ovarian cyst or cerebral tumour.

Hospital admission may be required if the situation deteriorates and loss of weight, ketosis and dehydration persist.

Medicolegal problems are paramount and an example is given by the antiemetic 'debendox', which is composed of doxylamine, dicyclomine and pyridoxine. This relatively benign drug was taken off the market by pressure from litigation.

Trial by media has resulted in therapeutic nihilism and promethazine theoclate (phenergan) has now been put on the drug data sheet as 'not to be taken in pregnancy' so that all patients will at least discuss the preparation

Table 2.10 Drugs used to control vomiting and nausea in pregnancy

Drug	Dosage
Antihistamines	
Cyclizine hydrochloride (50 mg)	One tablet three times daily
Cyclizine lactate (40 mg)	Intramuscularly three times daily
Promethazine theoclate (25 mg)	One to two tablets during the day and at night
Sedatives	
Prochlorperazine maleate (5 mg)	One tablet two to three times daily
Chlorpromazine hydrochloride	10–25 mg tablets every 4–6 hours; 100 mg as required every 6–8 hours; 25–50 mg intramuscularly every 3–4 hours
Tranquillizers	
Trifluoperazine hydrochloride	2–4 mg daily orally in divided doses; 1–3 mg daily intramuscularly
Thiethylperazine maleate	6.33 mg tablets three times daily; 6.5 mg intramuscularly; 6.5 mg suppositories night and morning
Vitamins	
Pyridoxine hydrochloride (50 mg)	50 mg intravenously three times daily in patients not responding to other preparations
Gastrointestinal sedative	
Metoclopramide hydrochloride (tablets 10 mg; syrup 5 mg/ml; injection 5 mg/ml)	10 mg three times daily

with their practitioner. Furthermore, the data sheet for promethazine theoclate states 'there is no epidemiological evidence for the safety of promethazine theoclate in pregnancy and animal studies have shown no hazard; nevertheless it should not be used in pregnancy unless the physician considers it essential': this statement protects the manufacturer but promethazine theoclate has been used for many years without harm to the fetus and can be used, if indicated, after full discussion with the patient.

OVER-THE-COUNTER MEDICINES

Herbal and homeopathic remedies have been recommended in pregnancy (Table 2.11) including raspberry leaf tea, which is reported to be 'uterotonic'.[32, 33] There appears to be no pharmacological evidence for this. Herbal medicines are not necessarily safe simply because they are natural; they may merit further detailed investigation in future years and they should – as all agents – be discouraged in pregnancy. Specialist information services on drugs in pregnancy, including herbal preparations, are available. In the UK, herbal preparations sold or supplied as 'medicinal products' have been controlled by the Medicines Act since its introduction in 1968. There are limited exemptions but all other herbal preparations, which fall within the definition of a 'medicinal product' as defined by Directive 65/65 EEC, require product licences as laid down in the Medicines for Human Use (Marketing Authorisation etc.) Regulations of 1994.

Table 2.11 Over-the-counter medicines

Symptom	Over-the-counter therapy
Heartburn	Simple antacids may help
Constipation	Bulk forming agents, bran, Ispagula or Sterculia should be tried initially
Haemorrhoids	Local therapy with soothing creams help
Cystitis	Urinary tract infections should be excluded
Leg cramps	Massage of the calf muscles is the only therapy
Restless legs syndrome	This is described as a creeping or crawling sensation deep within the legs that is relieved by walking. Correction of anaemia which may be associated with the syndrome is recommended together with support stockings
Pain	Restrict intake to aspirin or paracetamol in minimal doses
Cough	Simple linctus, cough and throat lozenges
Herbal therapy	e.g. raspberry leaf tea is promoted as a uterine tonic

TROPICAL MEDICINES

Mebendazole

Mebendazole may be given inadvertently to pregnant women for worms. Whilst stated as 'contraindicated in pregnancy' there have, however, been no reports of mebendazole causing human teratogenesis.

Diethylcarbamazine

This drug has been used for leptospirosis; fleas from cattle cause leptospirosis and the patient presents with fever, hepatorenal failure and haemorrhage. The differential diagnosis includes malaria and pregnancy-induced hypertension.

LABOUR

Bacterial vaginosis has been linked with a variety of obstetric and gynaecological disorders.[34] There is an association with preterm labour; premature rupture of the membranes, post-Caesarian section, posthysterectomy, and post-termination infection. It is a common condition and a significant cause of vaginal discomfort. Oral metronidazole for 7 days or oral or vaginal clindamycin cream (2%) may be indicated. The syndrome is caused by the replacement of the lactobacillus-predominant flora by anaerobic bacteria, *Gardnarella vaginalis* and *Mycoplasma hominis*.

For preterm labour, tocolytic agents have been used, including β-sympathomimetic agents, but recently such therapy has been shown to be associated with more than a twofold increase in the incidence of neonatal periventricular and interventricular haemorrhage.[35]

Ritodrine hydrochloride has been associated with maternal pulmonary oedema, and predisposing factors that have been identified include preexisting cardiac disease, multiple pregnancy, pre-eclampsia, eclampsia, concomitant corticosteroid treatment and maternal infection. Fluid overload would appear to be the most important single factor, and the use of 5% w/v dextrose solution is indicated.

Other approaches to preterm labour include the use of prostaglandin (PG) synthetase inhibitors and calcium channel blockers. Side effects associated with these agents include closure of patent ductus arteriosus with the PG synthetase inhibitors.

If the patient does go on to deliver, the respiratory distress syndrome can be prevented by synthetic surfactant, administered in a multiple dose prophylaxis for babies of less than 30 weeks gestation or less than 1100 g at birth. It is thought that three doses are better than one and the concurrent use of corticosteriods is indicated.

For the medical induction of labour, Prostaglandin E2 has been used and clinical doctors need to balance the cost of an elective medical and surgical induction of labour against the cost of probabilities of labour starting, the length of labour, probability of Caesarean section, probability of instrumental delivery, postpartum haemorrhage requiring blood transfusion, level of staff monitoring during labour and the extent of resource savings from reduction in Caesarean section incidence.

The prostaglandin carboprost is an analogue of prostaglandin F2 and is licensed for hospital use for uterine atony and persistent bleeding, despite exclusion of retained products and optimum treatment with conventional oxytocic drugs.[36] A dose of 250 μg intramuscularly repeated after 19 minutes is indicated.

PUERPERAL PROBLEMS

Feeding

To stimulate breast milk metoclopramide is indicated, whilst to stop lactation bromocriptine mesylate is indicated (Table 2.12). Bromocryptine is an ergot-derivative and coronary spasm has been reported following use.

Table 2.12 Drugs interfering with lactation

Bromocriptine, dopamine, pyridoxine
Inhibit prolactin secretion, and milk production

Alcohol, nicotine, excessive fluid intake
Suppress oxytocin release from the posterior pituitary gland, and milk production

Oestrogens, androgens
Act directly on the breast and may cause gynaecomastia

Diuretics
Interfere with fluid transfer, and milk production

Postpartum depression

Depression is not unknown and comes in three categories: 'the blues' where 50–80% of women are affected; postnatal depression; Puerperal psychosis.

Postnatal depression

Postnatal depression occurs in 10% of women. Symptoms include despondency, sleep and eating difficulties, feelings of guilt and inadequacy and loss of sexual interest. Treatment includes support, practical and psychological, as well as antidepressant drugs: the use of prophylactic progestogens is not scientifically established and is not recommended. Transdermal oestrogen has more recently been advocated.[37,38]

Puerperal psychosis

Depressive symptoms usually dominate in women affected by puerperal psychosis, but rarely schizophrenic symptoms have been noted. Psychological support is indicated together with antidepressant drugs. Electroconvulsant therapy may also be indicated with psychiatric in-patient treatment.

Contraception

Many patients select hormone contraceptive therapy following the birth of their child; the combined oestrogen-progestogen pill is not contraindicated and may be given from day 5 when clotting factors are at a level that reduce the risk of thromboembolism. Starting the preparation at this time helps to improve the lochia, and the patient is provided with contraception and also knows exactly when her first period will be. Many women prefer to wait until the 6 week stage and then start the progestogen-only pill but menstrual irregularities may be noted.

Alternative forms of contraception, including the intrauterine contraceptive devices and long acting contraceptives containing levonorgestrol, e.g. 'Norplant', may be elected at the postnatal phase.[39]

Neonates

In the puerperium, vitamin K is indicated for the neonate. There has been justified concern regarding new cases of cancer in children, and therefore intramuscular vitamin K1 is not offered routinely, but all normal term infants now receive oral vitamin K1, 1 mg at birth, 1 mg at the end of week 1 and 1 mg at the end of week 3. For at-risk infants, i.e. preterm, and those affected by severe asphyxia, cerebral birth trauma, extensive bruising, sepsis and illness, probable liver problems, epilepsy and others to be identified, then an injection of vitamin K1 0.5 mg is given at birth or in the first 24 hours if possible followed by oral vitamin K1 1 mg at 1 week and 3 weeks following birth.

Table 2.13 Indications for fetal drug therapy

Congenital adrenal hyperplasia
Fetal thyroid disease
Congenital toxoplasmosis
Congenital syphilis
Rh isoimmunisation
Symptomatic polyhydramnios
Fetal growth retardation
Fetal arrhythmias
Intrapartum fetal distress
Neonatal sepsis
Neonatal respiratory distress syndrome
Neonatal intraventricular haemorrhage

FETAL DRUG THERAPY

Fetal drug therapy is defined as the administration of any drug for the treatment of a fetal disorder to improve the capacity for later interuterine or postnatal adaption; indications are listed in Table 2.13.

The subject of fetal drug therapy has been well reviewed. Following the thalidomide tragedy there was therapeutic nihilism; however, the pendulum is now rebalanced with a number of fetal conditions listed which may benefit from maternal drug therapy. These include oral digitalis controlling fetal supraventricular tachycardia, or maternal corticosteroids stimulating enzyme activity for the biosynthesis of surface active phospholipids in the type II alveolar cells, thereby reducing the incidence of respiratory distress syndrome especially when coupled with fetal endotracheal surfactant.

Indications for fetal therapy

Prophylaxis

Folic acid therapy prior to conception is recommended to prevent neurotubal defects. A low-risk patient should receive 0.4 mg folic acid in her diet or by supplementation and high-risk patients should receive 4 mg folic acid and this should be started prior to conception. This is especially important for patients who are epileptic and receiving appropriate therapy.

Aspirin therapy has been advocated to prevent pregnancy-induced hypertension but is only really indicated for those who are at very high risk.

SUMMARY

Prophylactic therapy is definitely indicated in the prevention of neural tube disease and may be indicated for patients at very high risk of developing pregnancy-induced hypertension. In other conditions listed in Table 2.14 appropriate therapy is available.

BIBLIOGRAPHY

1 Beeley L, ed. Safer prescribing. Edinburgh: Blackwell Scientific Publications, 1994: pp 56–68
2 Eskes T K A B, ed. Neural tube defects: Pathogenesis and Prevention. Medicom, The Netherlands, 1992
3 Expert Advisory Group Report. Folic acid and the prevention of neural tube defects. Department of Health UK, 1997
4 Hawkins D F, ed. Drugs in pregnancy. Edinburgh: Churchill Livingstone, 1987
5 Krauer B, Krauer F, Hytten F. Drug prescribing in pregnancy. In: Lindt T et al, eds. Current reviews in obstetrics and gynaecology 7. Edinburgh: Churchill Livingstone, 1984, pp. 1–83
6 Ledward R S et al. Drug treatment in obstetrics. London: Chapman & Hall Medical, 1991
7 Rayburn W G. Fetal drug treatment. Obstet Gynaecol Surv 1992; 47: 1–19
8 While you are pregnant: Safe eating and how to avoid infection from food and animals. London: HMSO, 1993

REFERENCES

1 Luke B. Nutrition during pregnancy. Curr Opin Obstet Gynaecol 1994; 6: 402–407
2 Barker D J P et al. Fetal nutrition and cardiovascular disease in adult life. Lancet 1993; 341: 938–941
3 Khouzam M B, Scott G M. Neonatal listeriosis; a model for potential prenatal diagnosis and treatment. J Obstet Gynaecol 1989; 9: 263–270
4 Joynson D H M. Screening for toxoplasmosis in pregnancy. Contemp Rev Obstet Gynaecol 1991; 3: 61–68
5 Poggel H A, Giorzel P. Neural tube defects. In: Eskes T K A B. Neural Tube Defects: Pathogenesis and prevention. Medicom, The Netherlands, 1992
6 Wills L, Mehter M M. Studies in 'Pernicious Anaemia' in pregnancy: Part 1 Preliminary Report. Int J Med Res 1930; 17: 777–792
7 Smithells R W et al. Possible prevention of neural tube defects by periconceptual vitamin supplementation. Lancet 1980; 1: 339–340
8 Wald N, Bower C. Folic acid and the prevention of neural tube defects. Br Med J 1995 310: 1019–1020
9 Cornel M C. In: Eshes T K A B, ed. Ovulation stimulation and neural tube defects: Pathogenesis and prevention. Medicom, The Netherlands, 1992
10 Herbst A L et al. Adenocarcinoma of the vagina: Association of maternal stilboestrol therapy with tumour appearance in young women. N Engl J Med 1971; 284: 878–881
10a Rossing MA et al. Ovarian tumours in a cohort of infertile women. N Engl J Med 1994; 331: 771–776
10b Hughes G R V. The antiphilosophical syndrome: ten years on. Lancet 1993; 342: 341–344
10c Lima F et al. Obstetric outcome in systemic lopus erythematosus. Seminars in Arthritis and Rheumatism 1995; 25: 184–192
11 Lees C et al. Arrest of preterm labour and prolongation of gestation with glyceryl trinitrate, a nitric oxide donor. Lancet 1994; 343: 1325–1326
11a Johnstone F D. Drug abuse in pregnancy. The Dilpomate 1994; 1: 24–29
12 Butler N R, Goldstein H. Smoking in pregnancy and subsequent child development. Br Med J 1973; 4: 573–575
13 Jones K L, Smith D W. Recognition of the fetal alcohol syndrome in early infancy. Lancet 1973; 2: 999–1001
14 Thow S L. Cocaine and its effects on pregnant women. Br J Midwif 1994; 2: 362–367
15 Macdonald M G et al. HIV infection in pregnancy. Epidemiology & clinical management. J Acquir Immune Deficien Synd 1991; 4: 100–108
16 Sperling R S et al. Survey of zidovudine use in pregnant women with human immunodeficiency virus infection. N Engl J Med 1992; 326: 857–861
17 Drug and therapeutics bulletin. Epilepsy v pregnancy. 1994; 32: 49–51
18 Editorial. Epilepsy & Pregnancy. Drug Ther Bullet 1994; 32: 49–51
19 Loudon T B. Psychotropic drugs. Br Med J 1987; 294: 167–168

20 Sims C J. Organ transplantation and immunosuppressive drugs in pregnancy. Clin Obstet Gynaecol 1991; 34: 100–111
21 Lowe S A, Rubin P C. The pharmacological management of hypertension in pregnancy. J Hyperten 1992; 10: 201–207
22 Beilie L. Leading articles. Br Med J 1994; 308: 1250
23 de Swiet M, Fryers G. The use of aspirin in pregnancy. J Obstet Gynaecol 1990; 10: 467–482
24 Editorial. Diabetes and pregnancy. Int J Gynaecol Obstet 1995; 48: 331–339
25 Vaughan N J A. Treatment of diabetes in pregnancy. Br Med J 1987; 294: 558–560
26 Uhari M et al. Sauna habits of Finnish women during pregnancy. Br Med J 1979; 1216
27 Stolkowski J, Cloukrown J. Garcon en fille le choix par selection pre-conceptionnelle. Chiron Limited 1993
28 McBride W G. Thalidomide & Congenital Abnormalities. Lancet 1961; 2: 1358
29 Gregg N. Congenital cataracts following german measles in the mother. Trans Opthalmol Soc Aust 1941; 3: 3536
30 McBride W G. Letter to Editor. Br Med J 1994; 308: 1635–1636
31 Read A P. Thalidomide may be a mutagen. Br Med J 1994; 308: 1636
32 Anderson L. Herbal medicine, education and the pharmacist. Pharmaceut J 1986; 236: 303–311
33 Editorial. Herbal medicines – Safe and effective? Drug Ther Bullet 1986; 24: 97–100
34 Ledward R S, Ahmed B. Common bacterial infections in pregnancy: Update. 1994; 914–920
35 Groome L J et al. Neonatal periventricular – intraventricular haemorrhage after maternal sympathomimetic. Am J Obstet Gynaecol 1992; 167: 873–879
36 Editorial. The Management of Postpartum Haemorrhage. Drug Ther Bullet 1992; 30: 23
37 Gregoire A J P, Kumar R, Everitt B, Henderson A F, Studd J W W. Transdermal oestrogen for treatment of severe postnatal depression. Lancet 1996; 347: 930–933
38 Murray D. Editorial: Oestrogen and postnatal depression. Lancet 1996; 347: 918–919
39 Mascarenhas L. Long acting method of contraception. Br Med J 1994; 308: 991–992

3 Safe motherhood – an achievable and worthwhile aim

R. Pittrof R. Johanson

Despite advanced communications technology and a worldwide hunt for exciting stories, some tragedies do not attract much attention. The (un)safe motherhood story has all the trappings of a good headline: sex, blood, injustice, suffering of the defenceless and guiltless. The reasons make good headlines too: greed, discrimination, poverty and apathy. Why then do the 585 000 women who die every year as a result of pregnancy or child birth[1] raise no interest in our press? Indeed, as maternal mortality rates in developing countries are frequently underestimated[2] by 50% the true incidence of maternal mortality might be closer to 1 million per year.[3] Whatever the accurate figures might be we need to ask ourselves at what level of suffering we are prepared to become active. Is it inevitable that women will have to continue to suffer and die while trying to fulfil their reproductive and social function? One reason for our inactivity might be resignation, as the challenge appears too enormous to be tackled. Would it be better to forget and accept what cannot be changed? This paper will show that not all is 'doom and gloom', and that changes are possible.

Over 98% of all maternal mortalities occur in the developing countries,[4] many of which have a health budget of less than 10 US$/capita/year. Effective obstetric care delivered under those conditions cannot aim to copy European or North American concepts. What is best under these circumstances has to be different from that which is considered to be ideal and can only be determined when social and economic conditions are taken into account and when cultural and religious backgrounds are respected.

The scale of the safe motherhood challenge is indeed enormous. The World Health Organization (WHO)[5] estimates that 150 million deliveries occur annually. Every year 585 000 women will die (equivalent to one every minute), 35–40 million will suffer serious acute complications, 15–20 million serious long-term complications as a result of pregnancy related complication,[6] and 10–20 million women will risk their lives every year by subjecting themselves to clandestine terminations of pregnancy.[7] Only about one-third of all births are assisted by trained attendants in Africa and South Asia, and 64% in Latin America, as opposed to 93% in East Asia and virtually 100% in North America.[8] The lifetime risk for women in sub-Saharan Africa of dying of pregnancy-related complications is about 1 in 22, which is several hundred

47

times higher than for women in North America (1 in 6000)[9] or Northern Europe (1 in 9850).[10] It is important to remember that all the above quoted figures are conservative estimates and that maternal mortality is only the tip of the iceberg and it has been estimated that for every mother who dies 15 to 20 (equivalent to 8.25 million/year) will suffer serious long-term complications and more than 100 will suffer acute morbidity episodes (equivalent to 62 million/year).[11] The scale of the safe motherhood challenge is thus still a matter of speculation.

The resources available or needed to solve the problem are similarly difficult to quantify. Human and financial resources in the developed world do not prevent maternal mortalities in the developing world. In developed and more so in developing countries the situation is further complicated by a distribution bias delivering medical care to those who need it least: members of the urban, and middle or upper class.[12] Health services are therefore frequently inaccessible to rural populations.[13]

At the Safe Motherhood Conference in Nairobi 1987 the world set itself the aim of reducing maternal mortality by 50% by the year 2000. As all conditions leading to maternal mortality are preventable and treatable using contemporary obstetric knowledge, a reduction of essentially 'unnecessary' carnage by 50% did not seem to be too presumptuous at the time.

Even where resources are very limited, addressing the issue of safe motherhood makes economic sense. Women in the developing world have multiple roles. They do not only look after the young, the sick and the old but also, for example in Africa, produce 80% of the food consumed domestically and at least 50% of export crops.[14,15] Sivard[16] estimated that unpaid household work by women alone is equivalent to 4 trillion US$/year, equivalent to one-third of the world economic production. A recent World Bank report,[17] ranked maternity as health problem number one, with young adult women (ages 15–44) in developing countries accounting for 18% of the total disease burden.[17] Investment into women's health is not only very important but can also be a cost-effective way of improving the health and wealth of a nation (Table 3.1).[18]

Health, and maternal health in particular, is more than the product of medical intervention. Five interlinked groups of causes affecting maternal

Table 3.1 Cost effectiveness comparison of social development programmes

Programme	Cost per life saves (US$)
Oral rehydration therapy	100–700
Immunization	120–490
Nutritional supplementation	1230–33 000
Breast-feeding	87–400
Water and sanitation	1250–20 000
Education	1400–5600
Safe motherhood (family planning and maternal health)	800–4000

health can be identified: poverty, low socioeconomic status of women, poor nutrition and general health of women, poor availability of good quality health services and inadequate contraceptive/reproductive choice. While integrated action to address all aspects of women's health would be ideal, interlinked causes have the advantage that positive changes in one area will lead to positive changes in other areas, too.

Even if the safe motherhood equation contains many unknown variables, there is enough knowledge and skill to solve parts of the problem, as the subsequent examples will show.

POVERTY AND ALLOCATION OF RESOURCES, NUTRITION, EDUCATION AND HEALTH

Of all the variables which influence maternal health, poverty of a nation or a family might be the most important and most difficult to tackle. About 50% of the population of sub-Saharan Africa and South Asia are poor and the number of poor people is not likely to decrease over the next decade.[19] Poverty of a family will reduce a woman's ability to utilize health care while poverty of a country can make it difficult to provide an adequate health care infrastructure. Economic adjustment as prescribed by the IMF and World Bank have a drastic impact on the availability of health care to poor people.[20-22] When charges were introduced for the provision of maternity service its uptake fell by more than 50%.[23] Harrison[24] reported that mothers who received antenatal care in northern Nigeria had a maternal mortality rate three times lower than those who did not receive antenatal care. Charges for obstetric services are likely to be partially responsible for the recent increase in maternal mortality rates observed in many African countries.

Allocation of resources to women's health is influenced by two factors, the availability of resources and the will to distribute them to a needy population. Services provided at low costs can be effective. In the 1920s and 1930s, women in Liverpool who could not afford delivery by a doctor were attended in labour by dedicated lay persons, who could appropriately be described as traditional birth attendants/midwives. Despite a high prevalence of obstetric risk factors in this group maternal mortality ratios were lower than for those of more affluent women who had been cared for by doctors.[25] The obstetric care delivered by semi-skilled midwives was superior to obstetric care delivered by doctors despite or because it did not utilize 'medical' obstetric skills. A relative lack of resources does not equal poor health. Kerala State in South West India has achieved some of the developing world's best rates of life expectancy, literacy and infant mortality, despite having one of the lowest per capita incomes. Especially notable is the nearly equal distribution of development benefits to urban and rural, male and female, high-caste and low-caste sections of the population. An even population distribution, a cosmopolitan trading history, less discrimination against women and the development of militant worker and small farmer organizations led by dedicated activists provide the main explanations for Kerala's achievements. Land reform has redistributed wealth and political power from a rich elite to smallholders and landless labourers. Public food distribution at controlled prices, large-scale public health actions, accessible medical facilities and widespread literacy combine with and reinforce each other to maintain and expand Kerala's achievements.[26] Kerala's major reforms were not specifically aimed at improving the situation of women but have still resulted in a vast improvement of their living conditions and health. This is reflected in Kerala's maternal mortality rate (2/1000 live births) which is about one-third of the all-India rate in 1987 (5.8/1000 live births).[27]

SOCIAL STATUS OF WOMEN

Poor appreciation of women's social and biological function and of their work contribution manifests itself in a poor allocation of resources to female education and health at all stages in their lives.[28] Women peasant farmers in the developing world generate most domestically consumed food and while they work regularly 15 hours per day during the rainy season,[29,30] their calorie consumption is frequently less than that of their not-so-active male partners. A maternal health status report from Lesotho shows how customs or tradition can contribute to the poor nutritional status of women. Men and boys are fed before women and girls. Female family members would only have the leftovers.[31] Only 55% to 80% of women in sub-Saharan Africa will have an adequate daily calorie intake.[32] Maternal undernutrition and hard physical work not only contributes to the poor perinatal outcomes frequently observed in developing countries[33] but also influences the risk of maternal mortality.[34] It has been estimated that 500 million women in developing countries are stunted as a result of chronic inadequate nutrition in childhood.[35] Many of these women will have an inadequate development of the bony pelvis. This, together with early pregnancies, will expose women to the risks of obstructed labour. One consequence of obstructed labour can be the development of vesico-vaginal fistulae (VVF). The prevalence of obstetric fistulae in the developing world is reaching endemic proportions.[36] Falandry and colleagues[37] estimated that 40 000 women suffer from VVF in francophone Africa alone. These women have more than a medical problem. They are frequently marginalized and abandoned by their partners, family and society.

An anaemia prevalence of 60% to 70% has been found repeatedly among pregnant women in developing countries.[38,39] Whilst malaria, frequent pregnancies and haemoglobinopathies contribute significantly to this high incidence, anaemia in developing countries is largely a manifestation of undernutrition.[40] Unless oxytoxic drugs are given, postpartum haemorrhage occurs in 10% to 20% of all deliveries,[41] and anaemic women are less able to tolerate this. As postpartum haemorrhage is responsible for approximately 50% of maternal deaths in Indonesia and Egypt and over 30% of maternal deaths in India[42] anaemia must therefore contribute to a significant proportion of maternal mortalities.

Maternal education has an important influence on maternal mortality.[43-45] Women without formal education in northern Nigeria had a risk of maternal mortality five times greater than that of educated women.[24] Sri Lanka and Nigeria are equally poor, but adult female literacy rates are 83% for Sri Lanka as compared to 31% for Nigeria, and maternal deaths per 100 000 deliveries are 50 for Sri Lanka and 800 for Nigeria.[46]

Although education and social welfare are not primarily aimed at improving maternal health, provision of these services as demonstrated in Kerala State, Sri Lanka, Costa Rica, Cuba or China does lead to a sustained reduction of maternal mortality and morbidity. If families and politicians decide to allocate resources to female education and nutrition, a major impact on maternal mortality can be expected without spending any more on maternal or reproductive health care.

POOR AVAILABILITY OF GOOD QUALITY HEALTH SERVICE

Health care has to be accessible to be effective. Obstetric complications can be fatal within hours, and access to adequate emergency obstetric care (EOC) can determine if a woman lives or dies (Table 3.2).[47,48]

Religion, traditions and social status of women can interfere with their access to medical care even in emergencies.[48] Women in northern Cameroon, for example, say that they would prefer to die rather than to seek unauthorized care in their husband's absence.[50] While lack of knowledge, traditional or religious barriers undoubtedly prevent women from seeking EOC, many do not reach EOC because of inadequate medical or transport infrastructure.

Only 55% of the world's deliveries are conducted by a trained attendant (including trained traditional birth attendants)[51] and traditional birth attendants (TBAs) are the one 'cadre of health personnel' attending most deliveries. Many programmes have centred on training TBAs, who frequently have a high social standing within their community and can act as a facilitator for change in other areas of health too.[52,53] TBA training can reduce perinatal and maternal mortality and morbidity, and where co-operation between hospitals and TBAs is possible, and backup can be guaranteed, excellent results

Table 3. 2 Estimated average interval from onset to death[a]

Condition	Interval
Postpartum haemorrhage	2 hours
Antepartum haemorrhage	12 hours
Ruptured uterus	1 day
Eclampsia	2 days
Obstructed labour	3 days
Sepsis	6 days

have been achieved.[54] The Federal University of Ceara, Brazil, pioneered such a scheme. Following meetings with community leaders and TBAs in a medically unserved rural town, a vacant building was converted to an 'obstetric unit'. Community participation kept costs minimal. TBAs received basic training and supervision through the University hospital. TBAs did not perform vaginal examinations and used no drugs. The obstetric unit was mainly a clean labour and delivery environment. A working referral system for high-risk patients was established. Out of 1798 deliveries which attended for delivery in such units only 12% to 15% were transferred. Fetal distress resulting from prolonged labour was virtually absent, as was puerperal infection. Maternal injury or distress and neonatal diarrhoea were all less common than at the University hospital. Caesarean section rate for all patients who presented to the TBA obstetric unit was less than 4% (compared with 65% for private patients at the University hospital). The reputation of one of the units became so good that patients with health insurance who could choose hospital delivery preferred to confine at the obstetric TBA unit.[55]

When provision of adequate but minimal obstetric care by trained TBAs can be coupled with the provision of good quality emergency obstetric services a significant reduction of maternal mortality can be achieved with little extra financial resources. Fauveau and colleagues[56] and Greenwood and colleagues[57] evaluated the impact of training traditional birth attendants on the outcome of pregnancy in Bangladesh and The Gambia. When comparing pregnancy outcomes in villages where TBAs had been trained with villages without trained TBAs, they found that maternal mortality rates were significantly lower in villages with trained TBAs. A 68% reduction in maternal mortality was observed in Bangladesh![56] Although they concluded that trained TBAs contributed to improving the outcome of pregnancy they felt that other factors may have been important. Training TBAs is certainly not a panacea. It would be an inefficient intervention in areas where TBAs attend relatively few deliveries and where a referral and supervision system cannot be maintained. As occurs so often in medical care, failures of programmes or projects are hardly ever published. Improving the standards of delivery care provided by TBAs might still offer a cost-effective halfway solution to meet obstetric needs in the developing world.

Obstetric haemorrhage, which can kill in hours, remains the single most common direct obstetric cause of maternal mortality[58] and access to EOC largely determines if maternal mortality and morbidity can be prevented. Delay of EOC can be fatal. Several factors delaying attendance for emergency obstetric care can be identified: lack of knowledge, low social status of women or poor quality of the service, geographical or financial inaccessibility of health care.[59] To reduce maternal mortality rates some form of EOC has to be accessible for all women. EOC can be provided without being comprehensive and such an approach towards solving the obstetric needs of the community has been described in Bangladesh.[60] It does not copy European or North American high-technology concepts. Delivering basic care to all women will produce more health than delivering specialist care to the urban middle and upper class. Most obstetric emergencies do not require a fully equipped obstetric unit but can and should be treated closer to the mother's home. Effective emergency obstetric care can be delivered by rural midwives.[61] There are many obstacles to introducing such a programme as it requires empowering non-medical personnel to administer some medical treatment. Obstetricians and their professional bodies are not always in the forefront of supporting changes which they conceive as undermining their position. Delegation of basic EOC responsibilities and provision of the necessary resources to non-medical personnel remains the best option for health services in developing countries. Many reports confirm that delegating responsibilities to non-medical personnel can be successfully practised in developing countries, and midwives or medical assistants routinely perform all types of obstetric surgery with excellent results in some hospitals.[62,63] Further experience from Bangladesh, where professional organizations support the changes, should demonstrate the importance of this EOC program.

There is no need to wait for more research to fully support one of the time-honoured obstetric services in developing countries – maternity waiting homes. These low-cost buildings usually resemble the patient's home and are attached to health centres or hospitals. Women in whom obstetric complications are anticipated and who could otherwise not gain access to adequate EOC will stay in these facilities during the last weeks of their pregnancies. Very limited input of health care resources is required and the expectant mothers will look after themselves. Maternity waiting homes offer an environment to educate pregnant women, to improve their general health and their access to obstetric care, and to provide something they would not usually get – a 'holiday' – a significant but temporary improvement of social status. Not surprisingly maternity waiting homes are one type of appropriate obstetric technology which is very popular among women. The introduction of maternity waiting homes in Ituk Mbang, Eastern Nigeria reduced maternal mortality rate from 10 in 1000 to less than 1 in 1000 deliveries.[64] Cuba built its first maternity waiting home in 1962; by 1984 there were 85 such homes and 99% of babies were delivered in hospital; maternal mortality fell from 118 to 31 per 100 000 live births.[65] While maternity waiting homes are an under-researched health facility there can be no doubt that they can increase access to obstetric care in rural areas and can prevent obstetric disasters.[66] Maternity waiting homes are primary health care in the very best sense. The concept of maternity waiting homes is therefore not restricted to the developing world.[67]

INADEQUATE CONTRACEPTIVE/REPRODUCTIVE CHOICE

Complications of pregnancy termination are likely to be responsible for half of maternal mortalities. More than 200 000 women are therefore thought to die every year from the consequences of unsafe abortion.[68–70] If all women

Table 3.3[71] Comparison of contraceptive use with other human resource elements in Pakistan and Bangladesh

	Pakistan	Bangladesh
Gross national product (1985)	$ 286	$ 150
Literacy (1980)	26%	26%
Urbanization (1980)	29%	18%
Total fertility rate (1988)	6.5	4.8
Contraceptive use (1990)	12%	40%

who wanted no more children were to stop bearing children, the birth rate would fall by 17% in Africa, 33% in Asia and 35% in Latin America.[4] By providing means to avoid pregnancies too early, too late, too close together or too many, contraception is the best preventive care a gynaecologist can offer. Contraception, like education, does not aim at improving maternal health but does so as a spin off by preventing unskilled terminations of pregnancy and their sequelae: haemorrhage, infection, infertility or death.

Contraceptive technology is well advanced and research into distribution methods shows that poor societies can afford good family planning programmes. More than anything else this requires the will to provide contraceptive services (Table 3.3).

Family planning is more than an issue of safe motherhood or population growth control. Family planning is about the right of every couple to determine the size of their family.

While further research would be desirable we can use the tools we have and know to continue working at our aim of a 50% reduction of maternal mortality by the year 2000. We did not intend to describe the organization of obstetric services or the management of obstetric complications in the developing world. These topics are covered by many excellent publications.[51,58,72–76] The purpose of this paper was to show that improvements are possible even with restricted resources.

We have the tools, skills and resources to reduce maternal mortality but do we have the will to use them? Dr Fathalla[77] defined our position in the struggle for better maternal health: 'We have only one place to stand: with women, beside women and behind women, and when the moment of truth is called, we will stand up to be counted'.

REFERENCES

1 Count C. World Health Organization claims maternal mortality has been underestimated. BMJ 1996; 312: 398
2 Boerma T. The magnitude of the maternal mortality problem in sub-Saharan Africa. Sco Sci Med 1987; 24(6): 551–558
3 Jacobson J L. Women's reproductive health, the silent emergency. World watch papers 102. Washington, D.C.: Worldwatch institute, 1991

4 AbouZahr C, Royston E, eds. Maternal Mortality: a fact book. Geneva: World Health Organization, 1991: pp 3–14

5 World Health Organization. Prevention of maternal mortality: report of World Health Organization International Meeting, November 11–15, 1985. Geneva: World Health Organization, 1986

6 Turmen T, AbouZahr C. Safe motherhood. Int J Gynecol Obstet 1994; 46: 145–153

7 Henshaw S K. Induced abortion: a world review. Fam Plann Perspect 1990; 22: 72–76

8 Starrs A. Preventing the tragedy of maternal deaths; a report on the international safe motherhood conference. Nairobi: World Health Organization, 1987

9 World Health Organization. Maternal mortality ratios and rates. A tabulation of available information. 3rd edn. Geneva: World Health Organization, 1991

10 Rochat R W. Table 2: Estimated lifetime chance of dying from pregnancy related causes, by region, 1975–85 In: Starrs A, ed. Preventing the tragedy of maternal deaths: a report of the international safe motherhood conference, Nairobi. Washington, D.C.: World Bank, 1987

11 Koblinsky M A, Campbell O M R, Harlow S. Mother and more: a broader pespective on women's health. In: Koblinsky M, Timyan J, Gay J, eds. San Francisco: Westview Press 1993; pp 33–63

12 Griffin C. The need to change health care priorities in LDCs. Finan Dev 1991; 28: 1

13 Winikoff B, Sullivan M. Assessing the role of family planning in reducing maternal mortality. Stud Fam Plann 1987; 18: 128

14 United Nations Department of International Economic and Social Affairs (UNDIESA). The world's women: trends and statistics 1970–1990. New York: United Nations, 1991

15 United Nations Development Program (UNDP). Human development report 1991. New York: Oxford University Press, 1991

16 Sivard R L. Women . . . a world survey. Washington, D.C.: World Priorities. In: Koblinsky M, Timyan J, Gay J, eds. The health of women, a global perspective. San Francisco: Westview Press, 1993

17 World Bank. World Development Report, 1992

18 Merrick T W. Safe motherhood: programme costs effectiveness and benefits in Family Planning, meeting challenges: promoting choices. In: Senanayake P, Kleinman R, eds. Proceedings of the IPPF family planning congress. Pearl River USA: Parthenon Publishing Group, Cranforth, UK, 1992: p 553

19 World Health Organization Global Advisory Group. The global burden of disease. Contribution to World Development. Geneva: World Health Organization, 1992

20 DeBethune X, Alfani S, Lahaye P. The influence of an abrupt price increase on health service utilization: evidence from Zaire. Health Policy Plann 1989; 4: 76–81

21 Yoder R A. Are people willing and able to pay for health service? Soc Sci Med 1989; 29: 76–81

22 Bennett S. The impact of the increase in user fees: a preliminary investigation. Lesotho Epidemiol Bull 1989; 4: 29–37

23 Ekwempu C C, Maine D, Olorukoba M B, Essien E S, Kisseka M N. Structural adjustment and health in Africa. Lancet 1990; 336(8706): 56–57

24 Harrison K A. Approaches to reducing maternal and perinatal mortality in Africa. In: Philpott R H, ed. Maternity services in the developing world – what the community needs. London: RCOG, 1980: pp 52–69

25 Bickerton T H. A medical history of Liverpool from the earliest days to the year 1920. London: John Murray, 1936

26 Franke R W, Chais B H. Kerala state, India: radical reform as development. Int J Health Services 1992; 22: 139–156

27 Government of Kerala. Economic review. Thiruvananthapuram: 1989 State Planning Board, 1990; p 93

28 Makinson C. Discrimination against the female child. Int J Gynecol Obstet 1994; 46: 119

29 Bleiberg F M, Burn T A et al. Duration of activities and energy expenditure of female farmers in dry and rainy season in Upper Volta. Br J Nutr 1980; 45: 505–515

30 Roberts S, Paul A A, Cole T J et al. Seasonal changes in activity, birth weight and lactation performance in rural Gambian women. Transact R Soc Trop Med Hyg 1982; 76(5): 668–678.

31 Government of Lesotho. Lesotho Country paper. Paper presented at the Conference on Safe Motherhood for the Southern African Development Coordinating Council (SADCC) countries. Harare, Zimbabwe: Health Ministry, 1990

32 Mhloyi M. Maternal mortality in the SADCC region. Background paper for the Conference on Safe Motherhood for the Southern African Development Coordinating Council (SADCC) countries. Harare, Zimababwe: 1990
33 Tafari N, Naeye R L. Effect of maternal undernutrition and heavy physical work during pregnancy on birth weight. Br J Obstet Gynaecol 1980; 87: 222–226
34 Paul B K. Maternal mortality in Africa: 1980–87. Soc Sci Med 1993; 37(6): 745–752
35 Leslie J. Women nutrition: the key to improving family health in developing countries. Food Nutrit Bullet 1991; 10(3): 4–7
36 Lawson J. Vaginal fistulas. Int J Gynecol Obstet 1993; 40: 13–17
37 Falandry L, Dumergier C, Scham A, Ivoulsou E, Picaud J. La fistule obstetricale eb Afrique. Med Armees 1989; 17: 571
38 DeMaeyer D, Adies-Tegman M. The prevalence of anaemia in the world. World Health Stat Quart 1985; 38: 302–316
39 Jordan E A, Sloan L S. The prevalence of anaemia in developing countries. 1979–89 an annotated bibliography. MotherCare Working Paper 7A. Arlington, VA: MotherCare, 1991
40 Baker S J, DeMaeyer E M. Nutritional anaemia: its understanding and control with special reference to the work of the World Health Organization. Am J Clin Nutr 1979; 32: 368–417
41 World Health Organization. The prevention and management of postpartum haemorrhage. Report of a technical working group. World Health Organization Report, 1990
42 UNFPA. State of the world population 1989. Investing in women: the focus of the nineties. United Nations Population Fund, 1989
43 Nylander P P, Adekunle A O. Antenatal care in developing countries. Baillières Clin Obstet Gynaecol 1990; 4(1): 169–186
44 Obermeyer C M. Culture, maternal health care, and women's status: a comparison of Morocco and Tunisia. Stud Fam Plann 1993; 24(6 Pt 1): 354–365
45 Okafor C B. Availability of services for maternal and child health care in rural Nigeria. Int J Gynaecol Obstet 1991; 34(4): 331–346
46 Briggs N. Illiteracy and maternal health: educate or die. Lancet 1993; 341(8852): 1063–1064
47 Thaddeus S, Maine D. Too far to walk: maternal mortality in context. Soc Sci Med 1994; 38(8): 1091–1110
48 Okafor C B. Women helping women, incorporating women's perspective into community health projects. Paper presented at the 18th annual NCIH International Health Conference. Arlington, VA: 1991
49 Maine D, Rosenfield A, Kimball A M, Kwast B, White S. Prevention of maternal deaths in developing countries: program options and practical considerations. Paper presented at the International Safe Motherhood Conference. Nairobi: February 10–13, 1987
50 Alexandre M. The role of gender, socio-economic, cultural and religious pressure on the health of women in Cameroon. Paper presented at the 18th annual NCIH International Health Conference Arlington, VA, 1991
51 World Health Organization. Coverage of maternity care. A tabulation of available information. 3rd edn. Geneva: World Health Organization, 1993: p 12
52 Sparks B T. A descriptive study of the changing roles and practices of traditional birth attendants in Zimbabwe. J Nurse-Midwifery 1990; 35(3): 150–161
53 Kargbo T K. Rural maternity care in Sierra Leone. Int J Gynecol Obstet 1992; 38(Suppl): S29–S31
54 Hyppolito S B. Alternative model for low risk obstetric care in Third World rural and peri-urban areas. Int J Gynaecol Obstet 1992; 38(Suppl): S63–S66
55 Araujo G. The traditional birth attendant in Brazil. In: Phillpott R H, ed. Maternity services in the developing world – what the community needs. London: RCOG, 1980: pp 293–311
56 Fauveau V, Stewart K, Khan S A, Chakraborty J. Effect on mortality of community-based maternity-care programme in rural Bangladesh. Lancet 1991; 338(8776): 1183–1186
57 Greenwood A M, Bradley A K, Byass P, Greenwood B M, Snow R W, Bennett S, Hatib-N'Jie A B. Evaluation of a primary health care programme in The Gambia. I. The impact of trained traditional birth attendants on the outcome of pregnancy. J Trop Med Hyg 1990; 93(1): 58–66
58 World Health Organization. Prevention and management of postpartum haemorrhage. Geneva: World Health Organization, 1989
59 Timyan J, Griffey Brechin S, Measham D M, Ogunleye B. Access to care: more than a problem of distance. In: Koblinsky M, Timyan J, Gay J, eds. The health of women, a global perspective. San Francisco: Westview Press, 1993: pp 217–234

60 Haque Y, Mostafa G. A review of the emergency obstetric care functions of selected facilities in Bangladesh. UNICEF, 1993
61 Taylor J E. Life-saving skills training for rural midwives: report on the Ghanian experience. Int J Gynecol Obstet 1992; 38(Suppl): S41–S44
62 Nasah B T. General principles in delegation of maternity functions to community-based health workers. Int J Gynecol Obstet 1992; 38(Suppl): S23–S27
63 Duale S. Delegation of responsibility in maternity care in Kawara rural health zone, Zaire. Int J Gynecol Obstet 1992; 38(Suppl): S33–S35
64 Lawson L B, Stewart D B. The organization of obstetric services. In: Lawson L B, Stewart, D B, eds. Obstetrics and gynaecology in the tropics and developing countries. London: Edward Arnold, 1968: p 309
65 Farnot Cardoso U. Giving birth is safer now. World Health Forum 1988; 9: 387–388
66 Poovan P, Kifle F, Kwast B E. A maternity waiting home reduces obstetric catastrophes. World Health Forum 1990; 11: 440–445
67 Yordan E E, Yordan R A. The maternity home for adolescents: a concept from the past fulfilling a contemporary need. Connecticut Med 1993; 57(2): 65–68
68 Coeytoaux F M. Induced abortion in sub-Saharan Africa: what we do and do not know. Stud Fam Plann 1988; 19(3): 186–190
69 McLaurin K E, Hord C, Wolf M. Health System role in abortion care: the need for a pro-active approach (Carrboro NC: International Projects Assistance Service (IPAS)), 1991
70 Royston E. Estimating the number of abortion deaths. In: Coeytaux F, Leonard A, Royston E, eds. Methological issues in abortion research. New York: Population Council, 1989: pp 23–28
71 Potts M. Costs, finance and human resources. In: Senanayake P, Kleinman R, eds. Family Planning, meeting challenges: promoting choices. Proceedings of the IPPF family planning congress, 1992. Pearl River USA: Parthenon Publishing Group, Cranforth, UK, 1992; pp 709–721
72 World Health Organization. Studying maternal mortality in developing countries – a guide book. Geneva: World Health Organization, 1987
73 World Health Organization. Prevention and management of severe anaemia in pregnancy. Geneva: World Health Organization, 1993
74 World Health Organization. Essential elements of obstetric care at first referral level. Geneva: World Health Organization, 1991
75 Guidotti R, Jobson D. Detecting pre-eclampsia: a practical guide. Geneva: World Health Organization, 1992
76 World Health Organization. An annotated bibliography of the document produced by the division of family health. Geneva: World Health Organization, 1994
77 Fathalla M F. Women's health: an overview. Int J Gynecol Obstet 1994; 46: 105–118

4 Practical risk management advice on the labour ward

L. M. Irvine

Medicolegal claims are a major problem in the National Health Service (NHS).[1] The number and size of claims have increased from £53 million in 1990/1991 to £125 million in 1994 and are set to top £150 million in 1995. To combat increasing litigation the NHS Executive is launching a risk management campaign to stop these claims from crippling the National Health Service. Obstetrics and gynaecology is considered to be a high-risk speciality, and accounted for the second largest settlement by the Medical Defence Union between August and October 1994.[2]

The aim of this chapter is to draw attention to the implications of obstetric patient management, the importance of clear documentation in the case notes, good communication with the patient, her partner, and other medical and midwifery staff. This will hopefully reduce the number of claims, and simplify the preparation of a defence should a claim arise. It does not encourage the practice of defensive medicine, and does not deal in detail with the surgical techniques, which have already been covered in terms of fetal,[3] and maternal[4] safety at Caesarean section.

The points raised in the paper may be considered to be common sense, but audit of practice and documentation in the unit in which you work may yield unexpected results. In a recent review of 50 consecutive instrumental vaginal deliveries, in only 7 cases was the swab count, and in 1 case the needle count noted to be correct (L M Irvine, unpublished). Of 100 consecutive obstetric cases settled 29% involved retained swabs or instruments.[5]

LABOUR WARD PROTOCOL

The Labour Ward Protocol will have been drawn up by the Consultants and are local guidelines for patient management. The importance of guidelines has been stressed in a recent report from the Royal College of Obstetricians and Gynaecologists;[6] these should be drawn up by an 'in-house committee' and regularly audited. With the changes in working patterns and the introduction of shift systems, the junior medical staff may not be aware of the Consultant's management of various conditions, without reference to the Labour Ward Protocol.

Different units may have different protocols, therefore it should be read carefully. Examples may be the method of induction, management of breech presentation, the use of fetal scalp sampling and the use of syntocinon in multigravid patients.

LABOUR WARD ROUNDS

It is important that regular ward rounds are performed and documented in the case notes, the times of which may be suggested in the Labour Ward Protocol. When performing a ward round it is important that you introduce yourself to every patient on the labour ward, so that you are familiar with them should a problem arise.

It is prudent to look at the previous obstetric history as a previous Caesarean section or other complication in a past pregnancy may not have been fully appreciated. It is important to carefully examine all the cardiotocographic trace as although it may be normal at present there may have been abnormalities previously.

DOCUMENTATION IN THE NOTES

A recurring problem in constructing a defence is poor standard of note keeping. When seeing a patient it is important to document whether you saw the patient on a ward round, or were called to see the patient, and if called in from home, this should also be documented.

The date and time should be recorded; although a 24 hour system has been proposed most clocks and watches are 12 hours and a consistent system should be used; if 12 hours am or pm should be used.[7] A black pen should be used for writing notes as this photocopies more clearly than blue. A plan of action should be written and all entries clearly signed.

It is important to write in the correct place in the notes, as if not, it could be claimed that the notes were not read when the patient was seen. If a continuation sheet is used a patient Identification Label, or patient's details should be written on it. Should a mistake be made it should be crossed through, but should still be able to be read. Correction fluid should not be used. It is much easier to defend a case based on what is written in the notes, rather than what is one's clinical practice. Even though vaginal and rectal examination was carried out after episiotomy repair, if not documented in the notes a doubt is cast.

If litigation is suspected, the Consultant should be informed and a summary written in the notes. This should be clearly written, timed and dated. If one is a member of a defence organization it is also wise to inform them of the potential problems.

As obstetric claims may occur many years after delivery, it is useful to keep copies of the Labour Ward protocols. As it is updated it is important to have copies of the old protocols, and the date at which they were changed. It is also important that old day timetables, and night on-call rotas are kept so that members of staff involved with a case many years previously can be identified. These documents should be stored in one place, usually on Labour Ward, and their collection and safekeeping should be the responsibility of a named individual, usually the Consultant in charge of Labour Ward.

MECONIUM

Meconium is often the reason for being called and this should be described in the notes. If the blanket term meconium is used should there be a problem in the future this would be taken as a sign of fetal distress. Thin, old meconium is of no prognostic significance for the later development of asphyxia.[8] However, thick fresh meconium may be a marker of fetal hypoxia,[9] and the Labour Ward Protocol may suggest either fetal scalp blood sampling or emergency Caesarean section.

FETAL SCALP SAMPLING

Although the use of fetal scalp sampling has been shown to reduce the Caesarean section rate for fetal distress,[10] units may differ in the protocol for scalp sampling. When considering fetal scalp sampling the full clinical situation should be considered. If the patient is primigravid with a cervix which is only 2–3 cm dilated and an abnormal cardiotocographic trace, clearly delivery is some way off. Multiple scalp samples may be required, which may not be appropriate or acceptable to the patient and a Caesarean section should be considered.

If a scalp sample is taken the result should be acted upon. It is unwise to ignore a low result as it was unexpected. The result of the sample should be handwritten in the notes, and the hard copy, with the patient's name and hospital number recorded on it, fixed in the notes also. Clear adhesive tape should be avoided as it fades the result, which may become illegible within a few weeks.[11]

As the aim of fetal scalp sampling is to exclude suspected fetal distress, failure to obtain a sample should lead to emergency Caesarean section as fetal distress has not been excluded.

BREECH PRESENTATION

If a trial of vaginal breech delivery has been decided, usually estimated fetal weight, and CT or X-ray pelvimetry will have been carried out. The obstetrician on Labour Ward should review these and personally look at the films. It is possible that the measurements have been incorrectly reported or an abnormal sacral curve missed.

INSTRUMENTAL VAGINAL DELIVERY

When an instrumental delivery for delay is considered it is important to review the obstetric case notes. If the patient is multigravid, having spontaneously delivered infants of reasonable weights, the reason for the delay should be considered. It is possible that the fetus is macrosomic, and should a forceps delivery be undertaken there is a risk of shoulder dystocia, and Caesarean section should be considered.

In the case of instrumental vaginal delivery it is important that the amount of head palpable abdominally is clearly noted, the station, the position, and whether there is caput or moulding. If Kjelland's forceps are used it is suggested that this is done as a trial in theatre with preparations made for Caesarean section should there be a problem.

A trial of forceps means that the patient is assessed and forceps delivery attempted; if there is any problem, the forceps are removed and a Caesarean section carried out. If the patient is delivered by Caesarean section, it does not mean that the trial has failed, but rather that the trial showed that Caesarean section was appropriate. The term failed or abandoned trial of forceps is incorrect and should not be used.

VENTOUSE DELIVERY

With the development of silicone rubber cups and electronic suction equipment, the rate of ventouse delivery is increasing. There are, however, several basic principles that should be considered. The delivery should be completed within 15 minutes, and the cup should not be reapplied more than twice. If the patient is not delivered by ventouse, forceps should not be used and a Caesarean section should be performed.[12]

When writing the operation note of an instrumental delivery it is also important to document that the swab and needle count is correct and that rectal and vaginal examination have been performed. One of the most frequent claims in obstetrics is for retained swabs or instruments.

ELECTIVE CAESAREAN SECTION

The surgeon should review the case notes and see the patient preoperatively. The reasons for Caesarean section should be considered. It may be that the presentation is no longer breech, and if there is any doubt on clinical examination, an ultrasound scan should be performed to confirm presentation. In the case of elective repeat Caesarean section, if an ultrasonic scan in late pregnancy has been performed it should be studied.

The incidence of placenta praevia or acreata increases with the number of previous Caesarean sections, from 0.42% with an unscarred uterus to 22.2% with four previous Caesarean sections.[13] It may therefore be appropriate to delay the case until an ultrasonic scan has been performed for placental localization. In the case of placenta previa it is Royal College guidelines that a senior obstetrician should directly supervise or perform the Caesarean section themself.

If sterilization at Caesarean section has been agreed it is important to discuss other forms of contraception, the failure rate and irreversibility of the procedure. At delivery a paediatric opinion should be sought to see if there are any concerns with the infant, and if there is any doubt the procedure should be deferred.

EMERGENCY CAESAREAN SECTION

When the decision has been made to perform a Caesarean section, it is important that you write in the notes and on the cardiotocographic trace the time when the decision was made. If at emergency Caesarean section there is delay between the decision and the delivery of the fetus it is wise to state these reasons in the notes. It may be that the delay was caused by anaesthetic problems or by a lack of operating department assistance. Analysis of data of high value claims from the Medical Protection Society show over 70% of these cases were related to a delay in delivery.[14]

It is easy to be lulled into a false sense of security at emergency Caesarean section for fetal distress. The vast majority of infants delivered are in good condition, and it could be said that Caesarean section was unnecessary. It can, however, be argued that fetal distress had been diagnosed early and the infant delivered before severe acidosis has occurred. Once fetal distress has been diagnosed, Caesarean section should be carried out without delay. It is thought that there is individual vulnerability to the development of hypoxic damage, although all infants will suffer if the insult is of sufficient severity and duration.[15] As we do not have accurate means of predicting vulnerability, cardiotocographic abnormalities should be acted upon.

It is possible to perform a classical Caesarean section through a Pfannenstiel incision, although some operators prefer a midline skin incision.[2] If a midline skin incision is to be used it is wise to explain the reasons to the patient. If not adequately explained the patient may feel aggrieved that most of the other women on the ward had a Pfannenstiel incision, which they may find more cosmetically acceptable. After the Caesarean section the operation note should be written by the surgeon and any further thoughts on future pregnancies should be documented. It is also important to write in the notes that the swab and needle counts were correct.

COMMUNICATION WITH THE PATIENT

One of the possible reasons for litigation is that the patient may feel that she has been misled or let down. The patient should not be promised what cannot be delivered. A patient may request an epidural anaesthetic, but may have anaesthetic complications that are not apparent to the obstetrician. An

Table 4.1 Problems and solutions in medicolegal claims or patient complaints

Problem	Solution
Claim difficult to defend because of lack of documentation	Clear entries in notes of problem and management, timed, dated and signed. Operation notes written by surgeon
Difficulty in staff identification	Timetables, night rotas and specimen signatures kept on Labour Ward
Claims for problems after episiotomy repair	Documentation of materials used, method of repair, and vaginal and rectal examination
Claims for retained swabs or needles	Swabs and needles counted by surgeon and documented in the notes
Claims for retained placental tissue after Caesarean section	Check placenta before closing uterus
Claims for cerebral palsy	Regular teaching on cardiotographic interpretation. Once fetal distress has been diagnosed, delivery without delay. Cord pH performed and written in the notes
Complaints about patient management	Clear explanation about reasons for intervention. Follow-up visit next day

epidural does not always remove all pain sensation, so pain-free labour should not be promised.

A partner may wish to be present at instrumental delivery or Caesarean section. This is at the discretion of the obstetrician and also the paediatrician and anaesthetist, and should not be agreed to without their consent.

Many cases of litigation in obstetrics result from the fact that the patient wants an explanation as to what happened. It is suggested that on the following day the surgeon should see all the patients that he performed an instrumental vaginal delivery or Caesarean section on. An explanation can be given as to their management, and any questions which the patient or her partner have may be answered. It is possible that this alone may reduce the chances of a claim and it is also rewarding and satisfying for the surgeon.

Table 4.1 summarizes problems and solutions in medicolegal claims or patient complaints.

By taking these precautions it is hoped that preparation of a case should a claim be brought would be easy and involve less administrative time. Good documentation is vital to the construction of a defence and may well lead to an unjustified claim being dropped at an early stage.

ACKNOWLEDGEMENTS

I would like to thank Professor R.W. Shaw and Mr Martin Stone for their advice on the preparation of this chapter. I would also like to thank Miss Lillian Robertson. This paper has been partly funded by the Royal Gwent Gynaecological Research Fund.

REFERENCES

1 Sylvester R. Cost of medical errors threatens to cripple the NHS. The Sunday Telegraph, January 15th 1985, p 14
2 Top 10 Settled Cases. J Med Defen Union 1995; 11(2): 27
3 Roberts G. If only a Caesarean had been carried out. J Med Defen Union 1993; 9: 76–78
4 Irvine L M. Reducing maternal complications at Caesarean section. J Med Defen Union 1994; 10: 28–29
5 Medical Defence Union Data, 1991
6 Minimum standards of care in labour. Report of a Working Party of the Royal College of Obstetrics and Gynaecology, 1994
7 Woolfson J. Medicolegal risk management. The Diplomate 1994; 1(3): 228–229
8 Schulze M. The significance of the passage of meconium during labour. Am J Obstet Gynecol 1925; 10: 83–85
9 Desmond M M, Moore J, Lindley J E, Brown C A. Meconium staining of the amniotic fluid. Obstet Gynaecol 1957; 9: 91–103
10 Irvine L M, Shaw R W. Fetal blood sampling and Caesarean section for fetal distress: Results of a pilot study. J Obstet Gynaecol 1989; 10: 120–123
11 Irvine L M, O'Brien P M S, Shaw R W. A cause of medicolegal complications. J Med Defen Union 1989; 5: 23
12 Johanson R. Ventouse delivery. The Diplomate 1994; 1(3): 186–191
13 Couri J A, Sultan M G. Previous Caesarean section and the rising incidence of placenta previa and acreata. J Obstet Gynaecol 1994; 14: 14–16
14 Brown A D G. Medicolegal aspects of fetal monitoring. In: Spencer A J D, ed. Fetal monitoring physiology and techniques of antenatal and intrapartum fetal assessment. Turnbridge Wells: Caste House Publication, 1989
15 Hull D M B. Intrapartum events and cerebral palsy. Br J Obstet Gynaecol 1994; 101: 745–747

5 Prediction and prevention of preterm labour

J. J. Morrison

Preterm labour and delivery, before 37 weeks gestation, is the major cause of perinatal morbidity and mortality in developed countries and is the single most important complication of pregnancy in the absence of congenital abnormality.[1] The incidence of preterm delivery varies between 5 and 10% of pregnancies but 70–80% of perinatal deaths occur in preterm infants.[1-4] Despite advances in perinatal medicine in recent decades, the problem of preterm delivery continues to frustrate satisfactory reproductive outcome, with little progress having been made in reducing the frequency of preterm births.[5] Recent reports from a large multicentre trial have demonstrated that 83% of neonatal deaths occured in pregnancies ending before 37 completed weeks of gestation, and 66% of neonatal deaths were in infants delivered before 29 weeks gestation.[6] The long-term medical and public health implications of handicap among the survivors has raised more questions than answers.[7] In addition, the associated economic impact of preterm births is a major burden on resources.[8] The problem of preterm delivery has actually been magnified in recent years as other causes of adverse perinatal outcome have decreased and it remains one of the most serious problems facing obstetricians and other perinatal health care professionals.

PRETERM LABOUR

Incidence

The incidence of preterm labour must be considered separately from overall preterm delivery rates. The figures for preterm delivery rates are arrived at after consideration of all causes of spontaneous preterm labour and deliberate intervention to achieve elective delivery. Preterm delivery rates have been reported as 5.1% in Oxford[3] and 7.6% in New York[2] in the 1970s. During the years 1981–1989, in the USA, the proportion of births before 37 weeks gestation actually increased from 9.4% in 1981 to 10.6% in 1989.[1] The black population experienced a dramatically higher preterm delivery rate than the caucasian (18.9% versus 8.8% in 1989, for example) and the incidence of preterm births has risen in both races in recent years. During the 9 year period from 1985–1993 the preterm delivery rate for women booked at the

Rosie Maternity Hospital, Cambridge was 8.7%.[9] Therefore, the preterm delivery rate varies between populations, appears to be increasing recently and lies between 5 and 10% of all births in developed countries.

The incidence of preterm labour has not been so widely reported. In the context of predictive and preventative measures to improve the poor perinatal outcome associated with preterm labour, the pregnancies of interest are those in which there is no maternal (e.g. pre-eclampsia, antepartum haemorrhage, chorioamnionitis) or fetal (e.g. retarded growth, congenital malformation) reason for which delivery might confer some benefit. For many reasons, it is difficult to obtain comparable statistics for this proportion from reported literature. The distinction between true and spurious preterm labour is often unclear, and the criteria used for diagnosis vary widely in different studies. The most common problem is diagnosis of preterm labour on the basis of contractions only, without the added features of alteration in cervical effacement and dilatation. This can lead to ambiguity in incidence reporting and erroneous reports of treatment outcome. In addition, the medical features of pregnancies complicated by preterm labour are often presented without a clear outline of the potential applicability of tocolytic therapy. For example, published reports frequently refer to the proportion suitable for tocolysis as those in whom spontaneous idiopathic preterm labour occurred without due reference to other situations, of known cause, where tocolysis may be equally appropriate (e.g. cervical incompetence, congenital uterine malformation).

Rush et al[3] subdivided preterm deliveries into four groups: (1) spontaneous labour of unknown cause, (2) spontaneous labour with maternal and/or fetal complications, (3) multiple pregnancy and (4) elective delivery. They reported that preterm labour in singleton pregnancies, occuring for no apparent reason, accounted for 38% of all preterm deliveries and 35% of all preterm early neonatal deaths. The proportion of women with preterm labour suitable for tocolytic therapy varies widely with different reports. Arias et al[10] reported that 23.3% of preterm deliveries were spontaneous, unexplained and appropriate for treatment to defer labour. This figure did not include women with cervical incompetence, urinary tract infection or genital tract malformations who were also suitable for such treatment. A Tennessee study found that of 321 women delivering babies between 500 and 1000 g, 82 (25.5%) had been in 'idiopathic preterm labor'.[11] A Dundee study found that the most frequent precipitating cause of delivery was uncomplicated spontaneous preterm labour.[12] A Philadelphia study reported that 30% of all preterm deliveries represented a failure of tocolytic treatment.[13] Analysis of the incidence of unexplained preterm labour in two different socioeconomic groups in the USA, revealed that it accounted for 34% of all preterm deliveries in the group receiving private obstetric care and 55% of those receiving state funded care.[14]

In summary, therefore, it appears that between one-quarter and one-half of preterm deliveries are caused by spontaneous preterm labour for which effective predictive and preventative measures, if available, might confer perinatal benefit. This proportion varies with the socioeconomic status, and the medical and demographic features of the population being studied.

Perinatal mortality and morbidity

Rapid advances in perinatal and neonatal medicine in recent decades have led to improved survival of preterm infants. The majority of tertiary referral centres now report almost 100% survival for infants delivered after 32 weeks gestation. In the 1990s the contribution of preterm delivery to perinatal mortality is related to the 30–40% of preterm births that occur more than 8 weeks before the expected date of delivery. The perinatal statistics in a UK teaching hospital regional neonatal centre (Rosie Maternity Hospital, Cambridge) during the 8 year period 1985–1992 revealed survival between 23 and 29 weeks to be as follows: 20% at 23 weeks, 56% at 24 weeks, 41% at 25 weeks, 54% at 26 weeks, 65% at 27 weeks, 91% at 28 weeks and 94% at 29 weeks.[15] These survival figures are in agreement with published data from other centres in different parts of the world[16–19] and outline the importance of early delivery as a cause of perinatal wastage.

However, survival is not the only issue worthy of consideration. In fact, in developed countries statistics relating to intrauterine or neonatal deaths are of limited value as an index of the effectiveness of perinatal care in the early preterm gestation periods.[20] With the increased survival of these infants attention must be paid to short-term morbidity and long-term physical and intellectual handicap. Before the introduction of neonatal intensive care mortality was so high for early preterm infants that reliable follow-up data were scanty. In recent years morbidity in relation to preterm delivery, at all gestation periods, has been reasonably well documented. The problem with some of these reports is that confusion exists between preterm and growth-retarded fetuses, and that it is difficult to adjust for the potential confounding effects of medical complications of pregnancy on the fetus. A detailed report of 206 preterm infants with carefully determined gestational ages, and without any detectable maternal or fetal complications, in a predominantly caucasian population, was provided by Konte et al.[17] From 26–34 weeks gestation the incidence of major neonatal morbidity ranged from 81–23% for respiratory distress syndrome, 50–13% for patent ductus arteriosus, 31–5% for sepsis and 25–2% for necrotizing enterocolitis. Other major developmental insults attributed to preterm delivery include intraventricular haemorrhage, periventricular leukomalacia and retinopathy of prematurity.[21,22]

The long-term outcome for infants born preterm is an important health problem in society. Recently, rises in the incidence of cerebral palsy among preterm infants have been consistently reported.[23–25] The number of blind survivors of preterm delivery has reached epidemic proportions.[22,26] Refractive errors (astigmatism, myopia or hypermetropia) and strabismus are also common. Hearing loss has been reported to occur in 1.5–9% of preterm infants who require neonatal intensive care.[27] It may occur in children who have no other physical or neurological disabilities. Intellectual impairments, including difficulties in areas of learning and academic achievement, visual-motor integration, language performance and behavioural problems have all been noted in excess in children delivered at early periods of gestation.[28]

Other adverse consequences of preterm delivery extend beyond the neonatal period giving rise to long-term health problems. Growth in later childhood is often compromised.[29] Infants who suffered from hyaline membrane disease or required assisted ventilation may have long-term respiratory ill health and it has been shown that they may have abnormal airway function at school age.[30] Infants delivered preterm are between 2 and 4.5 times more likely to be hospitalized than term infants in the first year of life.[31] Male infants born early are at much greater risk of needing inguinal hernia repair by 8 years of age.[32] While it is hoped that progress in the care of preterm infants will give them the ability to contribute to their families, and the societies in which they live, there are many issues concerning the prediction and prevention of preterm labour for which scientific solutions are urgently required.

PREDICTION OF PRETERM LABOUR

Much research has been directed at identification of women in whom preterm labour is likely to occur so that prevention could be addressed. It is imperative that such a screening tool, for use in a random population of pregnant women, be sensitive and specific and have high predictive value in a population where the incidence of the condition is low. Such a screening test must also be safe and cost effective because it will be applied to a large number of individuals. Numerous methods of screening for preterm labour have been proposed but none has fulfilled all the necessary criteria. These methods include risk scoring, cervical assessment, uterine activity monitoring, cervico-vaginal fibronectin, biochemical markers and mediators of inflammation and infection.

Risk scoring

Preterm labour is a heterogenous condition with numerous associated social and medical risk factors. It is more common in black women,[1,33] in women of low socioeconomic class,[34] in those who have had a previous preterm birth,[35] in multiple pregnancy,[36] at the extremes of reproductive life,[37] in cigarette smokers,[38] in pregnancies resulting from assisted conception,[37] in abusers of alcohol[39] or cocaine,[40] in women who do manual work[41] or those who work long hours,[42] and in a host of general medical and obstetric disorders.[43] The hope that the epidemiology of preterm labour might help in the identification of high-risk pregnancies has not been borne out in practice. Papiernik in France was the first to prospectively assign objective factors to identify patients at risk of preterm labour.[44] In 1980 Creasy et al[45] reported that 64%

of spontaneous preterm births in a population of 966 women in New Zealand could be predicted by a scoring system. Later attempts to apply similar predictive methods in various American populations were not as successful and failed to identify approximately 50% of patients who deliver spontaneously before term while many are identified as being at high risk even though they do not subsequently have preterm labour.[5] The construction and validation of formal risk scores has been reviewed by Keirse[46] and appears to offer a low positive predictive value and shows poor reproducibility and large differences in performance among different populations.

Cervical assessment

Precocious cervical ripening has been shown to be associated with preterm labour and the largest published series has come from Papiernik's group in France.[47,48] Cervical assessment was performed prior to 37 weeks gestation and early cervical ripening noted in 30% of the pregnancies studied. The finding of dilatation of the internal cervical os was associated with a fourfold increase in the risk of preterm delivery. The sensitivity and positive predictive value of these findings were not reported. Mortensen et al[49] reported their findings from 1327 women who underwent regular cervical examinations at 24, 28 and 32 weeks gestation. They divided their subjects into those regarded as being at increased risk for preterm delivery and those without risk factors. The positive predictive values for abnormal cervical findings were disappointingly low at 25–30% for the high-risk group and 4% for the low-risk group.

It has been suggested that ultrasound, and particularly endovaginal ultrasound, has the potential to provide objective repeatable cervical length measurements, which could be used in prediction of preterm labour.[50] Andersen et al evaluated 113 patients at 30 weeks gestation by comparing transabdominal and endovaginal ultrasound to measure cervical length and manual vaginal examination of cervical length.[50] They showed that cervical measurement < 39 mm (the median length) was associated with a significantly increased risk of preterm delivery (25% versus 6.7%) and the sensitivity was 76%. They found that manual examination of cervical effacement detected 71% of preterm births, but transabdominal ultrasonographic measurement of cervical length was not predictive. They were unable to recommend an optimum cut-off point for cervical length to predict preterm delivery risk. It therefore appears that the sensitivity and positive predictive value of cervical assessment are too low for its use as a screening tool in an unselected population.

Uterine activity monitoring

Studies have shown that an increase in the number of uterine contractions precedes the onset of preterm labour and that women are often not aware of this until labour is advanced.[51] Hence it has been proposed that devices used for home uterine activity monitoring may allow earlier detection of the onset of preterm labour.[52] While benefit in terms of earlier diagnosis of preterm labour leading to earlier intervention with tocolytic treatment, and improved birth weight and neonatal morbidity, has been reported with monitored uterine activity,[53] it has also, conversely, been shown to achieve no statistically significant reduction in preterm birth[54] A review of various preterm delivery prevention programs in the USA concluded that a combination of uterine activity monitoring with daily intensive perinatal nursing support in relation to awareness of symptoms and signs of preterm labour led to its earlier detection.[8] There are no reliable UK data on this issue. It is controversial whether it is home uterine activity monitoring or the greater emphasis on patient education and the increased nursing support associated with it that account for the greater likelihood of diagnosis of preterm labour before advanced cervical dilatation.[8]

Fibronectin

The presence of fetal fibronectin in cervico-vaginal secretions has been proposed as a specific predictor of preterm labour.[55,56] The combined results from these studies demonstrated that the presence of cervical or vaginal fetal fibronectin between 21 and 37 weeks gestation predicted preterm labour with a sensitivity of 68–81.7%, a specificity of 72–82.5% and positive and negative predictive values of approximately 30% and 95%, respectively. This investigation is technically complicated by the fact that contamination with microscopic amounts of amniotic fluid[57] or cervico-vaginal blood staining[58] may also give a positive fibronectin result. However, of most concern is the high false positive rate.[59,60] There are as yet no reliable UK data on this screening method but investigations are apparently currently underway.[59]

Biochemical markers

Although the precise order of events leading to parturition in the human, at term or preterm, is unknown, it is clear that the state of excitability of the myometrium is controlled by a complex network of physiological mechanisms involving hormones, peptides, calcium, extracellular matrix, cell membrane receptors, intracellular signalling systems, neuronal and metabolic factors, gap junctions and ion channels.[61] On this basis much work has been devoted to identifying a biochemical marker for this process.

Measurement of total or free plasma progesterone or oestradiol, or the progesterone: oestradiol plasma ratio are of no predictive value for term[62] or preterm[63] labour. There is evidence, however, that the saliva oestriol to progesterone ratio may be increased prior to preterm labour and this needs further evaluation.[64] Salivary oestriol itself has recently been reported as a sensitive, timely and non-invasive marker for preterm labour.[63] For example, salivary oestriol $\geq$ 1.8 ng/ml before 34 weeks has a sensitivity of 68% and specificity of 76% for preterm labour before 35 weeks gestation. A prospective longitudinal trial is underway to confirm these findings.[65] While prostaglandins are intimately linked to uterine contractility during pregnancy and labour[66] plasma prostaglandin levels, including metabolites, do not show a recognizable trend which is of predictive value.[67]

Collagen is the main structural molecule in the uterine and cervical extacellular matrix.[68] Using an activity-based assay and a method of destroying serum inhibitors, an increase in serum collagenase activity has been noted at the onset of spontaneous labour at term and in association with preterm labour.[69] It was therefore suggested that serum collagenase might be a valuable marker for detecting preterm labour if a more rapid and easily reproducible assay were available. Using an enzyme-linked immunosorbent assay (ELISA) specific for tissue collagenase (as distinct from collagenase of neutrophil origin), which is rapid and reproducible, it was found that levels were elevated in pregnancy but not significantly altered at the onset of labour (term or preterm).[70] It was therefore speculated that measurement of neutrophil collagenase would be an interesting prospect for potential marker status for preterm labour, but resolution of this issue must await development of a specific and sensitive immunoassay for this enzyme. In addition, the enzyme which regulates the activity of metalloproteinases such as collagenase, tissue inhibitor of metalloproteinase (TIMP), was investigated and found to be significantly elevated in women in spontaneous preterm labour.[71] In fact, the altered collagenase activity previously reported[69] showed a pattern similar to that reported for tissue inhibitor of metalloproteinases,[69] but on a slightly advanced schedule, suggesting that the enzyme and inhibitor may be coming from the same source, and are being co-ordinately regulated during pregnancy and labour. Therefore, the possibility that changes in the extracellular matrix that occur in the uterus and cervix during pregnancy and labour may provide biochemical marker status of these events remains an exciting prospect which requires further evaluation.

Relaxin, which is structurally a member of the insulin and insulin-like growth factor family of hormones, is produced in the placenta, endometrium (and decidua) and ovary.[72] Its two major biological actions are rapid inhibition of myometrial activity, and a slow effect on connective tissue modelling in the reproductive tract. It is therefore thought to play a key role in the synchronization of events at parturition. Serum relaxin levels, as measured by ELISA, have been assessed for predictive value of preterm labour.[73] It was shown that there was a negative correlation between relaxin concentration at 30 weeks and the gestational age at parturition. However, the possibility that high relaxin concentrations are associated with preterm labour requires confirmation from larger studies, performed at earlier gestation periods, if it is to be of clinical value.

Corticotrophin releasing hormone (CRH) has been investigated as a predictive marker for preterm labour and other pregnancy complications.

Plasma levels of CRH are low or undetectable in the normal non-pregnant woman[74] but are measurable in normal pregnant women in the third trimester, and these higher levels are placental in origin.[75] CRH potentiates the contractile response to oxytocin of human gestational myometrium and this effect is dependent on prostaglandins.[76] Prospective measurements of plasma levels of CRH were performed sequentially from 24 weeks onwards in 80 normal and 88 abnormal pregnancies.[75] Women who delivered preterm had a steeper rise in plasma CRH. This difference was not, however, statistically significant, possibly because only 15 preterm deliveries occurred in the study. This finding has, however, been reported from other cross-sectional studies.[77,78] Further evaluation of the clinical efficacy of CRH as a marker for preterm labour will require a larger prospective study.

Mediators of inflammation and infection

Some cases of preterm labour are caused by systemic or intrauterine infection but the exact incidence, specific organisms and pathogenesis are poorly understood. Ascending infection from the lower genital tract, which may frequently be subclinical, is thought to be an important precipitating factor for preterm labour even in the presence of intact membranes.[79–81] However, as discussed above, in the majority of cases of preterm labour the pathophysiology is far from clear. For this reason tests that are based on the presence of inflammation or infection are unlikely to be generally helpful but attempts have been made to identify potential predictive value.

C-reactive protein (CRP) has been studied in women with preterm labour with and without preterm rupture of the membranes.[82–83] Elevated CRP is associated with clinical chorioamnionitis, but not consistently with histologically demonstrated chorioamnionitis.[83] While elevated CRP is also associated with delivery within 7 days, and infant death, it is not of predictive value for preterm labour.

Several vaginal organisms have been associated with preterm labour and delivery but none offer a posititve predictive value that would be practically useful for this condition. Much attention has been paid to bacterial vaginosis, a condition where there is an overgrowth of anaerobic and other bacteria in the vagina with a corresponding decrease in the number of lactobacilli. Hay et al analysed data from 718 women investigated for bacterial vaginosis in early pregnancy, of whom 27 women delivered before 37 weeks gestation.[84] In the group who delivered preterm there was an association between bacterial vaginosis and preterm delivery but there was a much greater association with previous preterm delivery. There is no definitive evidence of a causal relationship between bacterial vaginosis and preterm labour nor is it clear that screening for it will accurately help to identify subsequent cases of preterm labour. Similarly, carriage of other organisms detected in the early second trimester, such as *Trichomonas vaginalis*, *Ureaplasma urealyticum*, *Bacteroides fragilis* and *Mycoplasma hominis*, has been shown to be associated with preterm delivery[81] but is not useful as a predictive test.

In preterm labour associated with intrauterine infection, inflammatory mediators can be detected in the amniotic fluid. Many such mediators have been the subject of research including leukocytes,[85] leukocyte esterases,[86] cytokines (e.g. interleukin-1),[87] glucose concentration,[88] zinc[89] and lipocortin-1[90] as well as positive cultures,[91] but they are not practically helpful in the prediction of preterm labour.

PREVENTION OF PRETERM LABOUR

Efforts directed at preventing preterm labour, and hence the sequelae of preterm birth, can be divided into two major groups. The first potential approach is to prevent the initiation of preterm labour by the use of a predictive test with a high enough positive predictive value to warrant some sort of intervention or treatment. As discussed above, there is, as yet, no such optimum predictive test. The second approach is inhibition of the preterm labour process itself. The therapeutic interventions which have been evaluated include tocolytic agents, antibiotics and miscellaneous measures such as cervical cerclage, patient education and bed rest. Detailed analysis of all these measures is beyond the scope of this review so attention will be focused on the pharmacological methods of tocolysis that have been used clinically or are currently under evaluation for use.

Tocolytic agents

Throughout the years a variety of drugs with different pharmacological principles have been used to suppress unwanted uterine activity. As discussed previously, any proposed therapy should fulfil certain preconditions. There should be no maternal or fetal reason for which delivery might confer some advantage. The fetus should be at a gestational age at which it is expected to benefit from the treatment in excess of the potential risks imposed. Generally, this will correspond to gestations of less than 32 weeks duration or situations in which tocolytic therapy is limited to the time required to achieve maternal transport. Finally, contraindications to a particular tocolytic agent must be lacking and the fetal membranes should generally be intact.

The tocolytics used or under investigation for use include beta-adrenergic agonists, prostaglandin synthetase inhibitors, calcium channel blockers, magnesium sulphate, oxytocin antagonists, nitric oxide donors, potassium channel openers, and miscellaneous agents such as ethanol and progesterone derivatives.

Beta-adrenergic agonists

These include ritodrine, terbutaline, salbutamol, fenoterol and hexoprenaline. Unfortunately, in terms of clinical effectiveness, the inhibition of contractions by β-adrenergic agonists is often short-lived. Escape from their tocolytic effect is well described both in vitro and in vivo.[92-94] In their meta-analysis, King et al[95] reviewed 16 controlled trials in which tocolytic agents, chiefly ritodrine, were evaluated. β-adrenergic agonists were found to be effective in reducing the proportion of women who delivered within 24 hours and within 48 hours of treatment. However, this treatment did not decrease the likelihood of preterm delivery and had no effect on perinatal mortality or neonatal morbidity. A randomized, controlled, multicentre, Canadian trial, which involved 708 women receiving either ritodrine or placebo, concluded that the use of ritodrine in the treatment of preterm labour had no significant beneficial effect on perinatal mortality, the frequency of prolongation of pregnancy to term, or birth weight.[96] The accumulated evidence therefore shows that treatment with a β-adrenergic agonist reduces the rate of delivery within 48 hours, but that this immediate effect has not led to clinically significant reductions in the rates of preterm birth or low birth weight and, most importantly, has not resulted in an improvement in outcome in terms of severe neonatal respiratory distress syndrome or perinatal death.

Maternal side effects of the β-adrenergic agonists can be unpleasant and occasionally life-threatening;[97] the potentially fatal ones are cardiac arryth-mias, myocardial ischaemia and pulmonary oedema. The mechanism of development of pulmonary oedema with β-adrenergic agonist use is unknown but its incidence has been reported as being as high as 3–9%;[98] therefore their use requires close clinical monitoring. In addition, the reported fetal and neonatal side effects caused by β-adrenergic agonists include hypoglycaemia, hypocalcaemia, ileus, hypotension and death.[97] Despite these problems, β-adrenergic agonists remain as the primary, and most commonly used, method of tocolysis. Until more effective and safer tocolytic agents are available, appreciation of these cautions and limitations is mandatory for safe obstetric practice.

Prostaglandin synthetase inhibitors

Indomethacin is the most commonly used prostaglandin synthetase inhibitor for treatment of preterm labour. Some of the early studies, in the 1970s, reported good results for inhibition of preterm contractions but a review of these studies reveals that many were uncontrolled.[99] One prospective, ran-domised, double-blind study suggested that indomethacin was more effective than placebo in the first 24 hours of treatment, but there was no difference between the groups with respect to gestational age at delivery, birth weight, neonatal morbidity and perinatal mortality. In other studies, the success rates with indomethacin have been comparable to those achieved with β-agonists.[100,101]

As the use of prostaglandin synthetase inhibitors for preterm labour increased, questions arose regarding their safety for both mother and fetus.[99]

Recently it has been demonstrated that the incidence of serious neonatal complications (necrotizing enterocolitis, patent ductus arteriosus, intracranial haemorrhage and renal dysfunction), associated with antenatal indomethacin treatment, is significantly increased in infants born at or before 30 weeks gestation.[102] This had not previously been appreciated because of a preponderance of more mature infants in earlier studies concerning the safety of indomethacin. This introduces a dilemma for the future use of indomethacin as the fetuses most in need of tocolysis are those at most risk of serious complications from the treatment.

3 Calcium channel blockers

Myometrial contractility is intrinsically dependent on the availability of free intracellular calcium, hence, blockade of sarcolemmal calcium channels results in relaxation. Dihydropyridine derivatives, such as nifedipine, bind to the inside of the myometrial L-type voltage-dependent calcium channels, causing them to remain in the closed state.[103] They are potent inhibitors of tension development in uterine smooth muscle.[104] Published experience with these agents is limited to small series, and successful treatment of preterm labour has been reported in limited numbers of patients.[105] Attempts to combine their use with that of β-agonists, in order to modify the side effects of the latter agents, have not been successful. Of concern is the finding of reduced uterine blood flow, in parallel with decreased fetal oxygen saturation and a trend towards fetal acidosis, caused by these agents in sheep.[106] Nifedipine also affects placental vascularization and there is the unresolved question of embryotoxicity.[107] Their place and safety in preterm labour requires further evaluation.

4 Magnesium sulphate

For many years it has been recognized that magnesium sulphate inhibits myometrial contractility, because clinical use of magnesium for the treatment of pre-eclampsia frequently resulted in decreased uterine activity as a side effect. Its exact mechanism of action is unknown but it is believed that magnesium alters nerve transmission by affecting acetylcholine release and sensitivity at the motor end plate, and that it may displace calcium in transmission of the nerve impulse.[108] The reports concerning its tocolytic efficacy have been observational or have been comparisons with various β-adrenergic agents. Its success in the treatment of preterm labour appears to be, in general, comparable to that of β-adrenergic agonists.[109,110] It has been reported that the combination of the two treatments may be more effective but this approach requires great caution regarding the potential for cumulative side effects.[111]

Oxytocin antagonists

A series of oxytocin antagonists were synthesized and screened in both in vitro and in vivo animal pharmacology experiments in the early and mid 1980s.[112] Åkerlund et al[113] reported successful inhibition of contractions in an uncontrolled pilot study with 13 patients using [Mpa^{1}D-Tyr(Et)^{2}Thr^{4}Orn^8]OT (atosiban). The results from a more recent double-blind placebo-controlled study have revealed that atosiban diminished the mean frequency of contractions by −55.3% ± 36.3% as compared with placebo (−26.7 ± 40.4%) but no overall relationship between the effect of the drug and the length of gestation was apparent.[114] The fact that umbilical vein plasma levels are 12% of the maternal uterine vein plasma levels[112] is a concern which outlines the importance of follow-up studies on infants born to women receiving oxytocin antagonists. Further evaluation of these agents is currently required.

Nitric oxide donors

Recent reports from different animal species indicate that the L-arginine – nitric oxide (NO) system is central to inhibition of uterine activity during gestation but that its production, or effector mechanisms, are altered, or in some way inactivated, at parturition. It has been demonstrated that L-arginine is a potent in vitro inhibitor of spontaneous activity of isolated rat myometrium and that this effect was reversed by the addition of N^G-nitro-L-arginine-methyl-ester (L-NAME).[115,116] This inhibitory effect was significantly reduced at the time of parturition. In addition, application of NO gas to the tissue bath produced complete relaxation of spontaneous contractility of the rat myometrial strips. A similiar relaxant effect was achieved with the NO donor compound sodium nitroprusside, and this effect was antagonized by methylene blue, an inhibitor of soluble guanylate cyclase. Unlike the animal studies reported, L-arginine does not have an in vitro inhibitory effect on human pregnant myometrium but NO donor compounds are human myometrial relaxants under these circumstances.[117] While this raises questions regarding the role of endogenous NO in myometrial relaxation during human pregnancy the possibility of exogenous NO as a tocolytic agent is currently under investigation. Published reports to date, although as yet entirely provisional, have suggested possible benefits from NO compounds for prolongation of pregnancy after fetal surgery[118] and spontaneous preterm labour[119] but the results of prospective randomized trials are awaited.

Potassium channel openers

Research in potassium channels is an area of pharmacology that has expanded dramatically in recent years. Potassium (K) channel openers are a novel group of compounds which hyperpolarize excitable tissues and

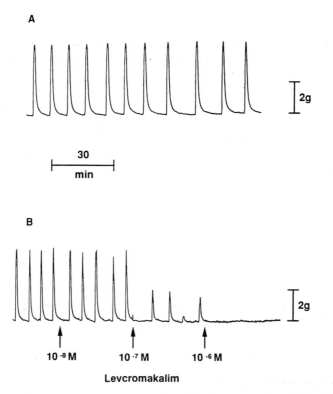

Fig. 5.1 Trace of in vitro spontaneous contractile activity in myometrium obtained at elective caesarean section is shown in A. Effects of cumulatively increasing concentrations of the potassium channel opener levcromakalim (10^{-8} to 10^{-6} M) on contractions are shown in B with maximal inhibition achieved at 10^{-6} M. Reproduced with permission from Morrison et al.[126]

function as potent smooth muscle relaxants.[120] For this reason K-channel openers have been used clinically for various conditions including hypertension, asthma, peripheral vascular disease, angina and congestive cardiac failure.[120–122] There is evidence that the physiological and pharmacological properties of potassium channels in human pregnant myometrium are markedly altered with the onset of parturition, suggesting that they have an intrinsic role in regulation of human uterine excitability.[123] K-channel openers are effective myometrial relaxants in vitro in the rat,[124] and in the human.[125–128] Maximal inhibition is achieved at micromolar concentrations, as shown in the trace in Fig. 5.1, and this has been shown in myometrium obtained before and after the onset of labour. This method of uterine inhibition is physiologically appealing because the outward current of potassium offsets depolarizing stimuli and so suppresses regenerative electrical activity, thereby rendering the myometrial cell quiescent.[126] The large number of K-channels, with different biochemical and biophysical properties of their gating mechanisms,[129] offers the exciting possibility that K-channel openers with myometrial selectivity can be developed.

Miscellaneous

Ethanol was the first widely used tocolytic agent in the late 1960s and early 1970s.[130] Its administration requires constant supervision because of the many associated side effects, which include intoxication, vomiting, restlessness, disorientation, hangover, lactic acidosis, dehydration and neonatal depression. The most serious of all is the risk of aspiration if the sleepy woman vomits. For all these reasons its use is no longer justified.

Pregnenolone sulphate, an immediate precursor of placental progesterone, has been reported in small trials to inhibit uterine activity.[97] The tocolytic effect of oral micronized progesterone was not as intense, nor as rapid, as that of β-sympathomimetics in a double-blind study of 57 women, of whom 29 received a single oral dose of 400 mg progesterone.[127] Progesterone is not routinely used in current obstetric practice.[131]

CONCLUSIONS

Preterm labour and delivery continue to have a significant impact on perinatal outcome in the 1990s. There is currently no satisfactory pharmacological method for the prevention or treatment of preterm labour. In spite of vigorous attempts to define the pathophysiology of this process and intervene therapeutically, the incidence of preterm birth is essentially unchanged. The epidemiology of this condition is such that an efficient therapeutic option would provide benefit in a significant proportion of preterm deliveries. The pursuit of a solution to this problem demands sound scientific investigation followed by rigorous clinical appraisal.

REFERENCES

1 Creasy R K. Preterm birth prevention: Where are we? Am J Obstet Gynecol 1993; 168: 1223–1230
2 Fuchs F. Prevention of prematurity. Am J Obstet Gynecol 1976; 126: 809–820
3 Rush R W, Keirse M J N C, Howat P, Baum J D, Anderson A B, Turnbull A C. Contribution of preterm delivery to perinatal mortality. Br Med J 1976; 2: 965–968
4 Hibbard B. The aetiology of preterm labour. Br Med J 1987; 294: 594–595
5 Iams J D, Peaceman A M, Creasy R K. Prevention of prematurity. Semin Perinatol 1988; 12: 280–291
6 Copper R L, Goldenberg R L, Creasy R K et al. A multi-center study of preterm birth weight and gestational age-specific neonatal mortality. Am J Obstet Gynecol 1993; 168: 78–83
7 Hack M, Fanaroff A A. Outcomes of extremely immature infants – a perinatal dilemma. N Engl J Med 1993; 329: 1649–1650
8 Morrison J C. Preterm birth: A puzzle worth solving. Obstet Gynecol 1990; 76: 5S–12S
9 Morrison J J, Rennie J M, Milton P J. Neonatal respiratory morbidity and mode of delivery at term: influence of timing of elective caesarean section. Br J Obstet Gynaecol 1995; 102: 101–106

10 Arias F, Tomich P. Etiology and outcome of low birth weight and preterm infants. Obstet Gynecol 1982; 60: 277–281
11 Amon E, Anderson G D, Sibai B M, Mabie W C. Factors responsible for preterm delivery of the immature newborn infant (≤1000 g). Am J Obstet Gynecol 1987; 156: 1143–1148
12 Walker E, Patel N. Aetiology and incidence. In: Harvey D, Cooke R W, Levitt G S, eds. The baby under 1000 g. London: Wright, 1990, pp. 68–79
13 Main D M, Gabbe S G, Richardson D, Strong S. Can preterm deliveries be prevented? Am J Obstet Gynecol 1985; 151: 892–898
14 Meis P J, Ernest J M, Moore M L. Causes of low birth weight in public and private patients. Am J Obstet Gynecol 1987; 156: 1165–1168
15 Rennie J M. Perinatal Statistics Report (1985–1992), Rosie Maternity Hospital, Cambridge, UK, 1993
16 Gilstrap L C, Hauth J C, Belle R E, Ackerman N B Jr, Yoder B A, Delemos R. Survival and short-term morbidity of the premature neonate. Obstet Gynecol 1985; 65: 37–41
17 Konte J M, Holbrook R H Jr, Laros R K Jr, Creasy R K. Short-term neonatal morbidity associated with preterm birth and effect of a preterm birth prevention program on expected incidence of morbidity. Am J Perinatol 1986; 3: 283–288
18 Yu V Y, Loke H L, Szymonowicz W, Orgill A A, Astbury J. Prognosis for infants born at 23–28 weeks gestation. Br Med J 1986; 293: 1200–1203
19 Allen M C, Donohue P K, Dusman A E. The limit of viability – neonatal outcome of infants born at 22 to 25 weeks' gestation. N Engl J Med 1993; 329: 1597–1601
20 Morrison J J, Rennie J M. Changing the definition of perinatal mortality. Lancet 1995; 346: 1038
21 Graham M, Levene M T, Trounce J Q, Rutter N. Prediction of cerebral palsy in very low birthweight infants: prospective ultrasound study. Lancet 1987; 2: 593–596
22 Gibson D L, Sheps S B, Schecter M T, Wiggins S, McCormick A Q. Retinopathy of prematurity: A new epidemic? Pediatrics 1989; 83: 486–492
23 Hagberg B, Hagberg G, Zetterstrom R. Decreasing perinatal mortality – increase in cerebral palsy morbidity. Acta Paediatr Scand 1989; 78: 664–670
24 Stanley F J, Watson L. Trends in perinatal mortality and cerebral palsy in Western Australia, 1967 to 1985. Br Med J 1992; 304: 1658–1663
25 Kuban K C K, Leviton A. Cerebral palsy. N Engl J Med 1994; 330: 188–195
26 Valentine P, Jackson J, Kalina R, Woodrum D. Increased survival of low birthweight infants: impact on the incidence of retinopathy of prematurity. Pediatrics 1989; 89: 359–364
27 Bergman I, Hirsch R P, Fria T J, Shapiro S M, Holzman I, Painter M J. Cause of hearing loss in the high-risk premature infant. J Pediatr 1985; 106: 95–101
28 Hack M, Breslau N, Weissman B et al. The effect of very low birth weight and social risk on neurocognitive abilities at school age. J Dev Behav Pediatr 1992; 18: 412–420
29 Hack M, Merkatz I R, Gordon D, Jones C K, Fanaroff A A. The prognostic significance of post-natal growth in very low birthweight infants. Am J Obstet Gynecol 1982; 143: 693–699
30 Riedel F. Long term effects of artificial ventilation in neonates. Acta Paediatr Scand 1987; 76: 24–29
31 McCormick M C, Shapiro S, Starfield B H. Rehospitalization in the first year of life for high risk survivors. Pediatrics 1980; 66: 991–999
32 Kitchen W H, Doyle L W, Ford G W. Inguinal hernia on very low birthweight children: a continuing risk to age 8 years. J Paediatr Child Health 1991; 27: 300–301
33 Paneth N. Recent trends in preterm delivery rates in the United States. In: Papiernik E, Breart G, Spira N, eds. Prevention de la naissance prematuree. Inserm, Colloque, 1986; 138: pp 15–30
34 Macfarlane A, Cole S, Johnson A, Botting B. Epidemiology of birth before 28 weeks of gestation. Br Med Bull 1988; 44: 861–891
35 Bakketeig L S, Hoffman H J. Epidemiology of preterm birth: results from a longitudinal study of births in Norway. In: Elder M G, Hendricks C H, eds. Preterm Labour. London: Butterworths, 1981: pp 17–46
36 Kingdom J C P, Morrison J J. Prediction, prevention and management of preterm labour in multiple pregnancy. In: Ward R H T, Whittle M J, eds. Multiple pregnancy. London: RCOG Press, 1995: pp 148–163
37 Lumley J. The epidemiology of preterm birth. Clin Obstet Gynaecol 1993; 7: 477–498
38 Meyer M B, Tonascia J A. Maternal smoking, pregnancy complications and perinatal mortality. Am J Obstet Gynecol 1977; 128: 494–498

39 Hingson R, Alpert J J, Day N et al. Effects of maternal drinking and marijuana use on fetal growth and development. Pediatrics 1982; 70: 539–549

40 Volpe J J. Effect of cocaine use on the fetus. N Engl J Med 1992; 327: 399–407

41 Launer L J, Villar J, Kestler E, de Onis M. The effect of maternal work on fetal growth and duration of pregnancy: a prospective study. Br J Obstet Gynaecol 1990; 97: 62–70

42 Klebanoff M A, Shiono P H, Rhoads G G. Outcomes of pregnancy in a national sample of resident physicians. N Engl J Med 1990; 323: 1040–1045

43 Niswander K C. Obstetric factors related to prematurity. In: Reed D M, Stanley F J, eds. The epidemiology of prematurity. Baltimore: Urban and Schwarzenburg, 1977

44 Papiernik-Berkhauer E. Coefficient de risque d'accouchement prématuré. Press Méd 1969; 77: 793–794

45 Creasy R K, Gummer G A, Liggins G C. System for predicting spontaneous preterm birth. Obstet Gynecol 1980; 55: 692–695

46 Keirse M J N C. An evaluation of formal risk scoring for preterm birth. Am J Perinatol 1989; 6: 226–233

47 Papiernik E, Bouyer J, Collin D et al. Precocious cervical ripening and preterm labor. Obstet Gynecol 1986; 67: 238–242

48 Bouer, J, Papiernik E, Dryfus J et al. Maturation signs of the cervix and prediction of preterm birth. Obstet Gynecol 1986; 68: 209–214

49 Mortensen O A, Franklin J, Lofstrand T et al. Prediction of preterm birth. Acta Obstet Gynecol Scand 1987; 66: 507–511

50 Andersen H F, Nugent C E, Wanty S D, Hayashi R H. Prediction of risk for preterm delivery by ultrasonographic measurement of cervical length. Am J Obstet Gynecol 1990; 163: 859–867

51 Newman R B, Campbell B A, Stramm S L. Objective tocodynamometry identifies labor onset earlier than subjective maternal perception. Obstet Gynecol 1990; 76: 1089–1092

52 Hill W C, Fleming A D, Martin R W et al. Home uterine activity monitoring is associated with a reduction in preterm birth. Obstet Gynecol 1990; 76: 135–175

53 Mou S M, Sunderji S G, Gall S et al. Multicenter randomized clinical trial of home uterine activity monitoring for detection of preterm labour. Am J Obstet Gynecol 1990; 165: 858–866

54 Iams J D, Johnson F F, O'Shaughnessy R W. A prospective random trial of home uterine activity monitoring in pregnancies at increased risk of preterm labor. Part II. Am J Obstet Gynecol 1988; 159: 595–603

55 Lockwood C J, Senyel A E, Renate Dische M et al. Fetal fibronectin in cervical and vaginal secretions as a predictor of preterm delivery. N Engl J Med 1991; 325: 669–674

56 Lockwood C J, Wein R, Lapinski R, Casal D, Berkowitz G, Alvarez M, Berkowitz R L. The presence of cervical and vaginal fetal fibronectin predicts preterm delivery in an inner-city obstetric population. Am J Obstet Gynecol 1993; 169: 798–804

57 Eriksen N L, Parisi V M, Daoust S, Flamm B, Garite T J, Cox S M. Fetal fibronectin: A method for detecting the presence of amniotic fluid. Obstet Gynecol 1992; 80: 451–454

58 Sadovsky Y, Friedman S A. Fetal fibronectin and preterm labour. N Engl J Med 1991; 326: 709

59 Leeson S, Maresh M. Fibronectin: a predictor of preterm delivery. Br J Obstet Gynaecol 1993; 100: 304–306

60 Morrison J J, Thornton S. Fibronectin: a predictor of preterm delivery? Br J Obstet Gynaecol 1993; 100: 969

61 Morrison J J. Physiology and pharmacology of human myometrium during pregnancy and labour, term and preterm. In: Studd J W, ed. Royal College of Obstetricians & Gynaecologists Yearbook 1996. London: RCOG Press, 1996 (in Press)

62 Anderson P J B, Hancock K W, Oakley R E. Nonprotein bound estradiol and progesterone in human peripheral plasma before labor and delivery. J Endocrinol 1985; 104: 7

63 Hanssens M C A J A, Selby C, Symonds E M. Sex steroid hormone concentrations in preterm labour and the outcome of treatment with ritodrine. Br J Obstet Gynaecol 1982; 92: 698–702

64 Darne J, McGarrigle H G, Lachelin G C L. Increased saliva oestriol to progesterone ratio before preterm delivery: A possible predictor for preterm labour? Br Med J 1987; 294: 270–272

65 Jackson G M, McGregor J A, Lachelin G C L, Goodwin T M, Artal R, Dullien V. Salivary estriol rise predicts preterm labour. Am J Obstet Gynecol 1995; 172: 406

66 Morrison J J, Smith S K. Prostaglandins and uterine activity. In: Chard T, Grudzinskas J G, eds. The uterus. Cambridge: Cambridge University Press, 1994: pp 230–251

67 Mitchell M D, Flint A P, Bibby J, Brunt J, Arnold J M, Anderson A B, Turnbull A C. Plasma concentration of prostaglandins during late human pregnancy. Influence of normal and preterm labour. J Clin Endocrinol 1978; 46: 947–951

68 Danforth D N, Buckingham J J, Roddick J W. Connective tissue changes incident to cervical effacement. Am J Obstet Gynecol 1960: 80: 939–945

69 Rajabi M, Dean D D, Woessner Jr J F. High levels of serum collagenase in premature labor – a potential biochemical marker. Obstet Gynecol 1987; 69: 179–186

70 Morrison J J, Clark I M, Powell E K, Cawston T E, Hackett G A, Smith S K. Tissue collagenase: serum levels during pregnancy and parturition. Eur J Obstet Gynaecol Rep Biol 1994; 54: 71–75

71 Clark I M, Morrison J J, Hackett G A, Powell E K, Cawston T E, Smith S K. Tissue inhibitor of metalloproteinases: serum levels during pregnancy and labor, term and preterm. Obstet Gynecol 1994; 83: 532–537

72 Bryant-Greenwood G D. Relaxin. In: Chard T, Grudzinskas J G, eds. The uterus. Cambridge: Cambridge University Press, 1994: pp 252–267

73 Petersen L K, Skajaa K, Uldberg N. Serum relaxin as a potential marker for preterm labour. Br J Obstet Gynaecol 1992; 99: 292–295

74 Linton E A, McLean C, Nieuwenhuyzen Kruseman A C, Tilders F J, Van der Veen E A, Lowry P J. Direct measurement of human plasma corticotrophin releasing hormone by 'two-site' immunoradiometric assay. J Clin Endocrinol Metab 1987; 64: 1047–1053

75 Wolfe C D A, Petruckevitch A, Quartero R et al. The rate of rise of corticotrophin releasing factor and endogenous digoxin-like immunoreactivity in normal and abnormal pregnancy. Br J Obstet Gynaecol 1990; 97: 832–837

76 Quartero H W, Noort W A, Fry C H, Keirse M J. Role of PG and leukotrienes in the synergistic effect of OT and CRH on the contraction force in human gestational myometrium. Prostaglandins 1991; 42: 137–150

77 Campbell E A, Linton E A, Wolfe C D A, et al. Plasma corticotrophin releasing hormone concentrations during pregnancy and parturition. J Clin Endocrinol Metab 1987; 64: 1054–1059

78 Warren W B, Patrick S L, Goland R S. Elevated maternal plasma corticotrophin releasing hormone levels in pregnancies complicated by preterm labour. Am J Obstet Gynecol 1992; 166: 1198–1204

79 McGregor J A, French J I, Lawelin D, Todd J K. Preterm birth and infection: pathogenic possibilities. Am J Reprod Immunol Microbiol 1988; 16: 123–132

80 Romero R, Major M, Wu Y K et al. Infection in the pathogenesis of preterm labor. Semin Perinatol 1988; 12: 62–79

81 Lamont R F, Fisk N M. The role of infection in the pathogenesis of preterm labour. In: Studd J W W, ed. Progress in obstetrics and gynaecology Vol 10. Edinburgh: Churchill Livingstone, 1993: pp 135–158

82 Farb H F, Arnesen M, Geistler P, Knox G E. C-reactive protein with premature rupture of membranes and premature labor. Am J Obstet Gynecol 1983; 62: 49–51

83 Cammu H, Goossens A, Derde M P, Temmerman M, Foulon W, Amy J J. C-reactive protein in preterm labour: Association with outcome of tocolysis and placental histology. Br J Obstet Gynaecol 1989; 96: 314–319

84 Hay P E, Lamont R F, Taylor-Robinson D, John Morgan D, Ison C, Pearson J. Abnormal bacterial colonisation of the genital tract and subsequent preterm delivery and late miscarriage. Br Med J 1994; 308: 295–298

85 Miller J M, Pupkin M J, Hill G B. Bacterial colonisation of amniotic fluid from intact fetal membranes. Am J Obstet Gynecol 1980; 136: 796–804

86 Hoskins I A, Johnson T R B, Winkel C A. Leucocyte esterase activity in human amniotic fluid for the rapid detection of chorioamnionitis. Am J Obstet Gynecol 1987; 157: 730–732

87 Romero R, Brody D T, Oyarzun E, Mazor M, Wu Y K, Hobbins J C, Durum S K. Infection and labor. III. Interleukin-1: A signal for the onset of parturition. Am J Obstet Gynecol 1989; 160: 1117–1123

88 Romero R, Jimenez C, Lohda A K et al. Amniotic fluid glucose concentrations: A rapid and simple method for the detection of intra-amniotic infection in preterm labor. Am J Obstet Gynecol 1990; 163: 968–974

89 Varner M W, Nuttall K, Hunter C, Dudley D, Mitchell M D. Amniotic fluid zinc levels

during term labor, preterm labor and chorioamnionitis. Chicago: Proceedings of Society for Gynecologic Investigation, 1994: 401

90 Romero R, Sepulveda W, Gomez R, Cotton D B, Goulding N J. Lipocortin-1 in term and preterm parturition. Chicago: Proceedings of Society for Gynecologic Investigation, 1993: 217

91 Armer T L, Duff P. Intraamniotic infection in patients with intact membranes and preterm labor. Obstet Gynecol Surv 1991; 46: 589–593

92 Caritis S N, Chiao J P, Kridgen P. Comparison of pulsatile and continuous itodrine administration. Effects on uterine contractility and β-adrenergic cascade. Am J Obstet Gynecol 1991; 164: 1005–1012

93 Lam F, Gill P, Smith M, Kitzmiller J L, Katz M. Use of the subcutaneous terbutaline pump for long-term tocolysis. Obstet Gynecol 1988; 72: 810–813

94 Ryden G, Andersson R G G, Berg G. Is the relaxing effect of β-adrenergic agonists on the human myometrium only transitory? Acta Obstet Gynecol Scand (Suppl) 1982; 108: 47–51

95 King J F, Grant A, Keirse M J N C, Chalmers I. Beta-mimetics in preterm labour: an overview of the randomized controlled trials. Br J Obstet Gynaecol 1988; 95: 211–222

96 Canadian Preterm Labor Investigators Group. Treatment of preterm labor with the beta-adrenergic agonist ritodrine. N Engl J Med 1992; 327: 308–312

97 Alger L S, Crehshaw M C. Preterm labour and delivery. In: Turnbull A, Chamberlain G, eds. Obstetrics. London: Churchill Livingstone, 1989: pp 749–770

98 Leveno K J, Cunningham F G. β-Adrenergic agents for preterm labour. N Engl J Med 1992; 327: 349–351

99 Niebyl J R. Prostaglandin synthetase inhibitors. Semin Perinatol 1981; 5: 274–287

100 Morales W J, Smith S G, Angel J L, O'Brien W F, Knuppel R A. Efficacy and safety of indomethacin versus ritodrine in the management of preterm labour: a randomized study. Obstet Gynecol 1989; 74: 567–572

101 Besinger R E, Niebyl J R, Keyes W G, Johnson T R. Randomized comparative trial of indomethacin and ritodrine for the long-term treatment of preterm labor. Am J Obstet Gynecol 1991; 164: 981–988

102 Norton M E, Merrill J, Cooper B A B, Kuller J A, Clyman R I. Neonatal complications after the administration of indomethacin for preterm labor. N Engl J Med 329: 1993; 1602–1607

103 Triggle D J, Janis R A. Calcium channel ligands. Annu Rev Pharmacol Toxicol 1987; 27: 369–374

104 Parkington H C, Coleman H A. The role of membrane potential in the control of uterine motility. In: Carsten M E, Miller J D, eds. Uterine function: Molecular and cellular aspects. New York: Plenum Press, 1990: pp 195–248

105 Leonardi M R, Hankins G D V. What's new in tocolytics? Clin Perinatol 1992; 19: 367–384

106 Harake B, Gilbert R D, Ashwal S, Power G G. Nifedipine: Effects on fetal and maternal hemodynamics in pregnant sheep. Am J Obstet Gynecol 1987; 157: 1003–1008

107 Richichi J, Vasilenko P. The effects of nifedipine on pregnancy outcome and morphology of the placenta, uterus, and cervix during late pregnancy in the rat. Am J Obstet Gynecol 1992; 167: 797–803

108 Petrie R H. Tocolysis using magnesium sulfate. Semin Perinatol 1981; 5: 256–273

109 Beall M H, Edgar B W, Paul R H, Smith-Wallace T. A comparison of ritodrine, terbutaline and magnesium sulfate for the suppression of preterm labor. Am J Obstet Gynecol 1985; 153: 854–859

110 Hollander D I, Nagey D A, Pupkin M J. Magnesium sulfate and ritodrine hydrochloride: A randomized comparison. Am J Obstet Gynecol 1987; 156: 631–637

111 Hatjis C G, Swain M, Nelson L H, Meis P J, Ernest J M. Efficacy of combined administration of magnesium sulfate and ritodrine in the treatment of preterm labor. Obstet Gynecol 1987; 69: 317–322

112 Melin P. Oxytocin antagonists in preterm labour and delivery. Clin Obstet Gynaecol 1993; 7: 577–600

113 Åkerlund M, Stromberg P, Hauksson A, Andersen L F, Lyndrup J, Trojnar J, Melin P. Inhibition of uterine contractions of premature labour with an oxytocin analogue. Results from a pilot study. Br J Obstet Gynaecol 1987; 94: 1040–1044

114 Goodwin T M, Paul R, Silver H et al. The effect of the oxytocin antagonist atosiban on

preterm uterine activity in the human. Am J Obstet Gynecol 1994; 170: 474–479

115 Yallampali C, Garfield R E, Byam-Smith M. Nitric oxide inhibits uterine contractility during pregnancy but not during delivery. Endocrinology 1993; 133: 1899–1902

116 Yallampali C, Izumi H, Byam-Smith M, Garfield R E. An L-arginine-nitric oxide guanosine monophosphate system exists in the uterus and inhibits contractility during pregnancy. Am J Obstet Gynecol 1994; 170: 175–185

117 Morrison J J, Perera D, O'Brien P, Marshall I, Rodeck C H. Effects of nitric oxide (NO) substrate, NO donors and NO synthase inhibitors on contractions of isolated human myometrium. Br J Obstet Gynaecol (in press)

118 Adzick N S, Harrison M R. Fetal surgical therapy. Lancet 1994; 343: 897–902

119 Lees C, Campbell S, Jauniaux E et al. Arrest of preterm labour and prolongation of gestation with glyceryl trinitrate, a nitric oxide donor. Lancet 1994; 343: 1325–1326

120 Duty S, Weston A H. Potassium channel openers: pharmacological effects and future uses. Drugs 1990; 40: 785–791

121 Frampton J, Buckley M M, Fitton A. Nicorandil: a review of its pharmacology and therapeutic efficiency in angina pectoris. Drugs 1992; 42: 625–655

122 Williams A J. Potassium channel openers: clinical aspects. In: Weston A H, Hamilton T C, eds. Potassium channel modulators. Oxford: Blackwell Scientific, 1992: pp 486–501

123 Khan R N, Smith S K, Morrison J J, Ashford M L J. Modification of large-conductance Ca^{2+}-activated K^+-channel properties of human myometrium during pregnancy and labour. Proc R Soc Lond (Biol) 1993; 251: 9–15

124 Piper I, Marshall E, Downing S J, Hollingsworth M, Sadrei H. Effects of several potassium channel openers and glibenclamide on the uterus of the rat. Br J Pharmacol 1990; 101: 901–907

125 Cheuk J M S, Hollingsworth M, Hughes S J, Piper I T, Maresh M J A. Inhibition of contractions of the isolated human myometrium by potassium channel openers. Am J Obstet Gynecol 1993; 168: 953–960

126 Morrison J J, Ashford M L J, Khan R N, Smith S K. The effects of potassium channel openers on the isolated human pregnant myometrium before and after the onset of labour: potential for tocolysis. Am J Obstet Gynecol 1993; 169: 1277–1285

127 Morrison J J, Smith S K, Khan R N, Ashford M L J. The effects of potassium channel opening (BRL38227) on human myometrium in pregnancy and labour. Toronto: Proceedings of Society for Gynecologic Investigation, 1993: 131

128 Morrison J J, Ashford M L J, Khan R N, Smith S K. The effects of SO121 on the isolated human pregnant myometrium, prior to and after the onset of labour. Br J Obstet Gynaecol 1993; 100: 773–774

129 Weston A H, Edwards G. Recent progress in potassium channel opener pharmacology. Biochem Pharmacol 1992; 43: 47–54

130 Fuchs A-R, Fuchs F. Ethanol for prevention of preterm birth. Semin Perinatol 1981; 5: 236–251

131 Erny R, Pigne A, Prouvost C et al. The effects of oral administration of progesterone for premature labour. Am J Obstet Gynecol 1986; 154: 525–529

6 Breech presentation: is external cephalic version worthwhile?

R. W. Burr   R. B. Johanson

Although only 3–4% of pregnancies at term have a breech presentation, the mode of delivery has aroused much debate. Since Wright,[1] amongst others, recommended routine Caesarean section for the breech presentation in 1959, in view of the reported increase in perinatal mortality and morbidity, the rate of vaginal breech delivery has decreased sharply as the rate of Caesarean section has risen.[2] In 1970, 11.6% of breech presentations were delivered by Caesarean section, and this had risen to 79.1% by 1985.[3] Although the reasons for this change in practice are not necessarily supported by the data, the end result is that Caesarean section is now the normal mode of delivery for the breech presentation. In England in 1993 69% of breech presentations were delivered by Caesarean section (RCOG Annual Statistical Return 1993), and this accounted for 15.5% of the 93 715 Caesarean sections performed at this time. The data supporting either mode of delivery is less than ideal, and must be considered against the changing background of professional practice in this country.

BREECH PRESENTATION

The two issues to consider in the management of the term breech presentation are the neonatal and the maternal outcome. Advocates of Caesarean section highlight the increased perinatal mortality and morbidity of vaginal breech delivery, but this is achieved with an increase in maternal morbidity. However, this increase in perinatal mortality and morbidity is not only related to mode of delivery but other factors such as prematurity, congenital malformations, twin pregnancies, preterm prelabour rupture of membranes and intrapartum events such as intracranial haemorrhage and cord prolapse. The incidence of perinatal mortality as a sole concern is an insufficient measure to assess the obstetrical management of breech presentations.[2] The perinatal morbidity rate, increased in all weight categories of vaginally delivered breeches, seems to be dependent on the quality of birth management and criteria for admission to a trial of labour.[2]

Vaginal breech delivery

Antenatal diagnosis of a breech presentation allows a considered decision to be made on the mode of delivery. In spite of antenatal surveillance, breech presentations are still diagnosed for the first time when the woman presents in labour, although these babies are more likely to deliver vaginally with no excess morbidity and mortality.[4] Routine ultrasound scanning in the third trimester could be used to diagnose breech presentations, as those found to be breech at 25 weeks gestation or greater have an increased risk of malpresentation at delivery.[5]

The major concern expressed by clinicians about a breech trial of labour is not the case in which the breech does not descend into the pelvis, but the case where the trunk delivers and the after-coming head becomes entrapped. To be able to predict and thus avoid this situation an accurate means of predicting disproportion in any individual patient is required. This requires some assessment of the size and shape of the pelvis together with an estimation of the size of the fetus. Radiological pelvimetry is the commonest method used to assess the size and shape of the maternal pelvis, although the efficacy of X-ray pelvimetry is controversial.[6] It also carries the risks inherent with ionizing radiation to the mother and fetus. Computerized tomography (CT) pelvimetry, although a more expensive procedure, offers a means of assessing the pelvic dimensions with similar accuracy as X-ray pelvimetry, but at a much reduced radiation dose.[7] An even more expensive and less widely available investigation is magnetic resonance imaging (MRI) pelvimetry, which has the advantage of no ionizing radiation. When also used to measure the size of the fetal breech this technique has predicted those women with disproportion.[8]

Ultrasound-derived estimates of fetal weight are commonly used to assess whether there is likely to be disproportion in any trial of labour. Although a valuable means of diagnosing congenital abnormalities and also for detecting fetal neck hyperextension,[9] the accuracy of the estimate decreases with increasing fetal size. In fact, the error margins in fetal weight estimations may be higher with breech presentations than with cephalic presentations.[10] For an ultrasound-derived estimate of fetal weight from 2400–2900 g the actual birth weight will range from 1500–3999 g.[10]

In spite of the limitations in antenatal selection, a number of studies[11–14] have shown vaginal breech delivery to be safe in selected cases. Other studies[15] have demonstrated a better outcome from an elective Caesarean section. A critical review of the literature[6] by the intended mode of delivery concluded that there may be an increase in neonatal morbidity and mortality in the planned vaginal delivery group compared with the planned Caesarean delivery group. However, it also highlighted that the majority of papers had selection biases such that the differences in outcomes may have been caused by factors other than the mode of delivery.

Caesarean section

This has now become the normal mode of delivery for the breech presentation in many countries in Northern Europe and in North America. The policy of delivering term breeches by Caesarean section was based on a number of studies that reported better neonatal outcome with abdominal delivery.[6] In conjunction with increasing litigation in obstetrics, many clinicians moved to delivering all breech pregnancies by Caesarean section. This policy has been criticized on the grounds that these studies were retrospective and did not differentiate elective from emergency Caesarean section, and included preterm deliveries. Reviewing the change in practice, one study noted that the increase in the Caesarean section rate did not significantly reduce the adverse perinatal outcome in breech presentation.[16] This change in practice will have led to an increase in maternal morbidity rates, and also increased economic costs to the health care provider.

More recently, studies looking at delivery mode of breech presentations, where fetal weight was >1500 g, showed that the route of delivery did not affect the perinatal outcome[12] or even that the outcome was poorer by abdominal delivery.[11]

However, most of the studies of either delivery policy are limited by flaws in the design of the study – many were retrospective or observational and therefore subject to selection biases and variations in management protocols.

The current data was summarized by FIGO[2] in its statement that 'well structured randomized and controlled studies of the mode of delivery which can affect the morbidity and mortality of breech presentations in unselected patients are not available'.

Such a study has been proposed by Hannah and co-workers in Canada (Term Breech Trial) to be an international multicentre randomized controlled trial of elective Caesarean section versus planned vaginal delivery of the term breech. This is due to start mid-1996 and is expected to take 3–4 years to complete. Whether such a study could ever be completed in a reasonable period of time is debatable – a number of authors have noted the difficulties in performing such large randomized controlled trials in this field.[17]

Other considerations

Uncertainty about the best mode of delivery of the term breech, together with both increasing litigation and the fear of litigation has contributed to the increase in the Caesarean section rate for term breeches.[18] Other changes in clinical practice may continue this trend, such as the decreasing opportunities to train junior doctors in the techniques of safe vaginal breech deliveries. This is a problem common to all sizes of units as in the larger units these breech deliveries are spread amongst more clinicians. The reduction in junior doctors' hours, changes in working practices and the absence of formal accreditation in clinical skills can only exacerbate this problem. Although a recommended technique,[19] how much more difficult will it be to teach symphysiotomy for the trapped after-coming head?

Therefore, even if vaginal breech delivery is shown to be safe by the Term Breech study, it is increasingly unlikely that it will be offered by clinicians with limited training in the technique. If an increase in the Caesarean section rate owing to routine abdominal delivery of the breech is to be avoided, alternatives to Caesarean section for the term breech presentation need to be considered.

EXTERNAL CEPHALIC VERSION (ECV)

History

External cephalic version, the transabdominal manipulation of a breech-presenting fetus into a cephalic presentation, has been practised for centuries. The earliest medical recordings of this technique date from the time of Hippocrates. Since then it has been an accepted technique, practised in a wide variety of cultures and societies. Within societies where medical cover is thin, or practitioners skilled in vaginal breech delivery are rare, there is little doubt as to its value.[20] Conversely, in societies where the medical services are more technologically sophisticated it is sometimes argued that ECV is associated with more risks than the surgical alternative. Within Europe and North America the practice of ECV has fallen from favour in recent times.

The true value of ECV is determined by whether ECV reduces the incidence of breech presentation at the time of labour, with less risk to the mother and neonate than the alternatives.

As one of the advocates of the gentle art of ECV, Ranney[21] claimed that not only did ECV reduce the incidence of breech presentation but that it also reduced the incidence of premature labour. In his series ECV was performed at repeated intervals from 24 weeks gestation, but without ultrasound scanning or electronic fetal monitoring. An overall success rate of 93.7% was achieved with 1240 external versions being performed on 860 single fetuses. This included 18 cases of previous lower-segment Caesarean section and seven procedures performed in labour. However, a poor outcome may be expected if the 'at-risk' fetus is not identified prior to any obstetric intervention. In this series two infants died of congenital abnormalities, two died of prematurity following an emergency Caesarean section for bleeding placenta praevia, and a further infant died of the complications of prematurity following a vaginal delivery.

Although shown in retrospective or observational studies to be effective in reducing the incidence of breech presentation, debate about both the safety and place of ECV in 'modern' obstetric practice continued. Bradley-Watson,[22] performing ECV either in clinic or under sedation or general anaesthetic from 32 weeks gestation, concluded that with a fetal mortality rate of 0.9% and an overall complication rate of 4.4% this technique could not be justified as a routine policy. Again this was a retrospective review of 1308 attempts at ECV in 866 patients without ultrasound scanning or routine electronic fetal monitoring prior to ECV. The value of assessing fetal well-being prior to ECV was highlighted in a paper by Berg & Kunze[23] where ECV was performed after an abnormal CTG at 37 weeks gestation and resulted in a stillbirth.

Although all the studies of this period were of limited value owing to their design being retrospective or observational, ECV rapidly fell from favour. Attitudes towards ECV were described at the time as: 'There are those who enthusiastically recommend it, others who violently oppose it, and still others who express a rather elegant distaste for it'.[1] Perhaps the increasing safety of Caesarean section and a more acute awareness of medical litigation may have contributed to this change in practice.

Current practice

The advent of routine ultrasonography and electronic fetal monitoring, together with tocolysis saw a safer approach towards ECV. Although no major maternal or fetal complications were reported with this approach, the success rates of unselected groups were less than 50%.[24] A review of studies performed in the 1980s[25] concluded that ECV was a safe and effective procedure given the careful selection of low-risk patients, screening by electronic fetal monitoring and ultrasound examination, use of tocolysis, fetal heart rate monitoring during version, electronic fetal monitoring after the version and administration of Rhesus immunoglobulin in appropriate cases. ECV before term was to be discouraged because of the high rate of spontaneous version, the risk of premature birth and the occasional need to perform premature delivery because of fetal distress associated with the procedure.

The best evidence for the safety and effectiveness of ECV at term is provided by the six randomized controlled studies summarized in the Cochrane database.[26] The pooled data from these trials showed a statistically significant and clinically meaningful reduction in the non-cephalic birth (odds ratio 0.14, 95% confidence intervals 0.10–0.20) and Caesarean section rates (odds ratio 0.42, 95% confidence intervals 0.28–0.62) where ECV was attempted. There was no significant difference in the incidence of Apgar score ratings below 7 at 1 or 5 minutes, or perinatal death.

ECV preterm

Although technically easier to perform preterm – relatively larger amniotic fluid pool and relatively smaller fetus – the two randomized controlled trials summarized in the Cochrane database[27] do not support the use of ECV preterm. As already noted there may be significant risks in attempting the procedure before term.

Effectiveness of ECV at term

The effectiveness of ECV at term varies: Hofmeyer achieved a success rate of 93% in black African women, although only 62% in white African women.[28] This was attributed to the known tendency for the presenting part in black African women not to engage prior to labour. A study from Zimbabwe achieved an 86% success rate with ECV.[29] Using tocolysis in a Dutch population van Dorsten et al[30] succeeded in 68% of attempted versions. Within the UK population a success rate of 48% has been reported.[31]

Spontaneous cephalic version

The argument that those fetuses, in whom ECV was successful, were those who would have undergone spontaneous version regardless has to be addressed. Certainly, before term the spontaneous version rate is higher as the incidence of breech presentation is about 20% at 28 weeks but only 3–4% at term. Westgren et al,[32] in a prospective longitudinal study of ultrasound-diagnosed breech presentations from 32 weeks onwards, noted that spontaneous cephalic version occurred in 57% after 32 weeks and 25% after 36 weeks of pregnancy.

In the randomized controlled studies of ECV at term the rate of spontaneous version in the control groups was 14–22%.[30,33,34] In these three trials there was a virtually constant ratio of 3:1 ECV success rate to spontaneous version rate. The rate of spontaneous reversion to breech presentation after one or more attempts at ECV ranged from 0%[33] to 3%.[29]

Tocolysis

Although used routinely by some authors[28,29,35,36] the two randomized controlled trials of tocolysis[37,38] do not demonstrate an increase in the probability of successful version. However, tocolysis may be of value in individual cases where the first attempt at version has been unsuccessful, with the probable reason being the uterine tone.

Factors affecting the success of ECV

Other than ethnic differences, a number of other variables have been studied in an attempt to improve the success rate of ECV at term by better case selection. A lateral or cornual placental site has been found by some investigators[39] to reduce the success rate, although others claim an anterior placental site[40] to reduce the success rate, whilst placental site has not affected the rates of other investigators.[41] Increased parity and a normal amniotic fluid volume[39–41] together with a frank rather than an extended breech[39,41,42] were found to increase the success rate. A scoring system similar to the Bishop scoring system has been derived to predict the likely success of ECV.[40]

Repeating the ECV procedure at a later date following an unsuccessful attempt will also increase the overall success rate, by an additional 17% in one study.[43]

To further increase the success rate, transabdominal amnioinfusion with 700–900 ml normal saline has been used successfully in six women.[44]

Fetal acoustic stimulation has been found to be a useful adjunct to ECV as it causes a shift in fetal position to spine lateral, which increases successful version of fetuses with midline spine presentations.[45]

Complications of ECV at term

Although no significant maternal or neonatal complications were noted in the randomized controlled trials of ECV, cardiotocographic changes after ECV have been noted.[28,42,46] These were all temporary episodes of fetal bradycardia, and none required operative intervention.

Concern about the risks of fetomaternal haemorrhage secondary to attempted and successful ECV has been expressed. However, the incidence in practice is low, in the order of 1.8%,[47] and not associated particularly with procedures described as difficult. Therefore, routine assessment of fetomaternal haemorrhage is not necessary, other than in Rhesus negative women to detect the 2% in whom the routine dose of 500 IU of anti-D immunoglobulin is insufficient.

The benefits to the mother from having a successful ECV are clear, with a marked reduction in the chance of having a Caesarean section, with the attendant increase in morbidity.

Outcome of labour after ECV

The outcome of labour after a successful ECV is not affected by the procedure; in particular there is no increase in dysfunctional labour requiring an increased rate of Caesarean section.[48] ECV has been performed in women who have had a previous lower segment Caesarean section[49,50] with no serious maternal or neonatal complications.

RCOG view

The evidence is so much in favour of ECV that the Royal College of Obstetricians and Gynaecologists (RCOG) has suggested that units audit their success in achieving the standard that 'all women at term with an uncomplicated pregnancy and breech presentation should be offered ECV'.[51]

Value of ECV in clinical practice

The impact of offering an ECV service in the UK has been estimated by Hofmeyr to give a reduction in the rate of breech births from 78% to 44%

and to reduce Caesarean section from 29% to 15% for those women in whom ECV is attempted.[52] If offered to 2% of pregnancies this would result in 15 000 ECV attempts, 5100 fewer breech births and 2100 fewer Caesarean sections.

Besides reducing the maternal morbidity from Caesarean sections, there will also be an economic benefit from avoiding an operation by performing an ECV instead. Within the UK such an evaluation is confounded by the paucity of information on the actual costs of either procedure. A study by Gifford et al in the USA[53] calculated the predicted outcomes and costs associated with four options for managing the term breech. The options considered were: (a) ECV to all term breeches without contraindications to labour or version, and allowing a trial of labour to those who failed version; (b) delivering unsuccessful versions by Caesarean section; (c) not using ECV but allowing a trial of labour for eligible women; and (d) routinely delivering all breeches by Caesarean section. Group (a) resulted in a Caesarean section rate of 25%, but was the cheapest option; group (b) had a 32% Caesarean section rate and was 3% more costly; group (c) had a 63% Caesarean section rate and was 8% more costly; whilst group (d) resulted in a Caesarean section rate of 89% and was 18% more costly per delivery.

OTHER METHODS OF CEPHALIC VERSION

Elkins[54] reported an uncontrolled, but successful, trial of adoption of the knee-chest position for 15 minutes, every 2 hours of waking, for 5 days. Subsequently, three small randomized controlled trials have been carried out to establish whether or not postural management is effective. Unfortunately, in these studies no significant benefits were found.[55]

An observational study[56] suggested that motivated subjects can be influenced by a skilled hypnotist in such a manner that their fetuses have a higher incidence of conversion from breech to vertex presentation.

CONCLUSIONS

Routine Caesarean section for the term breech fetus is not justified by the available data.[2,18] However, in reality a large percentage are delivered by Caesarean section and this is not likely to decrease as a result of an increased vaginal delivery rate. Delivering a healthy term baby in a healthy mother by Caesarean section is certainly more costly and is associated with an increased maternal morbidity. To avoid this unnecessary cost to the mother and health care provider alternatives to Caesarean section for the term breech must be considered. Currently, ECV is the only alternative adequately researched to be recommended.

REFERENCES

1 MacArthur J L. Reduction of the hazards of breech presentation by external cephalic version. Am J Obstet Gynecol 1964; 88: 302–306
2 Recommendations of the FIGO Committee on Perinatal Health on guidelines for the management of breech delivery. Eur J Obstet Gynecol 1995; 58: 89–92
3 Croughan-Minchane M S et al. Morbidity among breech infants according to method of delivery. Obstet Gynecol 1990; 75: 821–825
4 Nwosu E C, Walkinshaw S, Chia P, Manasse P R, Atlay R D. Undiagnosed breech. Br J Obstet Gynaecol 1993; 100(6): 531–533
5 Tadmor O P, Rabinowitz R, Alon L, Mostoslavsky V, Aboulafia Y, Diamant Y Z. Can breech presentation at birth be predicted from ultrasound examinations during the second or third trimesters? Int J Gynecol Obstet 1994; 46(1): 11–14
6 Cheng M, Hannah M. Breech delivery at term: a critical review of the literature. Obstet Gynecol 1993; 83(3): 478–479
7 Gimovsky M L, O'Grady J P, Morris B. Assessment of computed tomographic pelvimetry within a selective breech presentation management protocol. J Reprod Med 1994; 39(7): 489–491
8 Berger R, Sawodny E, Bachmann G, Herrmann S, Kunzel W. The prognostic value of magnetic resonance imaging for the management of breech delivery. Eur J Obstet Gynecol 1994; 55(2): 97–103
9 Rojansky N, Tanos V, Lewin A, Weinstein D. Sonographic evaluation of fetal head extension and maternal pelvis in cases of breech presentation. Acta Obstet Gynecol Scand 1994; 73(8): 607–611
10 Chauhan S P, Magann E F, Naef R W, Martin J R, Morrison J C. Sonographic assessment of birthweight among breech presentations. Ultrasound Obstet Gynecol 1995; 6: 54–57
11 Pajntar M, Verdenik I, Pestevsek M. Cesarean section in breech by birth weight. Eur J Obstet Gynecol 1994; 54(3): 181–184
12 Brown L, Karrison T, Cibils L A. Mode of delivery and perinatal results in breech presentation. Am J Obstet Gynecol 1994; 171(1): 28–34
13 Roumen F J, Luyben A G. Safety of term vaginal breech delivery. Eur J Obstet Gynecol 1991; 40(3): 171–177
14 Bingham P, Hird V, Lilford R J. Management of the mature selected breech presentation: an analysis based on the intended method of delivery. Br J Obstet Gynaecol 1987; 94: 746–752
15 Thorpe-Beeston J G, Banfield P J, StG Saunders N J. Outcome of breech delivery at term. Br Med J 1992; 305: 746–747
16 Bowes W A, Taylor E S, O'Brien M, Bowes C. Breech delivery: Evaluation of the method of delivery on perinatal results and maternal morbidity. Am J Obstet Gynecol 1979; 135(7): 965–973
17 Eller D P, Van Dorsten J P. Route of delivery for the breech presentation: a conundrum. Am J Obstet Gynecol 1995; 173: 393–398
18 Eller D P, Van Dorsten J P. Breech presentation. Curr Opin Obstet Gynecol 1993; 5(5): 664–668
19 Menticoglou S M. Symphisiotomy for the trapped aftercoming parts of the breech: A review of the literature and a plea for its use. Aust NZ J Obstet Gynaecol 1990; 30: 1–9
20 Jordan B. External cephalic version as an alternative to breech delivery and cesarean section. Soc Sci Med 1984; 18(8): 637–651
21 Ranney B. The gentle art of external cephalic version. Am J Obstet Gynecol 1973; 116: 239–251
22 Bradley-Watson P J. The decreasing value of external cephalic version in modern obstetric practice. Am J Obstet Gynecol 1975; 123: 237–240
23 Berg D, Kunze U. Critical remarks on external cephalic version under tocolysis. Report on a case of antepartum fetal death. J Perinat Med 1977; 5: 32–38
24 Hanss J W. The efficacy of external cephalic version and its impact on the breech experience. Am J Obstet Gynecol 1990; 162: 1459–1464
25 Zhang J, Bowes W A Jr, Fortney J A. Efficacy of external cephalic version: a review. Obstet Gynecol 1993; 82(2): 306–312
26 Hofmeyr G J. External cephalic version at term. In: Enkin M W, Keirse M J N C, Renfrew

M J, Neilson J P, eds. Pregnancy and childbirth module of the Cochrane database of systematic reviews, 1995. London: Br Med J Publishing Group, 1995

27 Hofmeyr G J. External cephalic version before term. In: Enkin M W, Keirse M J N C, Renfrew M J, Neilson J P, eds. Pregnancy and childbirth module of the Cochrane database of systematic reviews, 1995. London: Br Med J Publishing Group, 1995

28 Hofmeyr G J. Effect of external cephalic version in late pregnancy on breech presentation and caesarean section rate: a controlled trial. Br J Obstet Gynaecol 1983; 90: 392–399

29 Mahomed K, Seeras R, Coulson R. External cephalic version at term. A randomized controlled trial using tocolysis. Br J Obstet Gynaecol 1991; 98(1): 8–13

30 Van Dorsten J P, Schifrin B S, Wallace R L. Randomized control trial of external cephalic version with tocolysis in late pregnancy. Am J Obstet Gynecol 1981; 141(4): 417–424

31 Bewley S, Robson S C, Smith M, Glover A, Spencer J A D. The introduction of external cephalic version at term into routine clinical practice. Eur J Obstet Gynecol 1993; 52: 89–93

32 Westgren M, Edvall H, Nordstrom L, Svalenius E. Spontaneous cephalic version of breech presentation in the last trimester. Br J Obstet Gynaecol 1985; 92: 19–22

33 Brocks V, Philipsen T, Secher N J. A randomized trial of external cephalic version with tocolysis in late pregnancy. Br J Obstet Gynaecol 1984; 91: 653–656

34 Van Veelen A J, Van Cappellen A W, Flu P K, Straub M J P F, Wallenburg H C S. Effect of external cephalic version in late pregnancy on presentation at delivery: a randomized controlled trial. Br J Obstet Gynaecol 1989; 96: 916–921

35 Fall O, Nilsson B A. External cephalic version in breech presentation under tocolysis. Obstet Gynecol 1979; 53: 712–715

36 Morrison J C, Myatt R E, Martin J N et al. External cephalic version of the breech presentation under tocolysis. Am J Obstet Gynecol 1986; 154: 900–903

37 Robertson A W, Kopelman J N, Read J A. External cephalic version at term: is a tocolytic necessary? Obstet Gynecol 1987; 70: 896–899

38 Tan G W T, Jen S W, Tan S L, Salmon Y M. A prospective randomised controlled trial of external cephalic version comparing two methods of uterine tocolysis with a non-tocolysis group. Sing Med J 1989; 309: 155–158

39 Hofmeyr G J, Sadan O, Myer I G, Galal K C, Simko G. External cephalic version and spontaneous version rates: ethnic and other determinants. Br J Obstet Gynaecol 1986; 93: 13–16

40 Newman R B, Peacock B S, Van Dorsten J P, Hunt H H. Predicting success of external cephalic version. Am J Obstet Gynecol 1993; 169(2): 245–250

41 Hellstrom A C, Nilsson B, Stange L, Nylund L. When does external cephalic version succeed? Acta Obstet Gynecol Scand 1990; 69: 281–285

42 Donald W L, Barton J J. Ultrasonography and external cephalic version at term. Am J Obstet Gynecol 1990; 162: 1542–1547

43 Kilpatrick S J, Safford K L. Repeat external cephalic version. Is it worth the effort? J Reprod Med 1995; 40: 775–778

44 Benifla J L, Goffinet F, Darai E, Madelenat P. Antepartum transabdominal amnioinfusion to facilitate external cephalic version. Obstet Gynecol 1994; 84: 1041–1042

45 Johnson R L, Elliot J P. Fetal acoustic stimulation, an adjunct to external cephalic version: a blinded, randomized crossover study. Am J Obstet Gynecol 1995; 173: 1369–1372

46 Hofmeyr G J, Sonnendecker E W W. Cardiotocographic changes after external cephalic version. Br J Obstet Gynaecol 1983; 90: 914–918

47 Lau T K, Stock A, Rogers M. Fetomaternal haemorrhage after external cephalic version at term. Aust NZ J Obstet Gynaecol 1995; 35: 173–174

48 Egge T, Schauberger C, Schaper A. Dysfunctional labour after external cephalic version. Obstet Gynecol 1994; 83(5): 771–773

49 Schachter M, Kogan S, Blickstein I. External cephalic version after previous cesarean section – a clinical dilemma. Int J Gynecol Obstet 1994; 45: 17–20

50 Flamm B L, Fried M W, Lonky N M, Giles W S. External cephalic version after previous cesarean section. Am J Obstet Gynecol 1991; 165(2): 370–372

51 The effective procedures in obstetrics suitable for audit. RCOG audit unit, Manchester. July 1993.

52 Hofmeyr G J. External cephalic version at term: how high are the stakes? Br J Obstet Gynaecol 1991; 98: 1–7

53 Gifford D S, Keeler E, Kahn K L. Reductions in cost and cesarean section rate by routine use of external cephalic version: a decision analysis. Obstet Gynecol 1995; 85: 930–936

54 Elkins V H. Miscellaneous interventions in pregnancy: Rh immunization; Preparation for breast feeding; External cephalic version. In: Effectiveness and satisfaction in antenatal care. Enkin M, Chalmers, eds. London: Spastics International Medical Publishers, 1982: pp 216

55 Hofmeyr G J. Cephalic version by postural management. In: Enkin M W, Keirse M J N C, Renfrew M J, Neilson J P, eds. Pregnancy and childbirth module of the Cochrane database of systematic reviews, 1995. London: Br Med J Publishing Group, 1995

56 Mehl L E. Hypnosis and conversion of the breech to the vertex presentation. Arch Fam Med 1994; 3(10): 881–887

7 The cervix in pregnancy and labour

K. S. Oláh

The uterine cervix is a tubular, connective tissue structure that has generally been considered as an inert organ playing a passive role in labour to the more active body and fundus of the uterus. However, it must perform quite different functions in pregnancy and labour, the nature and control of which remain an enigma. Disorders of these functions can have a profound effect on pregnancy; preterm cervical ripening results in late miscarriage and preterm labour, and failure of adequate 'cervical ripening' at term may result in poor progress in labour. To fully understand the mechanism by which the cervix performs these functions, it is essential that the anatomy and physiology of that organ are first discussed.

ANATOMY

Differentiation of the cervix from the uterine body begins at the 10th week of intrauterine life and it is clearly recognized as a separate entity by the 20th week of life.[1] Within 2 weeks of birth the reduction of hormonal stimulation results in a reduction in length of the uterus to about 25 mm; two-thirds of this length is still the cervix. This infantile stage remains until about 2 years before the menarche when the uterus doubles its length and its weight increases tenfold. Maturation to the adult stage occurs over the next 2 or 3 years. In the nulligravida the cervix is usually 2.5 to 3 cm in length and only slightly less in diameter. It is supported by the pubocervical fascia, the uterosacral ligaments and the cardinal ligaments, which are attached to the marginal walls of the organ. The fibrous nature of the cervix has been well documented,[2-4] with up to 10% being composed of muscle fibres.[4,5] However, Hughesdon[3] claimed that Danforth,[4] using material obtained at hysterectomies, did not recognize an outer muscular layer because it was removed during the operation. This muscle is thought to correspond to the smooth muscle of the vagina, being a continuation of the outer longitudinal muscle of the corpus.[6]

The cervix has two openings, the internal os communicating with the uterine cavity, and the external os (Fig. 7.1). The cervical canal is spindle shaped and is lined by ciliated columnar epithelium. The mucosa is arranged in folds and has the appearance of a tree trunk with branches, hence the name 'arbor

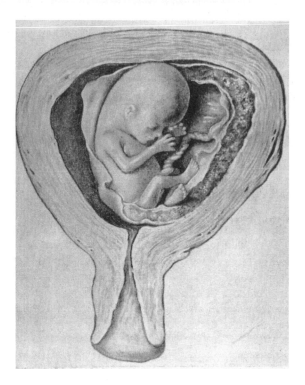

Fig.7.1 The cervix in a multiparous woman at 10 weeks gestation.

vitae'. This appearance is first noticed at 24–26 weeks of intrauterine life.[7] Squamous epthelium covers the external aspect of the cervix and is continuous with that of the vagina, ending at the external os at the 'squamo-columnar junction'.

HISTOLOGY

Light microscopic examinations of cervical tissue have shown that collagen dominates the cervical stroma.[4,8] According to Rorie and Newton[9] the muscle contents as determined by planometry is 29% in the upper third, 18% in the middle third and 6% in the lower third of the cervix, whereas it is 69% in the corpus. Schwalm and Dubrauszky[10] reported the cervical muscle content to be between 15% and 2%. The muscle cells are scattered in the tissue without regular orientation.[3] Often the most distal portion of the cervix is almost devoid of muscle.[11] The change from the fibrous tissue of the cervix to ne muscular tissue of the corpus is usually quite abrupt.

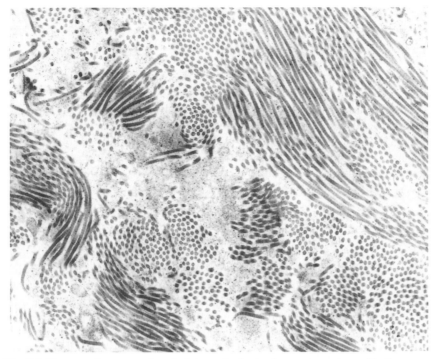

Fig. 7.2 Electron microscopy of cervical tissue obtained at hysterectomy (magnification ×
10 000). The collagen fibres are arranged in groups which traverse the tissue in all directions.

The collagen fibrils are uniform with a diameter of 57 nm.[12] They are
assembled in fibres which traverse the tissue in all directions (Fig. 7.2). Small
amounts of reticular fibres are also present.

Elastic fibres are difficult to demonstrate in cervical tissue, mainly because
of the rather non-specific staining methods available. Danforth et al[13] and
Krantz and Phillips,[11] found elastic fibres only in the walls of the larger blood
vessels. Pinto et al,[14] however, described elastic fibres in significant amounts.
The histological and electron microscopy studies by Leppert et al[15] are the
best to date. These authors described elastic fibres at 90° angles to the non-
vascular smooth muscle of the cervix, but did not try to quantitate them.[16]

Cervical fibroblasts are, at least in early pregnancy, characterized by long
'dendrites'.[17,18] Therefore, connective tissue components, proteolytic enzymes and other factors secreted by the cells through the 'dendrites' have a
relatively short diffusion distance to any point in the tissue, allowing fast re-
modulations of the organ. Furthermore, the fibroblasts have a well developed
rough endoplasmic reticulum, and numerous vesicles localized to the cell
membrane. Together, these details give the impression of an active cell type.
Smooth muscle cells, in general, share several properties with fibroblasts.
They have the same embryonic origin and synthesize collagen, proteoglycans

and elastin. The uterine cervix contains transitional forms between fibroblasts and smooth muscle cells.[19] Rather small numbers of mast cells[20,21] and neutrophilic polymorphonuclear leukocytes are also present.[12]

CERVICAL CONNECTIVE TISSUE

The extracellular matrix in fibrous connective tissues contains fibrillar components (collagen and elastin, proteoglycans, glycoproteins such as fibronectin and other proteins).[22,23] The non-fibrillar components are often designated as the 'ground substance'. The chemical compositions of the identified constituents are relatively well established. Except for collagen, however, their physiological significance is only partially known.

Collagen

Collagen, the most abundant protein in the body, determines the tensile strength of fibrous connective tissues. More than 10 genetically distinct forms of collagen have been reported,[24,25] and their distribution in different tissues described. The interstitial collagens (type I, II and III) which are cross striated, share many characteristics which will be discussed in more detail. Collagen types I and III are the main types found in the human cervix.

Tropocollagen, the characteristic subunit of the interstitial collagen, has a molecular weight of about 300 000 and a stiff, rod-like shape with unusual dimensions (300 nm long and 1.5 nm in diameter). It consists of three polypeptide chains, α-chains, joined together in a triple helix much like the strands of a rope. These chains are coiled into left-hand helices. Type I collagen consists of two identical chains (α1) and a distinct but homologous chain (α2). Therefore, the composition of type I collagen may be written $[\alpha1(I)]_2.\alpha2$. Type III collagen consists of three α1 chains which are genetically and chemically distinct from the type Iα1 chains. Therefore, type III collagen may be expressed as α1 (III)$_3$. The molecule itself is a right-handed superhelix (Fig. 7.3B) formed by these three chains.[26] At either end the α-chains contain short telopeptides, which do not participate in the triple helix formation. The amino acid composition of the triple helix is unique. The presence of glycine, the smallest amino acid, in every third position allows the very tight packing of the triple helix. Hydroxyproline, 13.4% by weight of type I collagen, is necessary for the stability of the tropocollagen. Small differences in hydroxyproline concentration exist between the different collagen types. The 60 nm thick collagen fibril is made up by tropocollagen molecules which are staggered (Fig. 7.3A) overlapping by one-quarter of their length, resulting in a periodicity of 640–700 Angstroms, thus creating the typical light and dark bands on electron microscopy (Fig. 7.4). Intra- and intermolecular covalent crosslinks are important for the physical strength of the fibril. There are two types of intermoleclular crosslinks; reducible and nonreducible. Reducible cross links may be studied in young tissues after mild

A

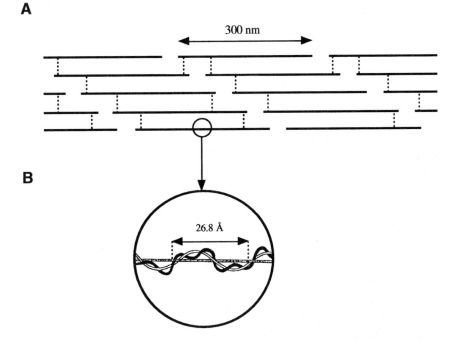

B

Fig. 7.3A Schematic diagram showing how the tropocollagens are composed of three α-chains, cross-linked and staggered to give rise to light and dark bands on electron microscopy. **B** The tropocollagen molecules are composed of polypeptide chains. There are three amino acid chains coiled into left-hand helices, the molecule constituted as a right-handed superhelix formed by these three chains. One of these chains (shown in black) is shown magnified to demonstrate it being wound round its own axis (white) and subsequently around that of the superhelix (dotted).

reduction utilizing tritiated borohydride.[27–29] The intermolecular crosslinks of 'old' tissue cannot be reduced by borohydride and are apparently stable at high temperatures, low pH and in the presence of pepsin. They are called non-reducible or mature crosslinks.

The reported ratios between type I and type III collagen found in the cervix are not very different from those found in skin.[30] Kleissl et al[31] found 62–80% type I collagen and 20–38% type III collagen. In another study Ito et al[32] found only 18% of the collagen to be of type III. Immunoperoxidase staining has revealed that type I and type III collagens are diffusely distributed in the cervical connective tissue with no remarkable differences shown in the distribution of these collagens.[33] Type IV collagens have been demonstrated in cervical basement membranes.[33,34]

Glycosaminoglycans

Glycosaminoglycans (GAGs) are large unbranched polysaccharide chains composed of disaccharide repeating units that contain a hexosamine residue

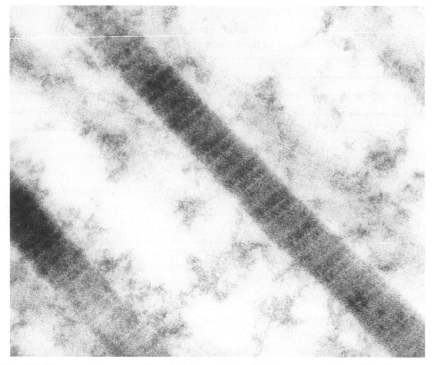

Fig. 7.4 Electron microscopy of cervical tissue obtained at hysterectomy (magnification ×
170 000). The striated appearance of the fibre resulting from the arrangement of the
tropocollagen is clearly visible.

and usually an uronic acid residue. Cervical GAGs constitute about 1% of
the dry defatted tissue, which is similar to other connective tissues. The
galactosaminoglycans dominate quantitatively, dermatan sulphates being the
most common (52–73%).[20,35–41] Chondroitin sulphate has been detected in
studies of cervical GAGs,[20,35,38–40] although more recent work would indicate
that little or no chondroitin sulphate is present,[19] and that previous analyses
were confused by the complexity of the dermatan sulphate (as they contain
'chondroitin sulphate-like' segments). Hyaluronic acid is found in smaller
amounts (8–22%).[20,35–41] The heparan sulphate found in the cervix
(6–13%)[20,35–42] has characteristics similar to that of heparan sulphate from the
human aorta,[40–42] and thus probably represents blood vessel connective tissue. Most authors have not detected keratan sulphate in cervical connective
tissue.[20,35,39–41]

Proteoglycans

A proteoglycan is made up of one or several GAGs connected to a protein
core. The chondroitin sulphate-rich proteoglycans in cartilage are well

characterized. A cervical dermatan sulphate proteoglycan has been isolated,[43] the average molecular weight ranging from 73 000 to 110 500. The amino acid composition is characterized by high contents of aspartic acid, glutamic acid and leucine. The GAGs are exclusively galactosaminoglycans with a co-polymeric structure similar to cervical dermatan sulphate. The function of the dermatan sulphate proteoglycan is unknown, although histological obser-vations suggest an interaction with collagen.[19] Scott and Orford[44] demon-strated a relationship between proteoglycans and collagen using an electron microscopic technique. They reported that the dermatan sulphate proteogly-cans were associated with the surface of the collagen fibre[45] and in particular to the so-called d-band, whereas chondroitin proteoglycans were found between the collagen fibres. The proteoglycans bind to collagen by low and high affinity binding sites. Danielsen[46] found altered biomechanical proper-ties of collagen membranes formed in vitro when dermatan sulphate was added. The maximum stress and the stiffness of the membranes were decreased in the presence of proteoglycan. In addition, collagen fibre thick-ness has been shown to be increased by dermatan sulphate proteoglycan. This increase in the diameter of collagen fibres is thought to be caused by lat-eral alignment of collagen fibrils as a result of the protein core of the proteo-glycan sticking to the collagen d-band, and the resulting dermatan sulphate 'side chains' interacting with other dermatan sulphate 'side chains' attached to other collagen fibrils.[47]

Glycoproteins

The protein cores of glycoproteins are combined with different amounts of oligosaccharides. Glycoproteins have been reported to be present in the uter-ine cervix.[40,41,48] It has been suggested that these glycoproteins originate from the mucus localized intracellularly and in crypts.[19]

Metabolism of cervical connective tissue

The turnover of cervical connective tissue is generally a slow process, but in pregnancy and as labour approaches dramatic changes occur. The synthesis of collagens and proteoglycans take place in both mesenchymal and epithelial cells. The collagens require a number of post-translational modifications for optimal function. These include hydroxylation of proline for stability of the fibre, and hydroxylation of lysine and oxidation by extracellular lysyl oxidase for cross link formation.

The degradation of collagen has been studied extensively.[49] The triple helix is resistant to most extracellular proteinases of vertebrate origin, exept the metalloproteinase collagenase which cleaves the collagen at only one site. The degradation products denature at 37°C and are then digested further by so-called gelatinases.[50] Leukocyte elastase degrades many proteins including elastin, proteoglycans and collagen telopeptides,[51] thus removing the cross links that are important for the stability of the collagen fibre. The activity of collagenase is considered to be essential for the regulation of collagen degradation under physiological conditions, whereas leukocyte elastase may primarily be concerned with collagen degradation in granulocyte-dependent inflammatory reactions, during which the two enzymes might act synergistically.[51,52] The intracellular enzymes cathepsin B and collagenolytic cathepsin may also contribute to collagen degradation. This implies phagocytosis of collagen fibrils that are possibly partly degraded by collagenase or leukocyte elastase.

It has been shown that a procollagenase is produced (latent collagenase), which may be activated immediately, or after storage in the extracellular matrix.[50] This latent collagenase may be stored in a way where it is bound to collagen. If so, the production of relatively small levels of activators could induce a dramatic increase in the collagen degradation. This might be important because fibroblasts contain no intracellular pool of collagenase. In addition, active collagenase may be inhibited by agents such as $\beta1$-anticollagenase and $\alpha2$-macroglobulin.[53] Studies of collagenase have shown 69% to be in complex with $\alpha2$-macroglobulin, 22% to be in free active form and 9% to be latent.[38,54]

PREGNANCY AND LABOUR

Historical aspects

Poor progress in labour because of 'rigidity' of the cervix was well recognized by previous generations of obstetricians. Smellie[55] gives an interesting account of four cases of prolonged labour caused by 'cervical rigidity' in which safe delivery was effected by a combination of attempting to allow time for the cervix to soften without undue force from the presenting part, followed by manual dilatation, a technique first described by Celsus in the 1st century AD.[56] Functional or spasmodic rigidity of the cervix was an entity recognized by obstetricians 50 years ago.[57] Although few obstetricians today would consider that the cervix could obstruct labour by a sustained 'spasm', recent biochemical evidence would support the view that the cervix may contribute to poor labour progress as a result of insufficient connective tissue remodelling.[58] Other conditions, such as conglutination of the external os or conglutinatio orificii externi is still encountered in modern obstetric practice. It is a condition whereby the cervix fails to dilate but is effaced, leaving the cervical opening as a 'pin-hole os' often with a ring of firm tissue around its margins. The lower uterine segment may be stretched across the head of the fetus, which may protrude from the vagina, the cervical os often being found behind the head in a sacral position. The thinned cervix and lower segment may even be mistaken for bulging membranes and an attempt may be made to rupture them. The condition may be congenital, but more commonly it is an acquired condition. In the past, abortifacients[59] and syphilitic chancre[60] have been major causes, although most recent cases are a result of cervical surgery.

In the 19th century rapid dilatation of the cervix was advocated as a means of inducing labour, and to improve labour progress where there was a risk to the life of the mother (usually eclampsia or cardiac decompensation) or the life of the fetus. *Accouchement forcé* was the term used for these latter procedures and methods included manual dilatation, fluid-filled bags, instrumental dilators and various operative techniques, including 'vaginal Caesarean section' and Dührssen's incisions of the cervix. All were associated with trauma to the cervix, lower uterine segment and vagina. With improvements in operative technique, transabdominal Caesarean section soon became the operation of choice and *accouchment forcé* was deemed an unnecessary and traumatic procedure.

Friedman's observations of the rate of cervical dilatation in labour, and his division of labour on the basis of these findings into the latent and active phases, were fundamental to a logical approach to labour management.[61,62] From the normal patterns it was possible to describe aberrant patterns, namely prolonged latent phase, primary dysfunctional labour and secondary arrest.[63] The subsequent development of the principles of the active management of labour[64] was based on the premise that the cervix, at least during the active phase of labour, was passive to the force generated by the myometrium – *accouchement forcé* resulting from forcible dilatation of the cervix by increasing myometrial activity! However, its application to the latent phase of labour is debatable.[65] The latent phase of labour is recognized as that period during which effacement of the cervix is being completed. This process is essential for the transition of the cervix from an obstruction to the passage of the fetus to a passive structure that will dilate without permanant deformity.[66] The onset of contractions before the process is complete will result in prolongation of the latent phase of labour and a poorer neonatal outcome.[67,68] Where the latent phase is prolonged, Friedman's advice to prescribe sedation and await the onset of the active phase of labour is similar to that of the exponents of the active management of labour,[64] and is probably, in essence, what Smellie was practicing.[55]

Changes in the physical properties of the cervix

The main function of the cervix is to retain the conceptus. However, it must allow the passage of the fetus at term and yet regain its retentative capacity within a short period. Dilatation to this degree in the non-pregnant, and even prior to the third trimester is often impossible; the non-pregnant cervix ruptures at strains of about 50%.[69] To enable this degree of dilatation to occur the cervix undergoes morphological and biochemical changes prior to the onset of labour. These features are incorporated into the scoring system described by Bishop for multiparous women as an index of the proximity of spontaneous labour, and included cervical position, consistency, dilatation and length or effacement.[70] Effacement is the process of thinning of the cervix which is usually accompanied by cervical softening or 'ripening'. Indeed, as discussed later, it may be the changes in the cervical connective tissues, which result in ripening, that allow effacement to occur. It is recognized that an uneffaced cervix may lead to prolongation of the latent phase of labour, and recent evidence would suggest that insufficient connective tissue remodelling may also lead to prolonged labour.[58]

Although the assessement of cervical consistency is rather subjective, the true consistency of the cervical tissue may be the most important change to have occurred, and may be a prerequisite for the other changes such as effacement and dilatation.[71] The lower stretch modulus of pregnancy and postpartum cervical tissue compared to non-pregnant tissue[69,72,73] and the increased viscoelastic creep properties of cervical tissue prior to delivery[73-76] are a direct measure of changes in the cervical consistency. It has been suggested that the measurement of cervical hydroxyproline concentration is an objective measure of cervical consistency.[19,77]

Changes in the connective tissue structure of the cervix

The histological appearance of the cervix has already altered by 9–14 weeks gestation. The collagen fibres become less densely packed and the waves are broader and deeper.[33,78] At term and immediately after delivery these changes are still more marked. The individual collagen fibres are separated by clear spaces and the fibrillar components appear to be dissociated.[79] Collagen fibres from the intrapartum cervix appear much thinner and more dispersed than those of non-pregnant controls.[12] In addition, the collagen fibres are irregular and are of variable thickness, suggesting that they were 'corroded'.[12] Electron microscopy has shown that at term the collagen fibrils become irregular and separated from one another and the average diameter decreases from 57 nm in the non-pregnant state to 42 nm at term.[12,80] This observation could reflect an increased turnover of collagen.[81] Cervical tissue oedema[14,79] and an increased vascularization have also been observed in late pregnancy and labour. Cervical fibroblasts in pregnancy share many of the characteristics of dendritic cells that are supposed to secrete collagenase in the synovial membrane from patients with rheumatoid arthritis.[82] They have long dendrites, a well-developed rough endoplasmic reticulum and vesicles under their plasma membrane.[17,78] Neutrophilic polymorphonuclear leukocytes are greatly increased in the pregnant cervix, and at term they are surrounded by a halo caused by the disappearance of collagen around the cells. The number of mast cells decreases in pregnancy.[14,20,21] However, mast cells may activate collagenase-secreting fibroblasts.[82]

Hydroxyproline, found only in collagen, is an indicator of the amount of collagen present in tissues. It is generally accepted that there is a decrease in the concentration of cervical hydroxyproline in pregnancy. At term and immediately after delivery the concentration is between 30–50% of that of non-pregnant controls.[32,48,77,79,83] The decrease in collagen in the cervix corresponds well with the increased softening of the tissues.[19] There is no significant difference between term and postpartum values, suggesting that no major break down and removal of cervical collagen takes place in labour. The importance of cervical hydroxyproline was demonstrated by Uldbjerg et al,[77] who showed that women with low concentrations of cervical hydroxyproline had a faster rate of cervical dilatation than those with high concentrations.

The absolute amounts of glycosaminoglycans (GAGs) increase by up to threefold during pregnancy,[84,85] the highest GAG level being found in cervical tissue obtained at the beginning of labour,[85] following which there is a progressive loss during parturition. However, dermatan sulphate has been reported to decrease by 30–45% towards the end of pregnancy, the lowest concentration being found in the active phase of labour,[38,39,85] and more recently it has been suggested that the onset of changes in dermatan sulphate concentrations in the cervix correspond to the process of cervical ripening in late pregnancy.[85] Dermatan sulphate proteoglycan, because of its ability to bind in orthogonal positions at the d- and e- bands of collagen fibrils, is the most important stabilizer of cervical consistency.[86] Furthermore, dermatan sulphate proteoglycan also binds to fibronectin,[87] which has a strong affinity to collagen.[88,89] These close interactions between collagen, fibronectin and dermatan sulphate proteoglycan is thought to account for the rigid consistency of the non-pregnant cervix.

The relative amounts of heparan sulphate in the cervix increases during parturition and becomes the dominant GAG in the second stage of labour.[38,85] However, this is probably caused by the increased vascularity of the cervix in pregnancy, and the absence of collagen degradation in the vessel wall.[90,91]

Chondroitin sulphate concentration in the cervix is relatively low in pregnancy, but peaks in the third trimester prior to labour, following which there is a decrease in the active phase of labour.[85] However, the relative changes are small.

Hyaluronic acid content of the cervix increases sharply at the onset of labour from a relative content of 5% in the third trimester to 49% in labour.[85] It is the most prominent GAG in the latent phase of labour, decreasing after delivery. It has been demonstrated that hyaluronic acid weakens the affinity of fibronectin to collagen,[92] thus contributing to the loosening of the collagenous framework. Hyaluronic acid itself has a high water-binding capacity,[91] and in comparison to a triple helical molecule of comparable weight a hyaluronic acid molecule has a much higher volume,[93] which may explain the increase in water content of the cervix at term.[85,91]

There is an increase in the water content of the cervix from 81% to 87% during pregnancy.[77] There is some evidence that the increase may be most marked just prior to delivery[94] which would correspond to those changes described above, regarding hyaluronic acid in the cervix. The increase is not explained by the rise in vascularity of the cervix because the water concentration of blood is almost identical to that of cervical tissue. It has been suggested that cervical ripening is similar to an inflammatory reaction.[95] If the capillary permeability is increased, as in inflammatory reactions, albumin would be expected to penetrate into the interstitial tissues. However, the concentration of albumin is not significantly increased in postpartum cervices compared to non-pregnant cervices.[19] Whatever the mechanism of the increase in water content of the cervix, the magnitude of the changes described do not suggest that cervical 'ripeness' is wholly dependent on the water content of the cervix.

THE MECHANISM OF CERVICAL CHANGE

The mechanism of cervical ripening or maturation remains an enigma. There is an increased level of collagenolytic activity in the cervix in pregnancy,[38,96,97] as well as an increase in leukocyte elastase[77] and other proteolytic enzymes.[32,98–100] The high level of such activity would destroy all of the cervical collagen long before term if the rate of collagen synthesis was unchanged, suggesting a marked increase in the rate of collagen biosynthesis. This would explain the shift from 'old collagen' to 'young collagen' suggested by the increase in hydroxyproline extractability in pregnancy[36,77] and the decreased diameter of the collagen fibrils seen in pregnancy.[81]

It has been suggested that the process of cervical maturation is similar to an inflammatory reaction, with neutrophil invasion of the cervix in labour.[12,97] Others have proposed that the changes are caused by collagenase and elastase produced not only by leukocytes, as would be found in an inflammatory reaction, but also by fibroblasts, which are known to produce collagenase.[77] The interleukins have been suggested to play an important role in the process because they are chemotactic for neutrophils and may represent the signal for the commencement of cervical ripening. It has been suggested that interleukin-8 (IL-8) is involved in neutrophil-mediated cervical ripening.[101] In vitro studies have shown that the cervix is capable of producing large quantities of IL-8 and production of IL-8 by the cervix may be influenced by steroid hormones.[101] However, studies of amniotic fluid and uterine vein IL-8 concentration (Fig. 7.5), recently conducted in Liverpool, have not demonstrated an increase in women in spontaneous labour undergoing emergency Caesarean section compared to elective controls (Oláh, Neilson & Johnson, unpublished observations). This suggests that if IL-8 is involved in the connective tissue changes in the cervix, it is isolated to cervical tissues alone.

Recent studies have indicated that amniotic fluid levels of interleukin-6 (IL-6) are elevated in the active phases of both preterm[102,103] and term[104] labour. Elevated levels of IL-6 can therefore be regarded as a marker of active

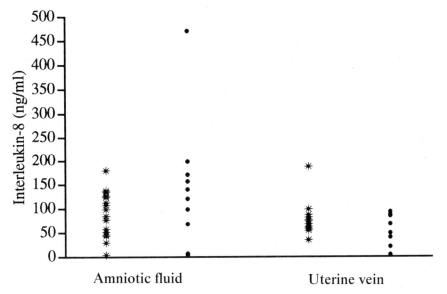

Fig. 7.5 Interleukin-8 levels in amniotic fluid and uterine vein blood in a) women in spontaneous labour requiring operative delivery with membranes ruptured ≤ 6 hours and b) women undergoing an elective Caesarean section.

labour, regardless of the number of weeks of gestation. In cases of preterm labour IL-6 is probably produced by an infective process; in term labour the process is yet to be elucidated. Interleukin-6 is known to stimulate the production of prostaglandin E_2 (PGE_2) by amnion and decidua[105] and may therefore be an important factor in the physiology of normal labour. It has been reported that concentrations of PGE_2 and IL-6 are higher in forewater compared to hindwater amniotic fluid samples.[106] Interleukin-6 is a pleiotropic cytokine, which is produced in response to other 'effector' cytokines such as IL-1α, IL-1β and TNFα.[107,108] The higher concentrations of IL-6 in the forewaters suggests that the production of IL-6, as a result of stimulation by its cytokine 'effectors', is greater at this site. In labour at term this may result from the effects of descent of the fetal head causing stretching of the lower segment of the uterus and fetal membranes.

The higher concentration of IL-6 in forewater compared to hindwater amniotic fluid samples parallels the reported levels of PGE_2.[109] It is therefore likely that if IL-6 is involved in the mechanism of labour it acts through the effects of the resultant PGE_2 release. However, IL-6 may have a direct effect on collagen formation and catabolism as well as other connective tissue components.[107,110,111] In addition, it also affects endothelial cell permeability,[112] which may result in an increase in extracellular fluid. There could therefore be a direct paracrine effect of IL-6 in normal labour.

Studies of the membranes at term have identified a zone of extreme altered morphology representing an area of structural weakness, likely to be present before membrane rupture during pregnancy.[113] These changes result from dissociation of membrane collagen and oedema in the spongy layer. Similar changes have been demonstrated in the fetal membranes that cover the cervix obtained at Caesarean section at term,[114] suggesting that such changes are localized to these membranes. Indeed, the changes described in the membranes at term and after delivery are similar to those in the cervix.[115] The synchronous changes in cervical and membrane morphology which precede normal labour may therefore occur as a result of the same or similar mechanisms, the consequence being that the membranes have weakened and the cervix is compliant when labour commences. This would imply a local mechanism resulting in these changes, and the high levels of IL-6 found in the forewaters suggests that this cytokine could be involved, either directly or indirectly though PGE_2.

The activity of the cervix in labour

The anatomical and histological studies of the cervix already described have shown that it is predominantly a connective tissue structure with a relatively sparse muscle content[3,4,8] Thus, the cervix has been considered passive in its response to the contractions of the fundus during labour, and the rate of cervical dilatation has been assumed to be directly dependent on myometrial activity. More recently it has been shown that the physical state of the cervix determines the rate of cervical dilatation and, in addition, modulates uterine wall tension and intrauterine pressure.[116] This effect has been termed the Cervical Attenuation/Augmentation of Pressure or CAP effect.[116,117] Therefore, a compliant cervix will result in rapid progress in labour, but owing to the compliance of the cervix and lower segment effectively reducing the wall tension, pressure will be attenuated. Conversley, a non-compliant cervix predisposes to slow labour progress, and myometrial activity will be directly translated into uterine wall tension and thus result in high intrauterine pressures.

It is generally accepted that the cervix dilates during contractions in labour, and studies that have measured the cervical response objectively[116–119] have confirmed this (Fig. 7.6). However, recent studies have indicated that the cervix may contract (Fig. 7.7) in response to oxytocic stimulation during the latent phase of labour.[120] The presence of cervical contractions appear to be a feature of the non-dilated, uneffaced cervix. Cervical contractions, when present, are observed only during the first 3–4 cm dilatation, the majority being synchronous with the contractions of the corpus. After this period there is a transition time, lasting up to 15 minutes, when no cervical response is seen. The cervix dilates in response to myometrial activity after this point, the appearance of this pattern corresponding to the point at which the rate of cervical dilatation increases, i.e., that time at which the 'active phase' of labour is thought to commence. The period where the cervix contracts is characterized by minimal residual dilatation and coincides with the latent

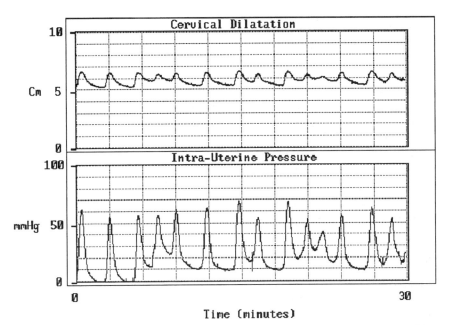

Fig. 7.6 Cervical dilatation (0–10 cm, upper chart) and intrauterine pressure (0–100 mmHg, lower chart) during the active phase of labour. The cervix dilates passively in response to uterine contractions.

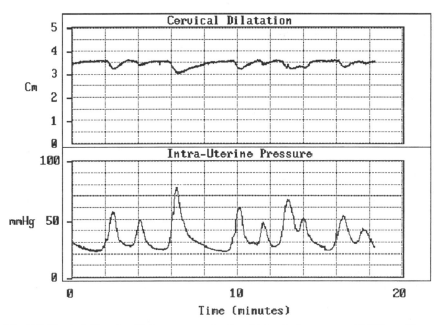

Fig. 7.7 Cervical dilatation (0–5 cm, upper chart) and intrauterine pressure (0–100 mmHg, lower chart) during the latent phase of labour. Cervical contractions synchronous with uterine activity are clearly visible.

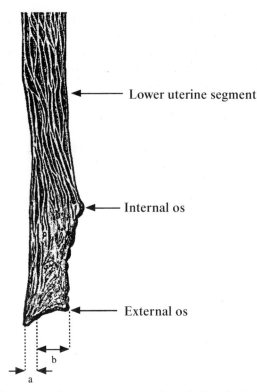

Fig. 7.8 Schematic diagram showing the arrangement of muscle fibres in the lateral third (a) of the cervix. In the inner 2/3 (b) there are generally no muscle fibres. The amount of muscle present in the cervix is very variable, and in fact may be absent (based on the work of Hofmeier, 1886).[131]

phase of Friedman's cervical dilatation curves. The transition period is followed by more rapid dilation, and corresponds to the acceleration and active phases.

Contractions of the cervix have been demonstrated in animals[121–124] and in humans.[125–127] Studies in pregnant women have shown that in the first and second trimesters of pregnancy the human cervix can contract in response to oxytocic agents[126,127] and at term the cervix can contract rhythmically, sometimes independently of activity in the uterine body.[125] Cervical contractions are thought to be caused by contractions of the sparse muscle content of the cervix. Hughesdon[3] and Wendell-Smith[128] ascribed a distinct architecture to the muscle in the cervix. Hughesdon[3] described an outer longitudinal muscle (the 'extrinsic muscle of the cervix'), which enhanced the tension transmitted to the outer part of the cervix by the muscle in the fundus (Fig. 7.8). The anatomy of the muscle layers in the cervix coupled with differential tension across the wall of the uterus would effectively induce differential movement of notional tissue layers, with the outer layers being most affected. The result is a gradual redistribution of cervical tissue, which may contribute towards the process of effacement.[116,129] Because movement of tissue would take place from the outer aspect of the cervix, this would result in thinning of the cervix from the external os upwards leaving the tissue of the upper cervical canal, i.e., in the region of the internal os to be effected last in the process. This would be in keeping with conventional obstetric teaching that it is the internal os which lends functional integrity to the cervix. Electromyographic recording from the human cervix in labour[130] has demonstrated functionally independent muscle activity consistent with Hughesdon's anatomical description. The commencement of the active phase is characterized by a change in electromyographic activity of the cervix, which may be explained by the removal of the muscle responsible for this activity, and is possibly a consequence of the mechanism of effacement described above.

CONCLUSIONS

The idea of the cervix as a passive, inert, connective tissue structure is no longer tenable. The cervix is in fact a dynamic structure, the control of which we still do not fully understand. A more comprehensive knowledge of this control mechanism may help us to manage preterm labour and mid-trimester pregnancy loss, and may help us to manipulate the cervical state at term. Indeed, pharmacological manipulation of the cervix to produce dilatation without inducing myometrial activity would be similar to surgically removing the resistance of the cervix – i.e., a vaginal Caesarean section. Similarly, reversing the process of ripening and effacement may be an effective method of preventing preterm birth. Studies of cervical collagen may also reveal the cause of recurrent midtrimester pregnancy loss in those women with no evidence of an infective aetiology. The apparent simplicity of the structue of the cervix belies its true complexity, and a greater knowledge of its function will allow us to understand and manage pregnancy and labour problems more effectively.

REFERENCES

1 Langman J. Genital system. In: Medical embryology, 3rd edn. Baltimore: Williams & Wilkins Co., 1974: pp 175–200
2 Benckiser A, Hofmeir M. Beiträge zur anatomie des schwangern und kreissenden uterus. Stuttgart: Verlag von Ferdinand Enke, 1887
3 Hughesdon P E. The fibromuscular structure of the cervix and its changes during pregnancy and labour. J Obstet Gynaecol Br Emp 1952; 59: 763–776
4 Danforth D N. The fibrous nature of the human cervix, and its relation to the isthmic segment in gravid and nongravid uteri. Am J Obstet Gynecol 1947; 53: 541–560
5 Buckingham J C, Buethe R A, Danforth D N. Collagen-muscle ratio in clinically normal and clinically incompetent cervices. Am J Obstet Gynecol 1965; 91: 232–237
6 Lierse W. Untersuchungen über die anordnung der längsverlaufenden muskulatur in der cervix uteri. Zeitsch Zellforsch 1960; 52: 739–747
7 Fluhman C F. The nature and development of the so-called glands of the cervix uteri. Am J Obstet Gynecol 1957; 74: 753–768

8 Danforth D N. The distribution and functional activity of the cervical musculature. Am J Obstet Gynecol 1954; 68: 1261–1271
9 Roric D K, Newton M. Histologic and chemical studies of the smooth muscle in the human cervix and uterus. Am J Obstet Gynecol 1967; 99: 466–469
10 Schwalm H, Dubrauszky V. The structure of the musculature of the human uterus-muscles and connective tissue. Am J Obstet Gynecol 1966; 94: 391–404
11 Krantz K E, Phillips W P. Anatomy of the human uterine cervix, gross and microscopic. In: Lang W R, ed. The cervix. Annals of the New York academy of sciences. New York: The New York Academy of Science, 1962: 551–563
12 Junquiera L C U, Zugaib M, Montes G S, Toledo O M S, Krisztán R M, Shigihara K M. Morphologic and histochemical evidence for the occurrence of collagenolysis and for the role of neutrophilic polymorphonuclear leukocytes during cervical dilatation. Am J Obstet Gynecol 1980; 138: 273–281
13 Danforth D N, Buckingham J C, Roddick J W. Connective tissue changes incident to cervical effacement. Am J Obstet Gynecol 1960; 80: 939–945
14 Pinto R M, Rabow W, Votta RA. Uterine cervix ripening in term pregnancy due to the action of estradiol-17β. A histological and histochemical study. Am J Obstet Gynecol 1965; 92: 319–324
15 Leppert P C, Keller S, Cerreta J, Mandl I. Conclusive evidence for the presence of elastin in human and monkey cervix. Am J obstet Gynecol 1982; 142: 179–182
16 Leppert P C, Cerreta J, Mandl I. Orientation of elastic fibres in the human cervix. Am J Obstet Gynecol 1986; 155: 219–242
17 Uldjberg N, Ekman G, Malmström A, Sporrong B, Ulmsten U, Wingerup L. Biochemical and morphological changes of human cervix after local application of prostaglandin E_2 in pregnancy. Lancet 1981; ii: 267–268
18 Joh K, Riede U N, Zahradnik H P. The effect of prostaglandins on the lysosomal function of the cervix uteri. Arch Gynecol 1983; 234: 1–16
19 Uldbjerg N. Cervical connective tissue in relation to pregnancy, labour and treatment with prostaglandin E2. Acta Obstet Gynecol Scand 1989; Supplement 148.
20 Iverson O H. Mast cells in the myometrium of the cervix uteri, and changes caused by androgenic and estrogenic hormones. Acta Path 1960; 49: 337–343
21 Iverson O H. Bindevaevsreaktioner i cervix uteri. Thesis. Copenhagen: Aarhus stiftbogtrykkerie, 1964
22 Paulsson M, Heinegård D. Radioimmunoassay of the 148-kilodalton cartilage protein. Biochem J 1982; 207: 207–213
23 Heinegård D, Larsson T, Sommarin Y, Franzén A, Paulsson M, Hedbom E. Two novel Matrix proteins isolated from articular cartilage show wide distribution among connective tissues. J Biol Chem 1986; 261: 13866–13872
24 Eyre D R. Collagen: Molecular diversity in the body's protein scaffold. Science 1980; 207: 1315–1322
25 von der Mark K. Localization of collagen types in tissues. Int Rev Connect Tissue Res 1981; 9: 265–324
26 Rich A, Crick F H C. Nature 1955; 176: 915
27 Robins S P, Bailey A J. The chemistry of the collagen cross-links. The characterization of fraction C, a possible artifact produced during the reduction of collagen fibres with borohydride. Biochem J 1973; 135: 657–665
28 Robins S P, Bailey A J. Relative stabilities of the intermediate reducible cross-links present in collagen fibres. FEBS Letts 1973; 33: 167–171
29 Robins S P, Shimokomaki M, Bailey A J. The chemistry of the collagen cross-links. Age-related changes in the reducible components of intact bovine collagen fibres. Biochem J 1973; 131: 771–780
30 Epstein E H. [α1 (III)]$_3$ human skin collagen, release by pepsin digestion and preponerance in fetal life. J Biol Chem 1974; 249: 3225–3231
31 Kleissl, H P, van der Rest M, Naftolin F, Glorieux F H, De Leon A. Collagen changes in the human uterine cervix at parturition. Am J Obstet Gynecol 1978; 130: 748–753
32 Ito A, Kitamura K, Mori Y, Hirakawa S. The change in solubility of type I collagen in human uterine cervix in pregnancy at term. Biochem Med 1979; 21: 262–270
33 Minamoto T, Arai K, Hirakawa S, Nagai Y. Immunohistochemical studies on collagen types in the uterine cervix in pregnant and non-pregnant states. Am J Obstet Gynecol 1987; 156: 138–144

34 Frappart L, Berger G, Grimaud J A, Chevalier M, Bremond A, Rochet Y, Feroldi J. Basement membrane of the uterine cervix: Immunofluorescence characteristics of the collagen component in normal or atypical epithelium and invasive carcinoma. Gynecol Oncol 1982; 13: 58–66
35 Nakaya T. Studies on acid mucopolysaccharides in the human cervix uteri. Nagoya Med 1973; 18: 295–319
36 Danforth D N, Veis A, Breen M, Weinstein H G, Buckingham J C, Manalo P. The effect of pregnancy and labor on the human cervix: Changes in collagen, glycoproteins, and glycosaminoglycans. Am J Obstet Gynecol 1974; 120: 641–651
37 von Maillot, K, Stuhlsatz H W, Mohanaradhakrishnan V, Greiling H. Changes in the glycosaminoglycans distribution pattern in the human uterine cervix during pregnancy and labour. Am J Obstet Gynecol 1979; 135: 503–506
38 Kitamura K, Ito A, Mori Y, Hirakawa S. Glycosaminoglycans of the human uterine cervix: heparan sulfate increases with reference to cervical ripening. Biochem Med 1980; 23: 159–166
39 Cabrol D, Breton M, Berrou E, Visser A, Sureau C, Picard J. Variations in the distribution of glycosaminoglycans in the uterine cervix of the pregnant woman. Eur J Obstet Gynecol Reprod Biol 1980; 10: 218–227
40 Shimizu T, Endo M, Yosizawa Z. Glycoconjugates (glycosaminoglycans and glycoproteins) and glycogen in the human cervix uteri. Tohoku J Exp Med 1980; 32: 1967–1976
41 Uldjberg N, Carlstedt I, Ekman G, Malmström A, Ulmsten U, Wingerup L. Dermatan sulphate and mucin glycopeptides from the human uterine cervix. Gynecol Obstet Invest 1983; 16: 199–209
42 Höök M, Lindahl U, Iverius P-H. Distribution of sulphate and iduronic acid residues in heparin and heparin sulphate. Biochem J 1974; 137: 33–43
43 Uldjberg N, Malmström A, Ekman G, Sheehan J, Ulmsten U, Wingerup L. Isolation and characterization of dermatan sulphate proteoglycan from human uterine cervix. Biochem J 1983; 209: 497–503
44 Scott J E, Orford C R. Dermatan sulphate-rich proteoglycan associates with rat tailtendon collagen at the d-band in the gap region. Biochem J 1981; 197: 213–216
45 Scott J E. The periphery of the developing collagen fibril. Biochem J 1984; 218: 229–233
46 Danielson C C. Mechanical properties of reconstituted collagen fibrils; influence of a glycosaminoglycan: dermatan sulfate. Connect Tiss Res 1982; 9: 219–225
47 Frannson L-Å, Cöster L, Malmström A, Sheehan J K. Self-association of scleral proteodermatan sulfate. J Biol Chem 1982; 257: 6333–6338
48 Karube H, Kanke Y, Mori Y. Increase of structural glycoprotein during dilatation of human cervix in pregnancy at term. Endocrinol Jap 1975; 22: 445–448
49 Woolley D E, Evanson J M, eds. Collagenase in normal and pathological connective tissues. Chichester: John Wiley & Sons Ltd., 1980
50 Sakyo K, Kobayashi J-I, Ito A, Mori Y. Partial purification and characterization of gelatinase and metal dependent peptidase from rabbit uterus and their synergistic action on gelatin in vitro. J Biochem 1983; 94: 1913–1923
51 Ohlsson K. Polymorphonuclear leucocyte collagenase. In: Woolley D E, Evanson J M, eds. Collagenase in normal and pathological connective tissues. Chichester: John Wiley & Sons Ltd., 1980: pp 209–222
52 Harris E D, Vater C A, Mainardi C L, Siegel R C. Degradation of cartilage collagen – factors affecting substrate and enzyme. In: Castpar H, ed. Biology of the articular cartilage in health and disease. Stuttgart: F. K. Schattauer Verlag, 1980: pp 175–187
53 Stricklin G P, Welgus H G. Human skin fibroblast collagenase inhibitor: purification and biochemical characterization. J Biol Chem 1983; 258: 122252–122258
54 Kitamura, K, Ito A, Mori Y, Hirakawa S. Changes in the human uterine cervical collagenase with special reference to cervical ripening. Biochem Med 1979; 22: 332–338
55 Smellie W. Collection XVII. Of tedious cases from the rigidity of the os internum, vagina, or os externum: also from the wrong position of the mouth of the womb. In: McClintock A H, ed. Smellie's treatise on the theory and practice of midwifery, Volume II. London: The New Sydenham Society, 1877: pp 200–207
56 Caldwell W E. Rapid methods of dilatation. Vaginal cesarean section. In: Curtis A H, ed. Obstetrics and gynecology, Vol. II. Philadelphia: W. B.Saunders Co., 1933: pp 304–318
57 DeLee J B, Greenhill J P. Anomalies of the passages. In: Principles and practice of obstetrics, 9th edn. London: W. B. Saunders Co., 1947: pp 597–600

58 Granström L, Ekman G, Malmström A. Insufficient remodelling of the uterine connective tissue in women with protracted labour. Br J Obstet Gynaecol 1991; 98: 1212–1216
59 Williams J W. Dystocia due to abnormalities of the generative tract. In: Obstetrics, 6th edn. New York: D. Appleton & Co., 1931: pp 828–843
60 Le Bigot P. De l'influence du chancre syphilitique du col de l'uterus sur l'accouchement. Thèse de Paris, 1899
61 Friedman E A. The graphic analysis of labor. Am J Obstet Gynecol 1954; 68: 1568–1575
62 Friedman E A. Primigravid labor. A graphicostatistical analysis. Obstet Gynecol 1955; 6: 567–589
63 Friedman E A, Sachtleben M R. Dysfunctional labor. I. Prolonged latent phase in the nullipara. Obstet Gynecol 1961; 17: 135–148
64 O'Driscoll K, Stronge J M, Minogue M. Active management of labour. Br Med J 1973; 3: 135–137
65 Oláh K S, Neilson J P. Failure to progress in the management of labour. Br J Obstet Gynaecol 1994; 101: 1–3
66 Oláh K S, Gee H. The functional response of the cervix in the first stage of labour. Br J Obstet Gynaecol 1992; 99: 1025
67 Cardozo L, Gibb D M F, Studd J W W, Vasant R V, Cooper D J. Predictive value of cervimetric patterns in primigravidae. Br J Obstet Gynaecol 1982; 89: 33–38
68 Chelmow D, Kilpatrick S, Laros R K. Maternal and neonatal outcomes after prolonged latent phase. Obstet Gynecol 1993; 81: 486–891
69 Rungren A. Physical properties of connective tissues as influenced by single and repeated pregnancies in the rat. Acta Physiol Scand 1974; 417: (suppl) 24
70 Bishop E H. Pelvic scoring for elective induction. Obstet Gynecol 1964; 24: 266–268
71 Oláh K S, Gee H, Brown J. The effect of cervical contractions on the generation of intra-uterine pressure during the latent phase of labour. Br J Obstet Gynaecol 1994; 101: 341–343
72 Conrad J T, Ueland K. Reduction of the stretch modulus of human cervical tissue by prostaglandin E$_2$. Am J Obstet Gynecol 1976; 126: 218–223
73 Harkness M L R, Harkness R D. Changes in the physical properties of the uterine cervix of the rat during pregnancy. J Physiol 1959; 148: 524–529
74 Harkness R D, Nightingale M A. The extensibility of the cervix uteri of the rat at different times of pregnancy. J Physiol 1962; 160: 214–220
75 Hollingsworth M, Gallimore S, Isherwood C N. Effects of prostaglandin F-2 alpha and E2 on cervical extensibility in the late pregnant rat. J Reprod Fertil 1980; 58: 95–99
76 Williams L M, Hollingsworth M, Dixon J S. Changes in the tensile properties and fine structure of the rat cervix in late pregnancy and during parturition. J Reprod Fertil 1982; 66: 203–211
77 Uldjberg N, Ekman G, Malmström A, Olsson K, Ulmsten U. Ripening of the human uterine cervix related to changes in collagen, glycosaminoglycans, and collagenolytic activity. Am J Obstet Gynecol 1983; 147: 662–666
78 Theobald P W, Rath W, Kühnle H, Kuhn W. Histological and electron-microscopic examinations of collagenous tissue of the non-pregnant cervix, the pregnant cervix, and the pregnant prostaglandin treated cervix. Arch Gynecol 1982; 231: 241–245
79 Danforth D N, Buckingham J C, Roddick J W. Connective tissue changes incident to cervical effacement. Am J Obstet Gynecol 1960; 80: 939–945
80 Berwind T. Elektronenmikroskopische untersuchungen am fasersystem der cervix uteri der frau. Arch Gynecol 1954; 184: 459–468
81 Svoboda E L A, Howley T P, Deporter D A. Collagen fibril diameter and its relation to collagen turnover in three soft connective tissues in the rat. Connect Tissue Res 1983; 12: 43–48
82 Wooley D E, Harris E D, Mainardi C L, Brinckerhoff C E. Collagenase immunolocalization in cultures of rheumatoid synovial cells. Science 1978; 200: 773–775
83 Danforth D N, Buckingham J C. The effects of pregnancy and labor on the amino acid composition of the human cervix. In: Blandau R, Moghissi K, eds. The biology of the cervix. Chicago: The University of Chicago Press, 1973: 351–451
84 Golichowski A M. Biochemical basis of cervical maturation. In: Huszar G, ed. The physiology and biochemistry of the uterus in pregnancy. Florida: C R C Press, 1986: 261–280
85 Osmers R, Rath W, Pflanz M, Kuhn W, Stuhlsatz H-W, Szeverényi M. Glycosaminoglycans in cervical connective tissue during pregnancy and parturition. Obstet Gynecol 1993; 81: 88–92

86 Scott J E. Proteoglycan-collagen interactions. Ciba Found Symp 1986; 124: 104–124
87 Isemura M, Sato N, Yamaguchi Y, Munakata H, Hayashi N, Yoshizawa M. Isolation and characterization of fibronectin-binding proteoglycan carrying both heparan sulfate and dermatan sulfate chains from human placenta. J Biol Chem 1987; 262: 8926–8933
88 Engvall E, Ruoslahti E. Binding of soluble form of fibroblast surface protein, fibronectin, to collagen. Int J Cancer 1977; 20: 1–5
89 Yamada K M. Cell surface interactions with extracellular materials. Annu Rev Biochem 1983; 52: 761–799
90 Rath W, Osmers R, Adelmann-Grill B C, Stuhlsatz H W, Szeverényi M, Kuhn W. Biophysical and biochemical changes of cervical ripening. In: Egarter C, Husslein P, eds. Prostaglandins for cervical ripening and/or induction of labor. Wien: Facultas Verlag, 1988; pp 32–41
91 Caplan A I, Hascall V. Structure and developmental changes in proteoglycans. In: Naftolin F, Stubblefield P G, eds. Dilatation of the the uterine cervix. Connective tissue biology and clinical management. New York: Raven Press, 1980: pp 79–98
92 Ruoslahti E. Structure and biology of proteoglycans. Annu Rev Cell Biol 1988; 4: 229–255
93 Comper W D, Caurent T C. Physiological function of connective tissue polysaccharides. Physiol Rev 1978; 58: 255–268
94 Oláh K S. Magnetic resonance imaging in the assessment of the cervical hydration state. Br J Obstet Gynaecol 1994; 101: 255–257
95 Liggins G C. Cervical ripening as an inflammatory reaction. In: Ellwood D A, Anderson A B M, eds. The cervix in pregnancy and labour. Clinical and biochemical investigations. Edinburgh: Churchill Livingstone, 1981: pp 1–12
96 Kitamura K, Ito A, Mori Y, Hirakawa S. Changes in the human uterine cervical collagenase with special reference to cervical ripening. Biochem Med 1979; 22: 332–338
97 Rath W, Adelmann-Grill B C, Pieper U, Kuhn W. Collagen degradation in the pregnant human cervix at term and after prostaglandin-induced cervical ripening. Arch Gynecol 1987; 240: 177–184
98 Ito A, Naganeo K, Mori Y, Hirakawa S, Hayashi M. PZ-peptidase activity in human uterine cervix in pregnancy at term. Clin Chim Acta 1977; 78: 267–270
99 Hutchins C J, Parkin E N. PZ-peptidase activity in the pregnant and non-pregnant human cervix. Br J Obstet Gynaecol 1981; 88: 150–152
100 Mori Y, Ito A, Hirakawa S, Kitamura K. Proteinases in the human and rabbit cervix. In: Ellwood D A, Anderson A B M, eds. The cervix in pregnancy and labour. Clinical and biochemical investigations. Edinburgh: Churchill Livingstone, 1981: 136–143
101 Barclay C G, Brennand J E, Kelly R W, Calder A A. Interleukin-8 production by the human cervix. Am J Obstet Gynecol 1993; 169: 625–632
102 Romero R, Avila C, Santhanam U, Sehgal P B. Amniotic fluid interleukin-6 in preterm labour: association with infection. J Clin Invest 1990; 85: 1392–1400
103 Hillier S L, Witkin S S, Krohn M A, Watts D H, Kiviat N B, Eschenbach D A. The relationship of amniotic fluid cytokines and preterm delivery, amniotic fluid infection, histologic chorioamnionitis, and chorioamnion infection. Obstet Gynecol 1993; 81: 941–948
104 Dudley D J, Hunter C, Mitchell M D, Varner M W. Clinical value of amniotic fluid interleukin-6 determinations in the management of preterm labour. Br J Obstet Gynaecol 1994; 101: 592–597
105 Mitchell M D, Dudley D J, Edwin S S, Lundin-Schiller S. Interleukin-6 stimulates prostaglandin production by human amnion and decidual cells. Eur J Pharmacol 1991; 192: 189–191
106 Oláh K S, Neilson J P, Johnson P M. Interleukin-6 in amniotic fluid obtained at forewater amniotomy compared with hindwater samples in women in spontaneous labour. Eur J Obstet Gynecol Reprod Biol 1995; 60: 65–67
107 Duncan M R, Berman B. Stimulation of collagen and glycosaminoglycan production in cultured adult dermal fibroblasts by recombinant human interleukin 6. J Invest Dermatol 1991; 97: 686–692
108 Ruef C, Kashgarian M, Coleman D L. Mesangial cell-matrix interactions. Effects on mesangial cell growth and cytokine secretion. Am J Pathol 1992; 141: 429–439
109 Romero R, Gonzalez R, Rittenhouse L et al. The effect of the sampling site (abdominal versus vaginal) on amniotic fluid concentrations of prostaglandins during human labour. 8th International Conference on Prostaglandins and Related Compounds, Montreal, Canada, 1992. Abstract 298

110 Ito A, Itoh Y, Sasaguri Y, Morimatsu M, Mori Y. Effects of interleukin-6 on the metabolism of connective tissue components in rheumatoid synovial fibroblasts. Arthrit Rheum 1992; 35: 1197–1201

111 Ishimi Y, Miyaura C, Jin C H et al. IL-6 is produced by osteoblasts and induces bone resorption. J Immunol 1990; 145: 3297–3303

112 Maruo N, Morita I, Shirao M, Murota S. IL-6 increases endothelial permeability in vitro. Endocrinology 1992; 131: 710–714

113 Malak T M, Bell S C. Structural characteristics of term human fetal membranes: a novel zone of extreme morphological alteration within the rupture site. Br J Obstet Gynaecol 1994; 101: 375–386

114 Malak T M, Mulhalland G, Bell S C. Structural characteristics and fibronectin synthesis by the intact term fetal membranes covering the cervix. Br J Obstet Gynaecol 1993; 100: 775–776

115 Yoshida Y, Manabe Y. Different characteristics of amniotic and cervical collagenous tissue during pregnancy and delivery: a morphological study. Am J Obstet Gynaecol 1990; 162: 190–193

116 Oláh K S, Gee H, Brown J S. Measurement of the cervical response to uterine activity in labour and observations on the mechanism of cervical effacement. J Perinat Med 1991; 19 (suppl 2): 245

117 Oláh K S, Gee H, Brown J S. The effect of cervical compliance on generation of intra-uterine pressure – The 'C.A.P.' effect. Proceedings of the 26th British Congress of Obstetrics & Gynaecology, Manchester, 1992, pp 429

118 Richardson J A, Sutherland I A, Allen D W. A cervimeter for continuous measurement of cervical dilatation in labour – Preliminary results. Br J Obstet Gynaecol 1978; 85: 178–184

119 Embrey M P, Siener H. Cervical tocodynamometry. J Obstet Gynaecol Br Commonwlth 1965; 62: 225–228

120 Oláh K S, Gee H, Brown J S. Cervical contractions: The response of the cervix to oxytocic stimulation in the latent phase of labour. Br J Obstet Gynaecol 1993; 100: 635–640

121 Newton W H. Reciprocal activity of the cornua and cervix uteri of the goat. J Physiol 1934; 81: 277–282

122 Newton W H. The insensitivity of the cervix uteri to oxytocin. J Physiol 1937; 89: 309–315

123 Bonnycastle D D, Ferguson J K W. The action of pitocin and adrenalin on different segments of the rabbit uterus. J Pharmacol 1941; 72: 90–98

124 Adler J, Bell G H, Knox J A C. The behaviour of the cervix uteri in vivo. J Physiol 1944; 103: 142–154

125 Karlson S. On the motility of the uterus during labour and the influence of the motility pattern on the duration of the labour. Acta Obstet Gynec Scand 1949; 28: 209–250

126 Schild H O, Fitzpatrick R J, Nixon W C W. Activity of the human cervix and corpus uteri. Lancet 1951; i: 250–252

127 Mackenzie I Z. The effect of oxytocics on the human cervix during midtrimester pregnancy. Br J Obstet Gynaecol 1976; 83: 780–785

128 Wendell-Smith C P. The lower uterine segment. J Obstet Gynaecol Brit Emp 1954; 61: 87–93

129 Gee H. M D Thesis. Uterine activity and cervical resistance determining cervical change in labour. England: University of Liverpool, 1981

130 Pajntar M, Roskar D, Rudel D. Longitudinally and circularly measured EMG activity in the human uterine cervix during labour. Acta Physiologic Hungaric 1988; 71: 497–502

131 Hofmeier, Das untere Uterinsegment in anat. und klin. Beiziehand. Schroeder's Der schwangere und kreissende Uterus. Bonn, 1886: pp 21–74

8 The intrapartum management of twin pregnancies

R.A. O'Connor   E. Hiadzi

P MR↑ 4 – 5 fold

P M L
14 G/1

It is usually stated that twin pregnancies are associated with four to fivefold increased perinatal mortality when compared to singletons.[1] This is said to be due in the main, to prematurity and intrauterine growth retardation. Various measures have been used in an attempt to reduce the incidence of prematurity, including bed rest,[2] oral tocolytics[3] and cervical circlage,[4] all of which have failed to significantly improve gestational age at delivery. It is generally accepted that regular antenatal ultrasound assessment should be undertaken to detect intrauterine growth retardation early and allow timely intervention.[5,6]

Many authorities have advocated delivery by Caesarean section in an effort to further improve perinatal outcome.[7,8] Since the mid-1970s there has been a dramatic increase in the incidence of Caesarean section for the delivery of twins. This arose because most of the statistical data from the early 1970s showed a significantly higher perinatal mortality and morbidity for the second twin, compared to the first, especially if the second was not presenting by the vertex. Taylor[7] in 1976, recommended that all twins, where the second was not presenting by the vertex, should be delivered by Caesarean section. Most of these studies, however, were performed at a time when the second twin was not monitored and often not diagnosed until after delivery of the first.

A number of epidemiological studies,[9-11] question whether there is really such a dramatic difference between twins and singletons in terms of mortality. These have not been published in the obstetric literature and are therefore largely ignored by obstetricians. It would appear, however, that weight-corrected mortality figures are similar for both twins and singletons.

Against this background, the more recent publications regarding the interpartum management of twins are reviewed to provide a protocol for the supervision of labour and the delivery of twin pregnancies.

EPIDEMIOLOGICAL BACKGROUND

John Kiely,[9] in his study of the epidemiology of perinatal mortality in multiple pregnancies, reviewed all twins born in New York between 1978 and 1984. A total of 15 902 twins were compared with 738 912 singletons. Twins had a perinatal mortality of 79 per 1000, more than four times that of

Table 8.1 Birth weight comparison between singletons and twins

Birth weights	Percentage of singletons	Percentage of twins
Less than 1001 g	0.6%	5%
Less than 1501 g	1.3%	12%
Less than 2001 g	2.8%	26%
Less than 2501 g	8%	53%

Table 8.2 Birth weight – specific neonatal mortality

Birth weight (g)	Relative risk: twins versus singletons
501–1000	1.26
1001–1250	1.07
1251–1500	0.69
1501–2000	0.39
2001–2500	0.41
2501–3000	1.21
>3000	3.32

singletons (19 per 1000). These statistics, however, warrant closer investigation. Twins tend to be born much earlier than singletons. The mean gestational age differed by 19 days; because of this, twins had a much lower birth weight than singletons. The mean difference was 870 g (Table 8.1). Comparison of birth-weight specific neonatal mortality rates among twins and singletons (Table 8.2) highlight a number of important points. Between 1250 and 2500 g mortality was much lower in twins. Above 3000 g the mortality was surprisingly much higher in twins.

Relating the mode of delivery to the mortality rate in breech presentations, those delivered vaginally had a death rate of about three times those delivered by Caesarean section. In twins delivering by the vertex, those delivered vaginally had a mortality rate that was 2.2 times higher than those delivered by Caesarean section. The problem again with these crude comparisons is that the vaginal delivery groups had a much lower birth weight than the Caesarean section group. Keily analysed birth-weight specific results for twins with a vertex presentation. Between 1001 and 2500 g, the neonatal mortality rate was slightly lower in the vaginal delivery group. (RR 0.81, 95% CI 0.55–1.18). In twins weighing more than 3000 the mortality rate was much higher in those delivered vaginally compared to those delivered by Caesarean section (RR 4.22, 95% CI 1.10–27.71). Unfortunately the same analysis was not carried out for breech presentations.

Fabre,[10] reporting from Spain, compared the outcome of 1956 twins with 110 734 singletons. The crude relative risk of perinatal death for twins compared to singletons was 4.92, but again, these statistics change with birth weight. The crude relative risk of perinatal death was similar when birth weight was between 500 and 1500 g. Twins fared better with birth weights between 1500 and 2499 g (RR 0.45), but with birth weights greater than 2500 g, the crude relative risk of perinatal death increased among twins (RR 2.27). The weight specific mortality rates described by Kiely and Fabre are supported by other studies from California and Georgia.[12,13] Surprisingly, all these studies confirm a markedly increased mortality among twins with birth weights greater than 2500 g, compared to singletons of the same weight, a fact not always appreciated. Furthermore, the higher overall mortality rate for twins is caused by the distribution of birth weights. An improvement in perinatal outcome will therefore be achieved by reducing the incidence of premature delivery. A dramatic increase in the Caesarean section rate would not appear to be justified.

The Magill University group,[14] showed quite conclusively that a liberal Caesarean section policy did not lead to an improvement in perinatal outcome. Their Caesarean section rate rose from 3.2% to 50.8% during a 10 year period. In the latter part of their study, when the first twin was not cephalic, the Caesarean section rate was 92%, and when the second twin was other than vertex, the rate was 57%. Despite this dramatic increase in the use of Caesarean section, the incidence of neonatal mortality did not change significantly. There was an improvement in the outcome of the very preterm infant, but this could be related to better neonatal intensive care facilities.

The epidemiological studies demonstrate the effect of weight on outcome. There are many other variables which need to be taken into account such as: the difference between twin I and twin II, the difference between spontaneous breech deliveries and breech extractions, and the delivery interval between twin I and twin II. We attempted to analyse the variables in some detail.

BIRTH WEIGHT GREATER THAN 1500 G

Vertex–vertex presentation

Both twins present by the vertex in about 43% of cases. There is a general consensus that vaginal delivery should be attempted in these circumstances, and vaginal delivery rates of 81% have been reported.[15] It is worth remembering that there is no guarantee that the vertex second twin will remain in that position following delivery of the first.

Vertex–non-vertex presentation

Vertex–non-vertex presentations account for about 38% of twins at term. Interpartum management remains controversial. Since Taylor's suggestion that all vertex, non-vertex presentations should be delivered by Caesarean section, this has increasingly become the preferred mode of delivery. Several recent studies have, however, supported the safety of vaginal delivery of the second twin in these circumstances. Radinovici[16] carried out the only randomized controlled trial of twin deliveries where the second twin presentation was non-vertex. Sixty twins at more than 35 weeks gestation were randomized between vaginal delivery and Caesarean section. The results showed no difference in 5 minute APGAR scores or in other indices of neonatal morbidity between the two groups. The small numbers in this study indicate the difficulties of trying to perform a randomized control trial to assess the risk of vaginal delivery in these circumstances.

A number of recent studies addressed the issue in the context of a modern neonatal intensive care unit. Greig and associates[17] recently reviewed 457 sets of twins delivered between 1985 and 1990. They looked at very detailed neonatal outcome measures, and their data is carefully weight stratified. The second twins were divided into four presentation/delivery groups: non-vertex/Caesarean section; non-vertex/vaginal delivery; vertex/Caesarean section; vertex/vaginal delivery. There was no significant difference in outcome between the groups. There were 11 cases of intraventricular haemorrhage, but none of these occurred in the vaginally delivered non-vertex group. Some might argue that a selection bias exists, with Caesarean sections being performed on the unwell babies. All emergency Caesarean sections were excluded to avoid this potential problem.

Adams and associates[18] were prompted by a Caesarean section rate, increasing from 25% to 40% during a 6 year period, to review 578 twin deliveries between 1980 and 1987. The perinatal outcome comparing the first twin (all vertex) with the second twin (vertex or non-vertex), with Caesarean section or vaginal delivery, was analysed. No statistically significant difference in perinatal mortality or morbidity was found when comparing non-vertex second twins delivered vaginally or by Caesarean section. One case of a twin with a fractured humerus, occurring in a second twin weighing 3300 g (600 g heavier than its sibling vertex delivery), and described as a difficult assisted breech delivery, illustrates the point that care needs to be exercised when dealing with large second twins. This is a point we will return to later.

Fishman and associates[19] reviewed 390 live-born vaginally delivered second twins, 207 delivered as vertex and 183 delivered as a breech. Ninety five per cent of breech deliveries were total breech extractions. There was no statistically significant difference between vaginal breech and vaginal vertex deliveries in any of the neonatal outcome measures studied, even when weight stratified. It is interesting to note the Caesarean section rate in this study is 47.8%, with 15.5% performed for the second twin alone.

The power of these studies is limited. The incidence of neonatal morbidity and mortality is low. It would take approximately 5000 mothers in each group to achieve a statistical significance with an alpha of 0.5 and a power of 80%. Accepting their limitations, these three recent studies do appear to indicate that it is safe to consider vaginal delivery of a non-vertex second twin weighing more than 1500 g.

When faced with a breech second twin the decision is often between external version and breech extraction. Many would opt for version because it is perceived as being less traumatic. In one series,[20] only 11 of 23 external versions succeeded. Of the 12 failures, 11 mothers were delivered abdominally. In the same series, only 1 of 43 breech extractions failed. There was no statistical difference in neonatal outcome between the 11 successful external versions, 29 deliveries by elective Caesarean section and 42 breech extractions. Grocke and associates[21] reporting a similar study comparing 41 external versions, 55 breech extractions and 40 elective Caesarean sections in babies weighing more than 1500 g, achieved only 46% successful vaginal deliveries following attempted external version. In the same study 96% of the breech extractions were successful. No statistical significant difference in scores, neonatal intensive care admissions, respiratory distress syndrome, birth trauma or intraventricular haemorrhage were noted between the three groups. This paper raises the point that more successful versions were achieved in those mothers with epidurals, although this did not reach statistical significance. Relaxation of the abdomen may improve the ability to move the fetal pole and improve success rates. This is an interesting observation which certainly needs further consideration. It is relevant because most authorities suggest epidural anaesthesia for all twin deliveries. However, the data that exists suggests that if attempted external version fails, one should resort to internal version and breech extraction without undue delay.

Non-vertex first twins

Most authorities[22,23] advocate delivery by Caesarean section, the main concern being interlocking of the fetal heads. Cohen[24] estimated the risk to be about 1% although accurate incidence reports are impossible to find.

A recent case report[25] suggested the use of the Zavanelli manoevre to revert the potentially catastrophic situation of locked twins. The first infant was delivered to the lower edges of the shoulder blades when interlocking was recognized. The partially delivered first twin was returned to the vagina with moderate force and an emergency Caesarean section performed. Babies weighing 2580 g and 2000 g were delivered; both subsequently did well. Few, we feel, would advocate this type of heroic measures in modern day obstetric practice, opting rather for an elective Caesarean section with a non-vertex first twin.

BABIES WITH LOW BIRTH WEIGHT (500–1499 G)

Twelve per cent of twin deliveries result in low birth weight infants weighing under 1500 g. This group accounts for about 75% of the overall neonatal mortality and morbidity for twins. In those who survive, long-term psychomotor and neurological outcome is closely associated with the occurrence and severity of intraventricular haemorrhages. Many have advocated increased use of Caesarean section to reduce the incidence of mortality and morbidity in this group, especially those presenting as a breech. Barrett and associates,[26] suggested that Caesarean section is the optimum route of delivery for all twins expected to have a birth weight of less than 1500 g. Second twins delivered vaginally, who weighed 601–990 g, had an increased risk of neonatal mortality compared to their sibling. Among twins weighing 1000–1499 g, vaginally delivered second twins had significantly lower APGAR scores and an increased risk of neonatal morbidity, compared with their siblings, whereas second twins delivered by Caesarean section had no increased morbidity.

The long-term outcome for very low birth weight babies is poor, especially those delivered before 28 weeks gestation,[27,28] but there is increasing evidence that delivery by Caesarean section does not confer significant improvement.

Doyle and associates[29] reported 124 sets of twins delivered at gestational ages of 32 weeks or less at the Royal Women's Hospital, Melbourne, of which 83.1% delivered vaginally. The crude mortality among those delivered vaginally was 26.7%, compared to only 14.3% among those delivered by Caesarean section, but when gestational age discrepancies were corrected, the trend favouring survival of those delivered by Caesarean section disappeared. Two hundred and fourteen infants survived beyond 24 h. Of these, 22 (10.3%) had moderate and 111 (51.9%) had severe respiratory distress. By logistic function regression, increasing gestational age was associated with proportionately fewer infants being depressed at birth, requiring active resuscitation or having moderate or severe respiratory distress ($P < 0.001$). Mode of delivery, birth order or presentation were not associated with any alteration in these outcomes, either alone or in any combination.

Moralis and associates[30] have produced the best study on low birth weight twins published to date. They investigated the effect of birth order, presentation and mode of delivery on neonatal outcome in non-discordant twin gestations under 1500 g. All 312 twins had echoencephalograms performed by the fourth day of life to diagnose the presence and severity of intraventricular haemorrhages. Among twins in which at least one of the babies was a non-vertex presentation, those born by Caesarean section demonstrated a lower incidence of both severe grades of intraventricular haemorrhage and mortality. However, after multivariant analysis to correct for differences in birth weight between the groups, no advantage for Caesarean section could be demonstrated. Therefore differences in birth weight, rather than the mode of delivery, accounted for the difference in neonatal outcome of non-vertex twins.

Rydhstrom,[31] in an effort to evaluate the impact of Caesarean section on long-term outcome in relation to the incidence of cerebral palsy and mental retardation, studied 265 twins born during two 4-year time periods, (1973–1976 and 1977–1980). The Caesarean section rate during the first period was 6%, while it had risen to 59.6% during the second study period. For twins born breech, the handicap rate during each period was the same. It is noteworthy that in this study 8–9% of all twins weighing less than 1500 g had cerebral palsy or mental retardation at follow-up 8 years or more after delivery. This incidence did not appear to be influenced by the mode of delivery, again emphasizing the point that the key to improving outcome is to reduce the incidence of prematurity.

A recent paper[32] compared 54 second twins, weighing between 750 and 2000 g and delivered by breech extraction, with their siblings and 43 sets of twins delivered by caesarean section. When the two groups were compared, there was no significant difference in: survival rates, the incidence of interventricular haemorrhages Grade III and IV, necrotizing entrocolitis, respiratory distress syndrome, duration of mechanical ventilation and oxygen therapy required. While the number of well-constructed studies in this birth weight is limited they do suggest that vaginal delivery is a safe option, even for a second twin presenting by the breech. Indeed, Caesarean section does not necessarily guarantee a good perinatal outcome. Chervench[15] reported a case of a neonatal death related to birth trauma in a 1000 g second twin of a breech–breech pair, both delivered by Caesarean section through a low vertical incision. The uterus clamped down around the head during breech extraction and extension of the uterus incision was necessary for delivery. The infant died after 12 hours.

There is really no conclusive information available if the first twin is a breech presentation.

DELIVERY INTERVAL   *15–30 min*

The accepted view for many years has been that the delivery interval between twins should preferably be less than 15 minutes, and certainly not more than 30 minutes. It has been felt that the risk of diminished placental perfusion increases with a prolonged birth interval. This dictum may lead to inappropriate intervention to expedite delivery. This fundamental issue has been addressed in only two papers during the last 10 years. Rayburn and associates[33] reported 115 twins delivered in a single institution during a 2 year period. A delivery interval of more than 15 minutes occurred in 45 cases. Excluding conditions associated with prematurity, all second twins did well despite the increased delivery interval. There was no significant increase in low 5 minute APGAR scores or perinatal trauma. Maternal complications were not increased except for an increased incidence of Caesarean section for the second twin: 8 of 45 compared to 2 of 70. The second study[34] used the Swedish Medical Birth Registry, from 1973–1985, to identify twin births, using a database of 7533 deliveries. They examined outcome in relation to delivery intervals of: less than 15 minutes, 15 to 30 minutes, 30 to 45 minutes and more than 45 minutes for different weight groupings of: less than 1500 g, 1501 to 2,499 g, and more than 2500 g. They compared deliveries between 1973 and 1978 with those delivered between 1979 and 1985. The only outcome measure that was reported was crude perinatal mortality. There were no details on the mode of delivery of the second twin. During the second 6 year study period there was no increased mortality with increased birth intervals. The incidence of combined vaginal and abdominal deliveries did, however, increase from 0.3% to 2% when the two time periods were compared. The overall Caesarean section rate also increased from 18.6% to 41.6%. While these two studies would suggest that perinatal mortality does not significantly increase with an increased delivery interval, they both have major shortcomings. It is difficult to envisage a good study addressing this issue being published in the forseeable future.

COMBINED VAGINAL-ABDOMINAL DELIVERY

With the rising tide of Caesarean sections for the delivery of twins, there has also been an increased incidence of Caesarean section for the second twin after vaginal delivery of the first, an incidence as high as 15% in one series.[35] Constantine and Redman[36] reported what they described as an alarming increase in the tendency towards Caesarean section for the second twin when the first twin had been delivered vaginally. During a 10 year period, 1974–1983, only three (0.6%) Caesarean sections were performed for the second twin. From 1984–1986, 12 Caesarean sections (6.5%) were performed for the delivery of the second twin. This increase mirrored an increase in the overall Caesarean section rate, between the two periods, from 18.5% to 40.8%, and was not associated with an improvement in perinatal mortality (63.5 per 1000, compared to 80.6 per 1000).

Sharma and associates,[37] reporting a series of 22 combined vaginal and abdominal deliveries from the Birmingham Maternity Hospital, looked at the time of delivery. Five occurred between 09.00 and 17.00 hours, two between 17.00 and 23.00 hours and 15 between 23.00 and 09.00 hours. They state that in all cases an experienced obstetrician was called only after the birth of the first twin. The intervals between the birth of the twins varies from 16 to 81 minutes. They conclude that if experienced personnel are summoned on time for the birth of the first twin, it would allow trainees to gain supervised practical experience in operative vaginal delivery techniques and reduce the incidence of Caesarean section for the second twin.

Blickstein and Associates,[38] reviewing their own experience and that of nine other papers, asked the question of whether a Caesarean delivery for the second twin after the vaginal birth of the first twin represents misfortune or mismanagement. They feel it cannot be answered at present since all series are essentially retrospective and relatively small. We have been able to locate 14 reports from the literature over the last 15 years (Table 8.3). From each we have extracted the total number of deliveries reported, the overall Caesarean section rate, and the incidence of Caesarean section for the second twin alone. It is apparent that in series with a high overall Caesarean section rate, the incidence of Caesarean section for the second twin alone is also high. This probably reflects the lack of experience in dealing with twin deliveries.

There are circumstances where Caesarean section for the delivery of the

Table 8.3 Caesarean section rate for the second twin

Reference	Total number of deliveries	Percentage Caesarean sections	Percentage Caesarean section for second twin only
Evard & Gold[39]	206	16.8	1.9
[c]Chervenak et al[40]	135	30	2.8
Eskes et al[41]	76	31	4
Rayburn et al[32]	186	37	9
Berglund et al[34]	120	34	6
Rattan et al[42]	352	38	6
[a]Constantine & Redman[35]	535	18	0.6
[b]Constantine & Redman[35]	186	41	6.5
[c]Gocke et al[21]	202	61	9
Bugalho et al[43]	254	26	2.3
Fleming et al[44]	114	54	2.6
O'Connor & Gaughan[45]	487	20	2.3
Samra et al[36]	510	36	4.3
Adam et al[18]	397	20	2.7
[c]Wells et al[20]	416	46	5.7
Fishman et al[19]	781	48	15.5

a. Period 1974–1983; b. period 1984–1986; c. non-vertex second twins only.

Table 8.4 Second twins delivered by Caesarean section at Northwick Park Hospital 1981–1990

Indication	Parity	Gestation	Weight (g)	APGAR score 1 min	5 min	Delivery/interval (min)
Transverse lie	2	39	2750	9	9	8
Transverse lie	2	37	2720	8	9	42
Transverse lie	1	34	2580	4	8	11
Transverse lie	1	38	2750	8	9	12
Shoulder presentation	1	35	2140	8	10	31
Cord prolapse	1	31	1335	4	6	16
Failed forceps	0	39	3500	8	9	38

second twin is justified. A 10 year review at Northwick Park Hospital identified seven Caesarean sections for the second twin alone, representing 2% of all twin deliveries (Table 8.4). Five of the Caesarean sections were performed for a transverse lie or shoulder presentation. In each case artificial rupture of the membranes was performed early, making subsequent internal version and breech extraction impossible. If the membranes were left intact it is possible that a successful extraction would have been achieved. The sixth Caesarean section was performed following a cord prolapse. It occurred in association with a cephalic presentation at 31 weeks gestation. At a later gestation a vacuum extraction might have been an alternative to Caesarean section. The final case clearly demonstrates that Caesarean section may be necessary. The first twin, weighing 2800 g delivered spontaneously. The second was also a cephalic presentation. Following artificial rupture of the membranes the vertex failed to descend. Forceps were easily applied but despite three moderate tractions the vertex still did not descend. A lower segment Caesarean section was performed and an infant weighing 3500 g was delivered. This case illustrates the point that safe passage of the first twin does not guarantee that the second twin will also deliver vaginally. Again, it emphasizes that caution is needed when dealing with twins weighing more than 3000 g, a group usually not felt to be at any increased risk of perinatal morbidity or mortality.

CONCLUSIONS

Twin deliveries should be undertaken in a fully equipped hospital unit. The mode of delivery should be based upon the presentation, rather than the estimated birth weight. The evidence presented suggests that all vertex–vertex pairs and all vertex–non-vertex pairs should be allowed a trial of labour. If the first twin presents by the breech, Caesarean section is probably the best delivery option; however, if the labour is supervised by an experienced obstetrician, attempted vaginal delivery may be entirely reasonable. One should not be complacent about bigger twins in the light of the epidemiological data. If the estimated fetal weight of the twins is greater than 3 kg, early recourse to Caesarean section may be advisable if there is any concern regarding fetal wellbeing in labour. If the second twin is considerably larger than the first, or more than 3000 g, it is worth considering performing a computer tomogram of the pelvis to ensure it is adequate to permit delivery of a second twin.

It is important to discuss the labour and delivery with the couple during the antenatal period, explaining the need to monitor both twins carefully during labour, even though this will restrict maternal movement. The advantages of epidural anaesthesia for the delivery of the second twin should be explained. It is worth mentioning the number of people normally present at all twin deliveries (Table 8.5). The sudden arrival of these can lead to a lot of unnecessary anxiety on the part of the couple who naturally assume their presence indicates a problem.

When labour is established, good intravenous access is needed. Blood should be sent for haemoglobin and serum saved in case cross-matched blood is necessary. An effective epidural should be set up early in labour provided the mother is agreeable. We perform 2-hourly vaginal examinations during labour. The indications to use syntocin augmentation are the same as with singletons. There is little data available on the use of intrauterine pressure monitoring in twin gestations. There is at least the theoretical risk of rupturing the second sac with the transducer.

Both fetal hearts should be monitored. Once the membranes are ruptured, a Copeland clip is applied to the first twin and the second twin monitored by an external transducer. Fetal blood sampling can be used to further assess any fetal heart rate abnormalities of the first twin. If the fetal heart of the second twin becomes abnormal during the first stage of labour, delivery should be expedited by Caesarean section. If discordant growth has been detected antenatally, early recourse to Caesarean section should be considered. This is particularly the case if the second twin is much smaller.

Table 8.5 Personnel required at a twin delivery

Two midwives

Two obstetricians – one of whom should be a consultant or experienced senior registrar to supervise

Anaesthetist

Operating department assistant

Paediatrician: one or two, depending on the gestation

Table 8.6 Delivery of the non-vertex second twin

Verts spontaneously
To cephalic	→	vaginal delivery
To breech	→	assisted breech delivery *or* breech extraction

Remains transverse
External version to cephalic and vaginal delivery
Internal version and breech extraction

If all fails, proceed to Caesarean section

It is important to have adequate personnel present for all twin deliveries (Table 8.5). Apart from the midwife looking after the mother, two obstetricians should be present if possible, one of whom is experienced and able to supervise the junior during the delivery. It is interesting to note that the recent Royal College of Obstetricians and Gynaecologists' guidelines on endometrial ablation,[46] suggest trainees should be carefully supervised before attempting any alone. How many of our Registrars who are often left to perform twin deliveries out-of-hours would have been involved in 10 cases of breech extraction? The need for adequate supervision is all too obvious but often lacking. It is imperative that the anaesthetist and paediatrician are also present at the delivery.

When the first twin presents by the vertex, the aim should be to allow spontaneous vaginal delivery. The indications to intervene are the same as in the singleton, undue delay or evidence of fetal distress. It is vitally important to obtain good quality fetal heart traces of both twins during the second stage of labour.

Once the first twin is delivered, abdominal palpation should be performed to assess the lie of the second twin (Table 8.6). This can be confirmed by ultrasound if necessary. If the lie is longitudinal and the presentation cephalic, one should wait until the head descends into the pelvis and perform an amniotomy during a contraction. A Copeland clip is applied to the vertex at this stage to ensure a good quality fetal heart recording. Occasionally contractions fail to continue after delivery of the first twin and it may be necessary to start an oxytocin infusion. If the fetal heart is satisfactory and the head descends with contractions, one can await a second spontaneous vaginal

per 15-30 minutes

delivery. If an assisted delivery becomes necessary, the vacuum extractor has a number of advantages. It may be applied at a higher station than the forceps and causes less vaginal and perineal trauma. Because the birth canal has been dilated by the first twin, its application does not necessarily need to be as perfect as in the case of a singleton presentation.

If the second twin presents by the breech, one can await a spontaneous assisted breech delivery or perform a breech extraction. Many will be happier expediting delivery in these circumstances and opt for a breech extraction, especially as the breech is often footling.

If the second twin remains transverse, an external version may be attempted. The version is performed by either forward or backward roll utilizing the shortest arc between the vertex and pelvic inlet first. If it is successful, the management is as for a vertex presentation. External version is probably the manoeuvre of choice when a transverse lie has its back dependant and the fetal parts are difficult to feel vaginally.

If the back is lying towards the fundus with the feet dependant, breech extraction may well be the best option. The technique described by Rabinovici and Associates[47] is certainly the method of choice. A fetal foot is identified by recognizing a heel through intact membranes. The foot is grasped and pulled gently and continuously lower into the birth canal. The membranes are ruptured as late as possible. Often they rupture spontaneously when the fetal foot is at the introitus. The rest of the breech delivery is performed using standard techniques.

After delivery of both the twins, the third stage should be managed actively. It may well be necessary to give intravenous ergometrine as there is an increased incidence of atonic uterus following twin deliveries.

The safe vaginal delivery of twins remains one of the most satisfying arts of obstetric practice. It beholds those of us who have been taught it to ensure that the endangered species of a vaginal delivered second twin does not become an object of obstetric folklore.

REFERENCES

1 MacGilvarry I. The maternal response to twin pregnancy. In: Studd J J, ed. Progress in obstetrics and gynaecology. Edinburgh: Churchill Livingstone, 1984: 4: 139–150
2 Komaromy B, Lampe L. Value of bedrest in twin pregnancies. Int J Obstet Gynaecol 1977; 15: 262–266
3 O'Connor M C, Murphy H, Dalrymple I J. Double blind trial of ritodrine and placebo in twin pregnancy. Br J Obstet Gynaecol 1979; 86: 707–709
4 Weeks A R L, Menzies D W, deBoer C W. The relative efficacy of bedrest, cervical suture and no treatment in the management of twin pregnancy. Br J Obstet Gynaecol 1977; 84: 161–164
5 O'Brien W F, Knuppel R A, Scerbe J C, Rattan P K. Birth weights in twins: an analysis of discordance and growth retardation. Obstet Gynaecol 1986; 67: 483–486
6 Gaughan B, O'Connor R A, Bonnar C, Dalrymple I J. Fetal biophysical profile in twin pregnancy. Ir J Med Sci 1990; 159: 256
7 Taylor E S. Editorial. Obstet Gynaecol 1976; 31: 535
8 Kelsick F, Minkoff H. Management of the breech second twin. Am J Obstet Gynaecol 1982; 144: 783–786

9 Kiely J L. The epidemiology of perinatal mortality in multiple births. Bull NY Med 1990; 66: 618–637

10 Fabre E, de Aguero R G, de Agustin J L, Perez-Hiraldo M P, Bescos J L. Perinatal mortality in twin pregnancy: An analysis of birth weight-specific mortality rates and adjusted rates for birth weight distributions. J Perinat Med 1988; 16: 85–88

11 Kleinman J C, Fower M G, Kessel S S. Comparison of infant mortality among twins and singletons: United States 1960 and 1983. Am J Epidemiol 1991; 133: 133–143

12 Williams R L, Creasy R K, Cunningham G C. Fetal growth and perinatal viability in California. Obstet Gynaecol 1982; 59: 624–632

13 McCartney B J, Sachs B P, Layde P M. The epidemiology of neonatal death in twins. Am J Obstet Gynaecol 1981; 141: 252–256

14 Bell D, Johansson D, McLean F H, Usher R H. Birth asphyxia, trauma, and mortality in twins: Has caesarean section improved outcome? Am J Obstet Gynaecol 1986; 154: 235–239

15 Chervenak F A, Johnson R E, Youcha S, Hobbins J C, Berkowitz R L. Intrapartum management of twin gestation. Obstet Gynaecol 1985; 65: 119–124

16 Rabinovici J, Barkai G, Reichman B, Serr D M, Mashiach S. Randomised management of the second non-vertex twin: Vaginal delivery or caesarean section. Am J Obstet Gynaecol 1987; 156: 52–56

17 Greig P C, Veille J, Morgan T, Henderson L. The effect of presentation and mode of delivery on neonatal outcome in the second twin. Am J Obstet Gynaecol 1992; 167: 901–906

18 Adam C, Allen A C, Baskett T F. Twin delivery: Influence of the presentation and method of delivery on the second twin. Am J Obstet Gynaecol 1991; 165: 23–27

19 Fishman A, Grubb D K, Kovacs B W. Vaginal delivery of the nonvertex second twin. Am J Obstet Gynaecol 1993; 168: 861–864

20 Wells S R, Thorp J M, Bowes W A. Management of the non-vertex second twin. Surg Gynaecol Obstet 1991; 172: 383–385

21 Gocke S E, Nageotte M P, Gariet T, Towers C V, Dorcester W. Management of the non-vertex second twin: Primary caesarean section, external version or primary breech extraction. Am J Obstet Gynaecol 1989; 161: 111–114

22 Chervenak F A. The controversy of mode of delivery in twins: The intrapartum management of twin gestation (Part II). Semin Perinatol 1986; 10: 44–49

23 Warenski J C, Kockenour N K. Intrapartum management of twin gestations. Clin Perinatol 1984; 16: 889–897

24 Cohen M, Kohl S G, Rosenthal A H. Fetal interlocking complicating twin gestations. Am J Obstet Gynaecol 1965; 91: 407–409

25 Swartjes J M, Bleker O P, Schutt M F. The Zavanelli Manoeuvre applied to locked twin. Am J Obstet Gynaecol 1992; 166: 532

26 Barrett J M, Staggs S M, Hooydonk J E, Growdon J H, Killam A P, Boehm F H. The effect of type of delivery upon neonatal outcome in premature twins. Am J Obstet Gynaecol 1982; 143: 360–367

27 Kitchen W H, Doyle L W, Rickards A L, Kelly E, Callanan C. Survivors of extreme prematurity – outcome at 8 years of age. Aust NZ J Obstet Gynaecol 1992; 31: 337–339

28 Brown L, Karrison T, Cibils B. Mode of delivery and perinatal results in breech presentation. Am J Obstet Gynaecol 1994; 171: 28–34

29 Doyle L W, Hughes C D, Guaran R L, Quinn M A, Kitchen W H. Mode of delivery of preterm twins. Aust NZ J Obstet Gynaecol 1988; 28: 25–28

30 Moralis W J, O'Brien W F, Knuppel R A, Gaylord S, Hayes P. The effect of mode of delivery on the risk of intraventricular haemorrhage in non discordant twins. Obstet Gynaecol 1989; 73: 107–110

31 Rydhstrom H. Prognosis for twins with birth weights < 1500 gm: The impact of caesarean section in relation to fetal presentation. Am J Obstet Gynaecol 1990; 163: 528–533

32 Davidson L, Easterling T R, Jackson J C, Benedetti T J. Breech extraction of low birth weight second twins: Can caesarean section be justified. Am J Obstet Gynaecol 1992; 166: 497–502

33 Rayburn W F, Lavin J P, Miodovnik M, Varner M W. Multiple gestation: Time interval between delivery of the first and second twins. Obstet Gynaecol 1984; 63: 502–506

34 Rydhstrom H, Ingemarsson I. Interval between birth of the first and the second twin and its impact on second twin perinatal mortality. J Perinat Med 1990; 18: 449–453

35 Berglund L, Axelsson O. Combined vaginal-abdominal delivery of twins. Ann Chirugiae et Gynaecol 1984; 73: 232–235

36 Constantine G, Redman C W E. Caesarean section for the second twin – an increasing trend? Lancet 1987; 618–619

37 Samra J S, Spillane H, Mukoyoko J, Tang L, Obhrai M S. Caesarean section for the birth of the second twin after vaginal delivery of the first twin. Br J Obstet Gynaecol 1990; 97: 234–236

38 Blickstein I, Zalel Y, Weissman A. Caesarean delivery of the second twin after the vaginal birth of the first twin. Misfortune or mismanagement. Acta Genet Med Gemellol 1991; 40: 389–394

39 Evard J R, Gold E M. Caesarean section for delivery of the second twin. Obstet Gynaecol 1981; 51: 581–583

40 Chervenak F A, Johnson R E, Berkowitz R L, Grannum P, Hobbins J L. Is routine caesarean section necessary for vertex–breech and vertex–transverse gestations. Am J Obstet Gynaecol 1984; 148: 1–5

41 Eskes T K A D, Timmer H, Kollef L A A, Jongsma H W. The second twin. Eur J Obstet Gynaecol Reprod Biol 1984; 19: 159–166

42 Rattan D K, Knuppel R A, O'Brien W F, Scerbo J C. Caesarean delivery of the second twin after vaginal delivery of the first twin. Am J Obstet Gynaecol 1986; 154: 936–940

43 Bugalho A, Strolego F, Carlomagno G. Outcome of twin pregnancies at the Hospital Central of Maputo: retrospective study of 315 consecutive twin deliveries, January 1–September 30 1987. Int J Gynaecol Obstet 1989; 29: 297–300

44 Fleming A D, Rayburn W F, Mandsager N T, Hill W C, Levine M G, Lawler R. Perinatal outcome of twin pregnancies at term. J Reproduct Med 1990; 35: 881–885

45 O'Connor R A, Gaughan B. Caesarean section for the birth of the second twin. Br J Obstet Gynaecol 1990; 97: 964

46 Report of the RCOG working party on training in gynaecological endoscopic surgery. RCOG 1994, pp. 1–36

47 Rabinovici J, Barkai G, Reichman B, Serr D M, Mashiach S. Internal podalic version with unruptured membranes for the second twin in transverse lie. Obstet Gynaecol 1988; 71: 428–4300

9 Antiphospholipid antibodies and adverse pregnancy outcome

R. Rai   L. Regan

Antiphospholipid antibodies (APA) are a group of autoantibodies which are clinically important because of their strong association with thrombosis, recurrent miscarriage (both first and second trimester) and thrombocytopenia – the primary antiphospholipid syndrome (PAPS).[1] The presence of APA has also been reported in association with early onset pre-eclampsia,[2] intrauterine growth retardation,[3,4] placental abruption[5] and infertility.[6] The two most studied APA are the lupus anticoagulant (LA) and the anticardiolipin antibodies (ACA), but other important APA are those directed against phosphotidylserine and phosphotidylethanolamine. Although both LA and ACA are often detected in individuals with systemic lupus erythematosus (SLE) a clear distinction must be made between SLE and PAPS. Individuals with PAPS do not have any of the major clinical or serological features of SLE.[7–9] Table 9.1 details some of the many clinical conditions associated with the presence of APA.

Antiphospholipid antibodies pose many difficulties for the clinician ranging from practical issues of detection and patient management to conceptual issues regarding the mechanism of fetal loss. A key question that remains unanswered is whether APA are a direct cause of adverse pregnancy outcome or merely an epiphenomenon. In this chapter we review the laboratory assays used to detect APA and the potential pitfalls in their diagnosis; the evidence that APA are associated with adverse pregnancy outcome; the mechanisms by which they may do this and the therapeutic strategies that have been used to counter their adverse effects.

HISTORICAL ASSOCIATIONS

In 1952, Conley and Hartman[10] first described an in vitro circulating anticoagulant, which occurred predominantly in patients with SLE. In 1972 Feinstein and Rapaport[11] termed this anticoagulant the 'lupus anticoagulant'; in vitro it caused a prolongation of the prothrombin time and the whole blood clotting time. These abnormalities could not be explained by a clotting factor deficiency. The paradoxical finding that individuals with LA are prone to thrombosis in vivo was reported by Bowie et al[12] and subsequently

135

Table 9.1 Clinical manifestations of antiphospholipid antibodies

Neurological
Transient ischaemic attacks
Cerebrovascular accidents
Chorea
Peripheral neuropathy
Migraine
Epilepsy

Obstetric
Recurrent miscarriage
Intrauterine growth retardation
Intrauterine death
Pre-eclampsia
Chorea gravidarum
Neonatal thrombosis

Dermatological
Livedo reticularis
Cutaneous necrosis

Haematological
Thrombocytopenia
Prothrombin deficiency

Vascular
Venous thrombosis
Arterial thrombosis
Mitral valve prolapse
Thrombotic endocarditis

confirmed by Lechner et al.[13] The association between LA and fetal loss was reported for the first time in 1975.[14]

Individuals with circulating LA have a high frequency of biological false-positive venereal disease research laboratory (VDRL) reagent tests. The VDRL reagent is composed of cholesterol, cardiolipin and phosphatidylcholine. Harris et al[15] using a solid-phase radioimmunoassay (RIA), sensitive and specific to ACA, reported a close, although not absolute concordance between LA and ACA. The RIA for the detection of ACA has subsequently been replaced by an enzyme-linked immunosorbent assay (ELISA).[16] It is now known that LA and ACA, although related antibodies, are separate and distinct.[17] In addition, most individuals with LA do not have ACA and vice versa.[18] Harris et al[15] reported the association between ACA and thrombosis and in 1985 Derue et al[19] reported the association between ACA and fetal loss.

APA AND THROMBOSIS

The presence of APA is associated with thrombosis. The fact that various mechanisms have been postulated to account for this association is not surprising as the APA are a heterogeneous family and are therefore likely to have different epitope specificities. The most common theories for their mechanism of action may be divided into (i) those that ascribe APA to disrupt platelet function and (ii) those that postulate that APA interfere with the function of endothelial cells. A major advance was made by the demonstration that both LA and ACA require plasma protein cofactors to exert their action. In the case of LA, prothrombin is the cofactor.[20] Beta 2 glycoprotein I (β_2GPI) plays this role for ACA.[21,22] It has also become apparent that APA do not bind directly to negatively charged phospholipids but to either the protein/phospholipid complex or to the protein modified to the phospholipid surface.[23,24]

The following have been proposed as modes of action of APA.

Effect on platelet function

Activation of platelets leading to release of the procoagulant thromboxane.[25]

However, the phospholipids to which APA bind are located on the inner leaflet of the platelet membrane and are only exposed once platelet activation has occurred.[25] Platelets must therefore have been activated before APA can bind to them and it is therefore unlikely that APA cause thrombosis by platelet activation.

Interference with the complex of phospholipid and β_2GPI.[21,26–28]

Beta 2 glycoprotein I is a plasma protein of 50 kDa, which has been demonstrated to have in vitro anticoagulant properties. It has been proposed that β_2GPI serves as a natural inhibitor of coagulation based on its properties of inhibiting contact activation of the intrinsic coagulation pathway,[29] platelet prothrombinase activity[30] and ADP-induced platelet aggregation.[31] It has been suggested that β_2GPI could bind to platelets and become the epitope for APA binding, leading to platelet aggregation and subsequent thrombosis. Antiphospholipid antibodies that are transiently present, for example after viral infections, and those that are drug-induced do not bind β_2GPI.

Effect on endothelial cell function

Inhibition of prostacyclin production by vascular endothelial cells.[32]

Endothelial cell damage leading to increased procoagulant activity or impaired fibrinolytic responses.[33,34]

Inhibition of the protein C/S anticoagulant system.[35,36]

Protein C is a vitamin K dependent protein which is responsible for the proteolytic degradation of coagulation factors Va and VIIIa. This action requires the presence of a cofactor — protein S. Impaired inhibition of factors Va and VIIIa leads to a prothrombotic state. Oosting et al[37] have recently demonstrated that some APA are directed against a combination of phospholipid-bound protein S and/or activated protein C.

Inhibition of antithrombin III activity.

Heparan sulphate is a physiological endothelial cell surface modulator of normal anticoagulation, containing a specific oligosaccharide sequence that binds antithrombin III with high affinity. By so doing it markedly enhances the inhibition of thrombin. Autoantibodies to vascular heparan sulphate could contribute to a thrombotic state by blocking the heparan sulphate-mediated activation of antithrombin III. In support of this theory, Cosgriff and Martin[38] described a patient with LA and recurrent thrombosis who had high antigenic, but low functional level of antithrombin III. More recently, Chamley et al[39] reported that IgM, purified from the serum of a patient with ACA, inhibited the heparin-dependent activation of antithrombin III. Interestingly, in 1994, Shibata et al[40] reported that IgG purified from sera obtained from seven patients with ACA bound heparin, whereas IgG obtained from controls did not. The IgG antiheparin antibodies were specifically reactive with a disaccharide region present on heparan sulphate that binds antithrombin III. Shibata et al[40] went on to conclude that APA with high affinity for heparin, or antiheparin antibodies may be an important cause of autoimmune vascular thrombosis in the antiphospholipid syndrome.

Not all APA are pathogenic. IgM ACA are often detected following viral infections, such as syphilis, adenovirus, chicken pox, mumps and the human immunodeficiency virus.[41] These antibodies are generally not associated with thrombotic complications and, unlike ACA associated with PAPS, do not bind β_2GPI. Similarly, APA induced by certain drugs such as procainamide, phenytoin, chlorpromazine, sodium valproate, hydralazine and propanalol do not appear to be thrombogenic.

LABORATORY DETECTION OF APA

Detection of LA and ACA is subject to widespread interlaboratory variation.[42] This can in part be accounted for by the heterogeneous nature of these antibodies, and by the lack of standardization of assays for their detection. This latter point has recently been addressed. The British Society for Haematology (BSH)[43] has published methodological guidelines for testing for the presence of LA, and attempts have been made to standardize the ELISA used for detection of ACA and the reporting of results.[44]

Detection of LA

Laboratory diagnosis of LA depends on demonstrating the following:

1. prolongation of in vitro phospholipid-dependent coagulation tests. Lupus anticoagulant acts at the level of the prothrombin activator complex to cause prolongation of such tests (Fig. 9.1)
2. that the abnormality is caused by an inhibitor (rather than a factor deficiency)

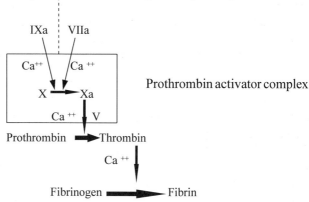

Intrinsic coagulation pathway

Extrinsic coagulation pathway

Prothrombin activator complex

Fig. 9.1 Lupus anticoagulant acts at the level of the prothrombin activator complex to cause prolongation of in vitro phospholipid-dependent coagulation tests.

3. that the inhibitor is directed against phospholipids.

A number of different coagulation tests have been used to screen for the presence of LA — the activated partial thromboplastin time (APTT), the kaolin clotting time (KCT), the tissue thromboplastin inhibition time (TTIT), and the dilute Russell's viper venom time (dRVVT). Each of these tests has its own proponents and it is now clear, because of the heterogeneous nature of LA, that no single test will detect all LAs. It has been our experience that the dRVVT, with a platelet neutralization procedure, detects LA significantly more often than either the APTT or the KCT in women with recurrent miscarriage.[45]

Detection of ACA

A standardized ELISA has been developed to detect both the IgG and IgM classes of ACA.[44] One-half of the wells on the ELISA plate are left blank to account for non-specific binding and all samples are run in duplicate. In addition, serial dilutions of a standard positive sample, calibrated against an international standard, are incorporated in each plate thus allowing the construction of a standard curve. A quality control sample, of known positivity, is also included in each plate. The units of measurement of IgG and the IgM ACA are GPL and MPL units, respectively. One GPL/MPL unit represents the binding activity of 1 μg/ml affinity-purified IgG/IgM ACA. An IgG ACA level of ≥ 5 GPL units and an IgM ACA level of ≥ 3 MPL units is considered positive.[44,46] Our protocol for the collection of samples and their processing when screening for LA and ACA is shown in Fig. 9.2.

It is important to remember that before a diagnosis of PAPS can be made

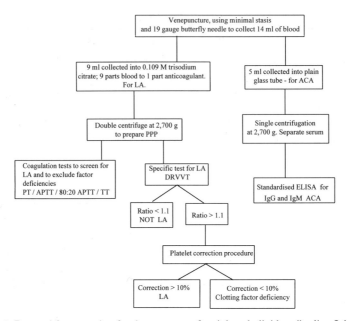

Fig. 9.2 Protocol for screening for the presence of antiphospholipid antibodies. LA = lupus anticoagulant; ACA = anticardiolipin antibody; PPP = platelet poor plasma; PT = prothrombin time; TT = thrombin time; APTT = activated partial thromboplastin time; DRVVT = dilute Russell's viper venom time.

the presence of either LA or positive levels of ACA must have been demonstrated on at least two occasions at least 8 weeks apart.[1] Our data demonstrates that a large number of women with a history of recurrent miscarriage have only transient positive results for APA, and therefore do not fulfil the criteria for a diagnosis of PAPS to be made.[45]

Prevalence of APA

Previous studies have reported that the prevalence of APA in women with three or more miscarriages is between 11% and 42%,[5,47–50] in contrast to a prevalence of 2% in women with a 'low-risk obstetric history'.[51,52] Available data is limited by the lack of standardization of laboratory methodology, the small numbers of women in individual studies, and the failure to perform confirmatory tests to exclude transient positive results.

Using nationally recognized laboratory protocols, we have screened 500 consecutive women, attending the St Mary's Hospital Recurrent Miscarriage Clinic, for the presence of LA and both the IgG and IgM classes of ACA.[45] All women had a history of at least three consecutive miscarriages (median 4; range 3–16) and none had either a genetic or anatomical cause to account for their recurrent pregnancy losses. All women with a positive test result had a

Table 9.2 Prevalence of LA and ACA in various conditions

Category	No of subjects	LA	ACA	Reference
Low risk obstetric population	737	0.27%	2.2%	Lockwood et al[51]
	933	1.0%	1.2%	Pattison et al[52]
Recurrent miscarriage (≥ 3)	500	9.1%	5.5%	Rai et al[45]
Early onset pre-eclampsia	43	16%		Branch et al[2]
Placental abruption	21	33%		Birdsall et al[5]
SLE	> 1000	34%	44%	Love and Santoro[93]

LA = lupus anticoagulant; ACA = anticardiolipin antibody; SLE = systemic lupus erythematosus.

second sample taken at least 8 weeks after the initial sample. In accordance with the definition of the PAPS only those women who tested positive on two occasions were classified as being positive. Using this criterion, the prevalence of LA among women with recurrent miscarriage was 9.1%, of IgG ACA 3.3% and of IgM ACA 2.2%. A large number of women had transient positive test results. Only 65.7% of those with an initial positive test for LA, 36.6% of those who were IgG ACA positive and 36.0% who were IgM ACA positive had a repeat positive test. Less than 2% of the women in this study were LA and ACA positive, emphasizing the importance of screening for both LA and ACA. Table 9.2 details the prevalence of APA in various conditions.

APA AND ADVERSE PREGNANCY OUTCOME

The prospective fetal loss rate in women with APA has been reported to be in the range of 50–75%,[51,53] and in women with SLE and circulating APA to be as high as 96%.[54,55] Although fetal demise can occur in any of the three trimesters of pregnancy, we have shown that first trimester pregnancy loss is the most common.[45] A typical history of a woman with pregnancy losses in association with APA is one with the first fetal loss occurring in the second or third trimester and subsequent losses invariably occurring in the first trimester.[56] A detailed history often elicits the fact that fetal heart activity was noted on ultrasound scanning prior to fetal demise.[45]

The actions of APA in causing adverse pregnancy outcome may be divided into their effects on implantation and their effects postimplantation.

Implantation

Implantation and trophoblast invasion of the maternal decidua and spiral arteries by the human blastocyst occurs in three stages: apposition, attachment and finally invasion of the endometrial epithelium by the trophectoderm. Defects in this process are the most important factor in early pregnancy loss following both natural conception and in vitro fertilization and are also implicated in the aetiology of pre-eclampsia and intrauterine growth retardation.[57,58]

There is accumulating evidence suggesting that APA impair trophoblast function via mechanisms unrelated to thrombosis, and have a direct effect on the placenta. Cytotrophoblast cells express phosphotidylserine on their surface, and binding of APA to these cells, leading to direct cellular injury and inhibition of syncytia formation, has been reported.[59,60] Sthoeger et al[61] reported that mice, which were both actively and passively immunized with monoclonal IgM ACA, experienced low fecundity and had a high rate of fetal resorption. This was associated with impairment of implantation and binding of ACA to the trophectoderm. Chamley et al[62] eluted IgG ACA from the placentae of four women with ACA and using immunohistochemistry demonstrated the presence of β_2GPI (a cofactor required for the binding of ACA) localized to the syncytiotrophoblast of placentae from both women with and without ACA. Increased deposition of β_2GPI on the trophoblast surface of placentae obtained from patients with persistently raised ACA titres has also been reported.[63]

POSTIMPLANTATION

The postimplantation effects of APA in causing adverse pregnancy outcome are related to their thrombogenic action leading to decreased placental perfusion.

Fetal loss in women with APA is often associated with thrombosis of the uteroplacental vasculature and placental infarction.[64,65] De Wolf et al[64] noted that in addition to intraluminal thromboses in the spiral arteries, there was decidual vasculopathy. This vasculopathy was characterized by fibrinoid necrosis, atherosis of decidual vessels and intimal thickening. In the largest reported series to date, Out et al[65] examined the placentae from 45 women with a history of intrauterine death between 16 and 39 weeks gestation. Sixteen of these women had APA. They reported that placentae obtained from women with APA and intrauterine death exhibited a significant decrease in vasculosyncytial membranes, an increase in fibrosis and in the number of hypovascular villi. These findings were consistent with prolonged hypoxia secondary to thrombosis or infarction. It should be noted, however, that these pathological findings are not universal and there have been reports showing no correlation between the degree of placental infarction and pregnancy loss.[3,66]

Evidence from murine models also supports the contention of a thrombotic diathesis in the mechanism of pregnancy loss in APA positive women. Branch et al[67] injected either purified IgG obtained from women with APA and a history of recurrent pregnancy losses or normal saline into the peritoneal cavity of pregnant BALB/c mice. In contrast to mice injected with control IgG or normal saline, each mouse injected with IgG from APA-positive women aborted and no live fetuses were found ($P < 0.05$). Histological examination of the uteroplacental interface showed decidual necrosis in the mice treated with IgG containing APA, and immunofluorescence studies showed prominent intravascular decidual IgG and fibrin deposition. Further evidence to support a thrombotic process as a cause of fetal loss was provided by Peaceman et al.[68] They reported that the IgG fraction obtained from patients with LA, when incubated with placental explants from normal human pregnancies, leads to a significant increase in thromboxane synthesis (prostacyclin synthesis being unchanged) when compared with the immunoglobulin fraction obtained from normal controls.

Several authors have addressed the question of which class of APA (LA, IgG ACA, or IgM ACA) is the best predictor of fetal loss. Results have been conflicting. Pattison et al[52] found that ACA had a higher predictive power than LA for fetal loss, and Lynch et al[69] reported that an elevated IgG ACA was the only APA to be significantly associated with fetal demise. In contrast, Out et al[70] reported that whilst the presence of LA could predict fetal loss, an elevated ACA titre was a risk factor for low birth weight in live born infants. In practice, as there is little crossover between LA and ACA positivity, women should be screened for both classes of APA.

TREATMENT OF APA-ASSOCIATED PREGNANCY LOSS

The successful treatment of women with lupus anticoagulant was first reported in 1983 by Lubbe et al[71] The previous 14 pregnancies in this series of six women had all resulted in intrauterine death. Treatment consisted of immunosuppressive doses of prednisolone (40–60 mg/day) together with low-dose aspirin (75 mg/day). Since this original report, a wide variety of therapeutic interventions have been used in order to improve the outcome of pregnancy in women with pregnancy losses associated with the presence of APA. Low-dose aspirin, steroids, heparin, immunoglobulin and plasma exchange have all been used either as single agents or as part of combination therapy. All studies reported to date have included only small numbers of women and have had different entry criteria. There is a paucity of prospective randomized trials, comparing the efficacy of various treatment regimens, of sufficient power to detect effect.

Steroids

The rationale behind the use of steroids in immunosuppressive doses is to normalize the prolongation of in vitro coagulation times and to decrease the titre of ACA. Since the initial account of the efficacy of steroid treatment by Lubbe et al[71] subsequent reports have been less promising. Lockshin et al[72] reported that 9 out of 11 pregnancies (82%) treated with prednisone (10–60 mg daily) ended in fetal death, compared with 5 out of 10 (50%) not treated with prednisone ($P < 0.01$). These authors concluded that prednisone does not improve, and indeed may worsen, fetal outcome in pregnant women with a high APA titre and prior fetal death. Subsequent work has confirmed a significant rate of complications in treatment protocols using prednisolone.

Cowchock et al[73] reported that women treated with prednisolone plus aspirin had a significantly increased number of preterm deliveries – often associated with preterm rupture of membranes or the onset of severe pre-eclampsia when compared to those treated with heparin plus aspirin. Similarly, Silver et al[74] reported a significant excess of preterm delivery in women treated with prednisone plus aspirin as opposed to aspirin alone and concluded that prednisone treatment was an independent risk factor for preterm delivery.

Some reports suggest that neither normalization of coagulation times and suppression of the ACA titre nor the levels of ACA correlate with pregnancy outcome.[54,70,75] This calls into question the rationale for the use of steroids in the treatment of pregnant women with a history of APA-associated pregnancy losses. In addition, the use of steroids is associated with the development of hypertension, Cushingoid features, vertebral body collapse, pre-eclampsia, and significant infections.

Low-dose aspirin (LDA)

Peaceman et al[68] have demonstrated that immunoglobulin G fractions from patients with LA consistently alters platelet thromboxane production without altering prostacyclin production. Increases in production of the procoagulant thromboxane may therefore be a cause of fetal demise in APA-positive women.

Low-dose aspirin has been shown to selectively inhibit platelet thromboxane synthesis without affecting prostacyclin production.[76] Lockshin et al (1989)[72] reported a fetal loss rate of 71% (five out of seven pregnancies) using 80 mg of aspirin daily. Conversely, Sánchez-Guerrero and Alacrón-Segovia[77] reported a live birth rate of 71% (five out of seven pregnancies) and Silver et al[74] reported a 100% success rate (22 pregnancies) using 81 mg aspirin daily. In this latter study, however, only a minority of patients had experienced at least three miscarriages, and most had low titres of ACA.

Heparin

Heparin is a mixture of polysaccharides with an average molecular mass of 15 000 Da. After administration, it has an immediate effect on the coagulation system potentiating the formation of irreversible complexes between antithrombin III and the activated serine protease coagulation factors (thrombin, XIIa, XIa, Xa, IXa, and VIIa).

Moe[78] administered 12 500 U of heparin subcutaneously twice daily to 15 pregnant women whose prior pregnancies had been complicated by extensive placental infarctions, intrauterine growth retardation, and/or stillbirth. With anticoagulant treatment, 15 live births were recorded. None of the infants were growth retarded. In 1990, Rosove et al[79] reported the first series of women with APA-associated pregnancy losses to have been treated with heparin. This group reported a live birth rate of 93% (14 out of 15 pregnancies) using full-dose subcutaneous heparin (mean dose 24 700 U daily; range 10 000–36 000). The dose of heparin was adjusted to maintain a mid-interval APTT ratio of 1.5–2 times that of the control.

Cowchock et al[73] compared twice daily heparin (mean daily dose 17 000 U) to a prednisone plus aspirin combination. The live birth weight in both treatment groups was 75%. However, pre-eclampsia and preterm delivery were significantly more common in the prednisone plus aspirin group. Therefore, in this small, but randomized series, low-dose heparin appeared preferable to a prednisone plus aspirin combination.

The use of heparin is associated with a number of potential complications including bleeding and immune thrombocytopenia. The most feared complication, however, is osteopenia. De Swiet[80] reported that heparin therapy during pregnancy was associated with significant bone demineralization. This effect was both dependent on the dose of heparin and the duration of its use. Dahlman et al[81] studied 39 women, during pregnancy, who were given a mean daily dose of 17 300 units of heparin daily for a mean of 28 weeks as thromboprophylaxis. Using single-photon absorptiometry of the distal forearm they reported a significant decrease in trabecular bone mass during pregnancy in those treated with heparin as compared to controls. Interestingly, this decrease in bone mass may be reversible upon cessation of treatment.[81]

More recently, low-molecular-weight heparins (LMWH) have become available. Like conventional, unfractionated heparin, they do not cross the placenta[82] and have the additional advantages of once-daily administration and of requiring less laboratory monitoring than conventional heparin.[83] It is also claimed that the long-term use of LMWH is associated with a lesser degree of osteopenia than conventional unfractionated heparin.[84]

Other treatments

Apart from aspirin, heparin and steroids a variety of other therapeutic agents – intravenous immunoglobulin,[85–87] plasmapharesis[88] and azathioprine[89,90] – have been used to treat women with APA-associated pregnancy losses. Available data on these treatment modalities is sparse and consists of individual case reports. Their efficacy has still to be determined in randomized prospective studies. The role of these alternative therapies is likely to be confined to the treatment of those cases which have been refractory to more conventional treatments.

No treatment

There have been no published trials of the prospective treatment of women with APA-associated recurrent pregnancy losses in which a placebo arm has been incorporated into the protocol. We have a cohort of 20 recurrent miscarriers (median 4 miscarriages; range 3–11), with persistently positive tests for APA, who declined pharmacological treatment in their next pregnancy.

None of the 20 women had a genetic, endocrine or anatomical cause to explain their pregnancy losses. Eighteen of the 20 women (90%) miscarried their subsequent pregnancy – 17 first trimester and 1 second trimester IUD at 20 weeks gestation. Of note is that fetal heart activity had been observed in 12 of the 17 women (71%) with first trimester loss prior to fetal demise.[91]

Current treatment strategy at St Mary's Hospital

In the light of our experience of the high pregnancy loss rate in women with a history of recurrent miscarriage in association with APA, we are conducting a prospective randomized therapeutic trial comparing the efficacy of treatment with low-dose aspirin (75 mg daily) versus low-dose aspirin plus 5000 U unfractionated heparin twice daily. We commence treatment as soon as the pregnancy test is positive, when the woman is randomized to one of the two treatment arms. Treatment continues until 34 weeks gestation. Both mother and fetus are intensively monitored. All women are encouraged to attend for weekly first trimester ultrasound scans. Thereafter, fortnightly scans for growth, liquor volume and Doppler studies are performed. Antiphospholipid antibody screens (looking for both LA and ACA) are performed monthly, and platelet counts fortnightly. The latter are particularly important as a drop in the platelet count may indicate a worsening of the disease process and the development of a consumptive coagulopathy. In view of the reported association between long-term use of heparin and the development of osteopenia, women randomized to the heparin arm of the study have serial bone mineral density scans performed. Postnatally, blood is taken for an APA screen and platelet count.

Unanswered questions

Although our knowledge of the relationship between APA and adverse pregnancy outcome has improved greatly over the last decade certain fundamental questions are still unanswered. Amongst these are:

1. whether these antibodies are a direct cause of pregnancy loss or merely an epiphenomenon
2. which women should be screened for the presence of APA
3. should all women in whom APA are detected be treated
4. does pharmacological intervention alter the outcome of pregnancy.

The evidence that APA are a direct cause of pregnancy loss comes from work, described above, using murine models.[61,67,92] However, although placentation in the mouse is haemochorial (as is human placentation), trophoblast invasion is not as deep. Consequently, it may not be possible to extrapolate the findings obtained from murine models of antiphospholipid syndrome to humans. More recent evidence, that human placental tissue when exposed to the IgG fraction of plasma from patients with LA increases

Table 9.3 Indications for testing for the presence of antiphospholipid antibodies

Recurrent miscarriage (≥ 3)
Second or third trimester pregnancy loss
Thrombosis (arterial or venous)
Intrauterine growth retardation
Early onset pre-eclampsia
Placental abruption
Systemic lupus erythematosus
Thrombocytopenia

placental thromboxane production,[68] provides a mechanism for a direct effect of APA on pregnancy outcome. In addition, the identification of β_2GPI on the trophoblast surface of placentae from women with pregnancy loss who are found to have APA lends credence to there being a direct effect of APA on pregnancy loss. This evidence has to be balanced against the fact that suppression of either LA activity and/or the ACA titre is not a prerequisite for successful pregnancy outcome. Indeed, there have been reports of successful pregnancies in women with APA who have received no specific treatment.[72]

This last point has should be borne in mind when deciding whom to screen for APA and who needs treatment. In a case control study, Infante-Rivard et al[93] reported that there was no justification for considering LA or IgG ACA to be risk factors for fetal loss among women who present with spontaneous abortion or fetal death and have no previous history of fetal loss. Indeed, a firm relationship between pregnancy loss and the presence of APA has only been established in patients with SLE, 'lupus-like conditions' and those with clinical features of PAPS.[94,95] Table 9.3 lists those who warrant screening for APA.

The final question of whether pharmacological intervention is of benefit, and if so which is the optimum treatment protocol, remains unanswered. To date, all reported studies have been based on small numbers of women and all have had different entry criteria – both clinical and laboratory. In addition, some have not been randomized and lack a proper control group. No treatment protocol has been shown to be superior to another.

CONCLUSIONS

Antiphospholipid antibodies are associated with recurrent miscarriage, early onset pre-eclampsia, placental abruption and infertility. Attention has traditionally focused on the association between APA and thrombosis, and indeed, the most consistently reported placental pathology in women with fetal loss in association with the presence of APA is thrombosis and infarction. However, as we have shown, the majority of pregnancy losses in women with APA are first trimester and the effects of APA on implantation of the blastocyst and trophoblast invasion deserves further attention. It is unclear whether APA are directly implicated in adverse pregnancy outcome or merely an epiphenomenon. Evidence for the former comes from murine models and more recently from in vitro studies using human tissue.

A variety of therapeutic interventions have been reported to improve the outcome of pregnancy in women with APA and a previous poor obstetric history. However, evidence to date has largely been based on small, non-randomized, uncontrolled trials. At present, low-dose aspirin, or low-dose aspirin in combination with low-dose heparin, are the most favoured therapies. In pregnancies progressing beyond 24 weeks gestation, close antenatal surveillance in the form of regular ultrasound scans to assess fetal growth, doppler studies of the uterine and umbilical artery blood flow, and a willingness to deliver early in order to salvage a pregnancy that might otherwise fail form the mainstay of current treatment.

REFERENCES

1 Harris E N. Syndrome of the black swan. Br J Rheumatol 1987; 26: 324–326
2 Branch D W, Andres R, Digre K B, Rote N S, Scott J R. The association of antiphospholipid antibodies with severe preeclampsia. Obstet Gynecol 1989; 73: 541–545
3 Lockshin M D, Druzin M L, Goei S et al. Antibody to cardiolipin as a predictor of fetal distress or death in pregnant patients with systemic lupus erythematosus. N Engl J Med 1985; 313: 152–156
4 Christensen K, Herskind A M, Junker P. Antiphospholipid antibodies and occlusive vascular disease. Ugeskr Laeger 1993; 155: 2896–2900
5 Birdsall M, Pattison N, Chamley L. Antiphospholipid antibodies in pregnancy. Aust NZ J Obstet Gynaecol 1992; 32: 328–330
6 Taylor P V, Campbell J M, Scott J S. Presence of autoantibodies in women with unexplained infertility. Am J Obstet Gynecol 1989; 161: 377–379
7 Tan E M, Cohen A S, Fries J F et al. The 1982 revised criteria for the classification of systemic lupus erythematosus. Arthritis Rheum 1982; 25: 1271–1277
8 Asherson R A, Khamashta M A, Ordi Ros J et al. The 'primary' antiphospholipid syndrome: major clinical and serological features. Medicine Baltimore 1989; 68: 366–374
9 Mackworth Young C G, Loizou S, Walport M J. Primary antiphospholipid syndrome: features of patients with raised anticardiolipin antibodies and no other disorder. Ann Rheum Dis 1989; 48: 362–367
10 Conley C L, Hartmann R C. A hemorrhagic disorder caused by circulating anticoagulant in patients with disseminated lupus erythematosus. J Clin Invest 1952; 62: 416–430
11 Feinstein D I, Rapaport S I. Acquired inhibitors of blood coagulation. Prog Hemost Thromb 1972; 1: 75–95
12 Bowie E J W, Thompson J H, Pascuzzi C A. Thrombosis in systemic lupus erythematosus despite circulating anticoagulant. J Lab Clin Med 1963; 62: 416
13 Lechner K, Pabinger Fasching I. Lupus anticoagulants and thrombosis. A study of 25 cases and review of the literature. Haemostasis 1985; 15: 254–262
14 Nilsson I M, Astedt B, Hedner U, Berezin D. Intrauterine death and circulating anticoagulant ('antithromboplastin'). Acta Med Scand 1975; 197: 153–159
15 Harris E N, Gharavi A E, Boey M L et al. Anticardiolipin antibodies: detection by radioimmunoassay and association with thrombosis in systemic lupus erythematosus. Lancet 1983; 2: 1211–1214
16 Loizou S, McCrea J D, Rudge A C, Reynolds R, Boyle C C, Harris E N. Measurement of anti-cardiolipin antibodies by an enzyme-linked immunosorbent assay (ELISA): standardization and quantitation of results. Clin Exp Immunol 1985; 62: 738–745
17 McNeil H P, Chesterman C N, Krilis S A. Anticardiolipin antibodies and lupus anticoagulants comprise separate antibody subgroups with different phospholipid binding characteristics. Br J Haematol 1989; 73: 506–513
18 Rosove M H, Brewer P M, Runge A, Hirji K. Simultaneous lupus anticoagulant and

anticardiolipin assays and clinical detection of antiphospholipids. Am J Hematol 1989; 32: 148–149

19 Derue G, Englert H, Harris E N, Gharavi A E et al. Fetal loss in systemic lupus erythematosus: association with anticardiolipin antibodies. J Obstet Gynaecol 1985; 5: 207–209

20 Bevers E M, Galli M, Barbui T, Comfurius P, Zwaal R F. Lupus anticoagulant IgG's (LA) are not directed to phospholipids only, but to a complex of lipid-bound human prothrombin. Thromb Haemost 1991; 66: 629–632

21 Galli M, Comfurius P, Maassen C et al. Anticardiolipin antibodies (ACA) directed not to cardiolipin but to a plasma protein cofactor. Lancet 1990; 335: 1544–1547

22 McNeil H P, Simpson R J, Chesterman C N, Krilis S A. Anti-phospholipid antibodies are directed against a complex antigen that includes a lipid-binding inhibitor of coagulation: beta 2-glycoprotein I (apolipoprotein H). Proc Natl Acad Sci USA 1990; 87: 4120–4124

23 Shoenfeld Y, Meroni P L. The beta-2-glycoprotein I and antiphospholipid antibodies. Clin Exp Rheumatol 1992; 10: 205–209

24 Wagenknecht D R, McIntyre J A. Changes in beta 2-glycoprotein I antigenicity induced by phospholipid binding. Thromb Haemost 1993; 69: 361–365

25 Khamashta M A, Harris E N, Gharavi A E et al. Immune mediated mechanism for thrombosis: antiphospholipid antibody binding to platelet membranes. Ann Rheum Dis 1988; 47: 849–854

26 McNeil H P, Simpson R J, Chesterman C N, Krilis S A. Anti-phospholipid antibodies are directed against a complex antigen that includes a lipid-binding inhibitor of coagulation: beta 2-glycoprotein I (apolipoprotein H). Proc Natl Acad Sci USA 1990; 87: 4120–4124

27 Bevers E M, Galli M. Beta 2-glycoprotein I for binding of anticardiolipin antibodies to cardiolipin. Lancet 1990; 336: 952–953

28 Matsuura E, Igarashi Y, Fujimoto M, Ichikawa K, Koike T. Anticardiolipin cofactor(s) and differential diagnosis of autoimmune disease. Lancet 1990; 336: 177–178

29 Schousboe I. Beta 2-Glycoprotein I: a plasma inhibitor of the contact activation of the intrinsic blood coagulation pathway. Blood 1985; 66: 1086–1091

30 Nimpf J, Bevers E M, Bomans P H et al. Prothrombinase activity of human platelets is inhibited by beta 2-glycoprotein-I. Biochim Biophys Acta 1986; 884: 142–149

31 Nimpf J, Wurm H, Kostner G M. Beta 2-glycoprotein-I (apo-H) inhibits the release reaction of human platelets during ADP-induced aggregation. Atherosclerosis 1987; 63: 109–114

32 Carreras L O, Vermylen J, Spitz B, Van Assche A. 'Lupus' anticoagulant and inhibition of prostacyclin formation in patients with repeated abortion, intrauterine growth retardation and intrauterine death. Br J Obstet Gynaecol 1981; 88: 890–894

33 Angles Cano E, Sultan Y, Clauvel J P. Predisposing factors to thrombosis in systemic lupus erythematosus: possible relation to endothelial cell damage. J Lab Clin Med 1979; 94: 312–323

34 Keeling D M, Campbell S J, Mackie I J, Machin S J, Isenberg D A. The fibrinolytic response to venous occlusion and the natural anticoagulants in patients with antiphospholipid antibodies both with and without systemic lupus erythematosus. Br J Haematol 1991; 77: 354–359

35 Cariou R, Tobelem G, Bellucci S et al. Effect of lupus anticoagulant on antithrombogenic properties of endothelial cells – inhibition of thrombomodulin-dependent protein C activation. Thromb Haemost 1988; 60: 54–58

36 Malia R G, Kitchen S, Greaves M, Preston F E. Inhibition of activated protein C and its cofactor protein S by antiphospholipid antibodies. Br J Haematol 1990; 76: 101–107

37 Oosting J D, Derksen R H, Bobbink I W, Hackeng T M, Bouma B N, de Groot P G. Antiphospholipid antibodies directed against a combination of phospholipids with prothrombin, protein C, or protein S: an explanation for their pathogenic mechanism? Blood 1993; 81: 2618–2625

38 Cosgriff T M, Martin B A. Low functional and high antigenic antithrombin III level in a patient with the lupus anticoagulant and recurrent thrombosis. Arthritis Rheum 1981; 24: 94–96

39 Chamley L W, McKay E J, Pattison N S. Inhibition of heparin/antithrombin III cofactor activity by anticardiolipin antibodies: a mechanism for thrombosis. Thromb Res 1993; 71: 103–111

40 Shibata S, Harpel P C, Gharavi A, Rand J, Fillit H. Autoantibodies to heparin from

patients with antiphospholipid antibody syndrome inhibit formation of antithrombin III–thrombin complexes. Blood 1994; 83: 2532–2540

41 Vaarala O, Palosuo T, Kleemola M, Aho K. Anticardiolipin response in acute infections. Clin Immunol Immunopathol 1986; 41: 8–15

42 Peaceman A M, Silver R K, MacGregor S N, Socol M L. Interlaboratory variation in antiphospholipid antibody testing. Am J Obstet Gynecol 1992; 166: 1780–1784

43 Lupus Anticoagulant Working Party on behalf of the BCSH Haemostasis and Thrombosis Taskforce. Guidelines on testing for the lupus anticoagulant. J Clin Path 1991; 44: 885–889

44 Khamashta M A, Hughes G R V. Detection and importance of anticardiolipin antibodies. J Clin Path 1993; 104–107

45 Rai R, Regan L, Clifford K, Pickering W, Dave Mackie I, McNally T, Cohen H. Antiphospholipid antibodies and beta 2 glycoprotein-I in 500 women with recurrent miscarriage: results of a comprehensive screening approach. Hum Reprod 1995; 10(8): 2001–2005

46 Naimi N, Plancherel C, Bosser C, Jeannet M, de Moerloose P. Anticardiolipin antibodies in HIV-negative and HIV-positive haemophiliacs. Blood Coagul Fibrinolysis 1990; 1: 5–8

47 Barbui T, Cortelazzo S, Galli M et al. Antiphospholipid antibodies in early repeated abortions: a case-controlled study. Fertil Steril 1988; 50: 589–592

48 Creagh M D, Malia R G, Cooper S M, Smith A R, Duncan S L B, Greaves M. Screening for the lupus anticoagulant and anticardiolipin antibodies in women with fetal loss. J Clin Path 1991; 44: 45–47

49 Parke A L, Wilson D, Maier D. The prevalence of antiphospholipid antibodies in women with recurrent spontaneous abortion, women with successful pregnancies, and women who have never been pregnant. Arthritis Rheum 1991; 34(10): 1231–1235

50 Unander A M, Norberg R, Hahn L, Arfors L. Anticardiolipin antibodies and complement in ninety-nine women with habitual abortion. Am J Obstet Gynecol 1987; 156: 114–119

51 Lockwood C J, Romero R, Feinberg R F, Clyne L P, Coster B, Hobbins J C. The prevalence and biologic significance of lupus anticoagulant and anticardiolipin antibodies in a general obstetric population. Am J Obstet Gynecol 1989; 161: 369–373

52 Pattison N S, Chamley L W, McKay E J, Liggins G C, Butler W S. Antiphospholipid antibodies in pregnancy: prevalence and clinical associations. Br J Obstet Gynaecol 1993; 100: 909–913

53 Perez M C, Wilson W A, Brown H L, Scopelitis E. Anti-cardiolipin antibodies in unselected pregnant women in relationship to fetal outcome. J Perinatol 1991; 11: 33–36

54 Branch D W, Scott J R, Kochenour N K. Obstetric complications associated with lupus anticoagulant. N Engl J Med 1985; 313: 1322–1326

55 Lubbe W F, Liggins G C. Lupus anticoagulant and pregnancy. Am J Obstet Gynecol 1985; 153: 322–327

56 Lubbe W F, Butler W S, Palmer S J, Liggins G C. Lupus anticoagulant in pregnancy. Br J Obstet Gynaecol 1984; 91: 357–363

57 Khong T Y, Liddell H S, Robertson W B. Defective haemochorial placentation as a cause of miscarriage: a preliminary study. Br J Obstet Gynaecol 1987; 94: 649–655

58 Khong T Y, De Wolf F, Robertson W B, Brosens I. Inadequate maternal vascular response to placentation in pregnancies complicated by pre-eclampsia and by small-for-gestational age infants. Br J Obstet Gynaecol 1986; 93: 1049–1059

59 Rote N S, Walter A, Lyden T W. Antiphospholipid antibodies – lobsters or red herrings? Am J Reprod Immunol 1992; 28: 31–37

60 Lyden T W, Vogt E, Ng A K, Johnson P M, Rote N S. Monoclonal antiphospholipid antibody reactivity against human placental trophoblast. J Reprod Immunol 1992; 22: 1–14

61 Sthoeger Z M, Mozes E, Tartakovsky B. Anti-cardiolipin antibodies induce pregnancy failure by impairing embryonic implantation. Proc Natl Acad Sci USA 1993; 90: 6464–6467

62 Chamley L W, Pattison N S, McKay E J. Elution of anticardiolipin antibodies and their cofactor beta 2-glycoprotein 1 from the placentae of patients with a poor obstetric history. J Reprod Immunol 1993; 25: 209–220

63 La Rosa L, Meroni P L, Tincani A et al. Beta 2 glycoprotein I and placental anticoagulant protein I in placentae from patients with antiphospholipid syndrome. J Rheumatol 1994; 21: 1684–1693

64 De Wolf F, Carreras L O, Moerman P, Vermylen J, Van Assche A, Renaer M. Decidual vasculopathy and extensive placental infarction in a patient with repeated thromboembolic

accidents, recurrent fetal loss, and a lupus anticoagulant. Am J Obstet Gynecol 1982; 142: 829–834

65 Out H J, Kooijman C D, Bruinse H W, Derksen R H. Histopathological findings in placentae from patients with intra-uterine fetal death and anti-phospholipid antibodies. Eur J Obstet Gynecol Reprod Biol 1991; 41: 179–186

66 Hanly J G, Gladman D D, Rose T H, Laskin C A, Urowitz M B. Lupus pregnancy. A prospective study of placental changes. Arthritis Rheum 1988; 31: 358–366

67 Branch D W, Dudley D J, Mitchell M D et al. Immunoglobulin G fractions from patients with antiphospholipid antibodies cause fetal death in BALB/c mice: a model for autoimmune fetal loss. Am J Obstet Gynecol 1990; 163: 210–216

68 Peaceman A M, Rehnberg K A. The effect of immunoglobulin G fractions from patients with lupus anticoagulant on placental prostacyclin and thromboxane production. Am J Obstet Gynecol 1993; 169: 1403–1406

69 Lynch A, Marlar R, Murphy J et al. Antiphospholipid antibodies in predicting adverse pregnancy outcome. A prospective study. Ann Intern Med 1994; 120: 470–475

70 Out H J, Bruinse H W, Christiaens G C et al. A prospective, controlled multicenter study on the obstetric risks of pregnant women with antiphospholipid antibodies. Am J Obstet Gynecol 1992; 167: 26–32

71 Lubbe W F, Butler W S, Palmer S J, Liggins G C. Fetal survival after prednisone suppression of maternal lupus-anticoagulant. Lancet 1983; 1: 1361–1363

72 Lockshin M D, Druzin M L, Qamar T. Prednisone does not prevent recurrent fetal death in women with antiphospholipid antibody. Am J Obstet Gynecol 1989; 160: 439–443

73 Cowchock F S, Reece E A, Balaban D, Branch D W, Plouffe L. Repeated fetal losses associated with antiphospholipid antibodies: a collaborative randomized trial comparing prednisone with low-dose heparin treatment. Am J Obstet Gynecol 1992; 166: 1318–1323

74 Silver R K, MacGregor S N, Sholl J S, Hobart J M, Neerhof M G, Ragin A. Comparative trial of prednisone plus aspirin versus aspirin alone in the treatment of anticardiolipin antibody-positive obstetric patients. Am J Obstet Gynecol 1993; 169: 1411–1417

75 Norberg R, Nived O, Sturfelt G, Unander M, Arfors L. Anticardiolipin and complement activation: relation to clinical symptoms. J Rheumatol 1987; 14 (Suppl 13): 149–153

76 Tohgi H, Konno S, Tamura K, Kimura B, Kawano K. Effects of low-to-high doses of aspirin on platelet aggregability and metabolites of thromboxane A2 and prostacyclin. Stroke 1992; 23: 1400–1403

77 Sanchez Guerrero J, Alarcon Segovia D. Course of antiphospholipid antibodies in patients with primary antiphospholipid syndrome before, during and after pregnancy treated with low dose aspirin. Relationship of antibody levels to outcome in 7 patients. J Rheumatol 1992; 19: 1083–1088

78 Moe N. Anticoagulant therapy in the prevention of placental infarction and perinatal death. Obstet Gynecol 1982; 59: 481–483

79 Rosove M H, Tabsh K, Wasserstrum N, Howard P, Hahn B H, Kalunian K C. Heparin therapy for pregnant women with lupus anticoagulant or anticardiolipin antibodies. Obstet Gynecol 1990; 75: 630–634

80 De Swiet M, Dorrington Ward P, Fidler J et al. Prolonged heparin therapy in pregnancy causes bone demineralisation. Br J Obstet Gynaecol 1983; 90: 1129–1134

81 Dahlman T C, Sjoberg H E, Ringertz H. Bone mineral density during long-term prophylaxis with heparin in pregnancy. Am J Obstet Gynecol 1994; 170: 1315–1320

82 Harenberg J, Schneider D, Heilmann L, Wolf H. Lack of anti-factor Xa activity in umbilical cord vein samples after subcutaneous administration of heparin or low molecular mass heparin in pregnant women. Haemostasis 1993; 23: 314–320

83 Hirsh J, Levine M N. Low molecular weight heparin. Blood 1992; 79: 1–17

84 Melissari E, Parker C J, Wilson N V et al. Use of low molecular weight heparin in pregnancy. Thromb Haemost 1992; 68: 652–656

85 Parke A, Maier D, Wilson D, Andreoli J, Ballow M. Intravenous gamma-globulin, antiphospholipid antibodies and pregnancy. Ann Intern Med 1989; 110: 495–496

86 Scott J R, Branch D W, Kochenour N K, Ward K. Intravenous immunoglobulin treatment of pregnant patients with recurrent pregnancy loss caused by antiphospholipid antibodies and Rh immunization. Am J Obstet Gynecol 1988; 159: 1055–1056

87 Carreras L O, Perez G N, Vega H R, Casavilla F. Lupus anticoagulant and recurrent fetal loss: successful treatment with gammaglobulin. Lancet 1988; 2: 393

88 Frampton G, Cameron J S, Thom M, Jones S, Raftery M. Successful removal of anti-

phospholipid antibody during pregnancy using plasma exchange and low-dose prednisolone. Lancet 1987; 2: 1023–1024

89 Chan J K H, Harris E N, Hughes G R V. Successful pregnancy following suppression of anticardiolipin antibody and lupus anticoagulant with azathioprine in systemic lupus erythematosus. J Obstet Gynecol 1986; 7: 16

90 Steier J A, Akslen L A, Flesland O, Askvik K. Fetal heart block, anti-SSA and anti-SSB antibodies. Association with intra-uterine growth retardation, fetal death and lupus anticoagulant. Acta Obstet Gynecol Scand 1987; 66: 737–739

91 Rai R, Cohen H, Clifford K, Regan L. High prospective fetal loss rate in women with recurrent miscarriage and antiphospholipid antibodies. Hum Reprod 1995; 10(12): 3301–3304

92 Blank M, Cohen J, Toder V, Shoenfeld Y. Induction of anti-phospholipid syndrome in naive mice with mouse lupus monoclonal and human polyclonal anti-cardiolipin antibodies. Proc Natl Acad Sci USA 1991; 88: 3069–3073

93 Infante Rivard C, David M, Gauthier R, Rivard G E. Lupus anticoagulants, anticardiolipin antibodies, and fetal loss. A case-control study. N Engl J Med 1991; 325: 1063–1066

94 Love P E, Santoro S A. Antiphospholipid antibodies: anticardiolipin and the lupus anticoagulant in systemic lupus erythematosus (SLE) and in non-SLE disorders. Prevalence and clinical significance. Ann Intern Med 1990; 112: 682–698

95 Out H J, Bruinse H W, Derksen R H. Anti-phospholipid antibodies and pregnancy loss. Hum Reprod 1991; 6: 889–897

10 Congenital abnormalities of the fetal brain

J. K. Gupta   F. A. Chervenak   R. J. Lilford

With the development of high resolution real-time ultrasonography, an accurate anatomical antenatal diagnosis of many fetal brain abnormalities can be made, but this has led to the identification of features whose significance is still unclear. While there are many isolated reports of specific anomalies, very few surveys include patients where the abnormality has been followed up long-term after birth. It is, therefore, very difficult to advise prospective parents about the probabilities of the various outcomes for their child.

If one congenital abnormality has been detected then extracranial defects should be sought by an expert ultrasonographer as their presence will usually affect the prognosis adversely. If the outcome is expected to be good and counselling can reflect this optimistic forecast, then full support should be given to the parents throughout pregnancy because, despite reassurances, parents continue to have anxieties about the normality of their child, even after delivery and a normal paediatric assessment. Some question whether parents should be informed of such an abnormality in these circumstances. Clearly, a delicate interplay between the ethical obligations and autonomy and possible future medico-legal implications will need to be carefully considered.

It is much more difficult to provide probabilistic information for parents whose child falls into the usually poor or variable prognosis groups. This group presents the most challenging counselling problem for the obstetrician. Frequently, the information regarding prognosis is not available and much of it is based on neurosurgical series, which is potentially biased towards patients with a better prognosis than might be expected for cases diagnosed antenatally. Antenatal diagnosis, however, does enable arrangements to be made for the future management of the pregnancy, timing and place of delivery and, if necessary, availability of intensive neurosurgical care.

There are several management options for pregnancies complicated by fetal brain anomalies: aggressive management, abortion, termination of pregnancy after fetal viability (usually during the third trimester) and non-aggressive management. However, complex obstetric ethical issues have to be considered.[1] Before viability (presently defined as 24 weeks of gestational age in the UK), the management of a pregnancy complicated by fetal brain anomalies is ethically straightforward, where counselling should be rigorous and non-directive. The woman should be given the choice between continuing her pregnancy to viability, and thus to term, or offered an abortion. If the woman elects to continue her pregnancy, she should be apprized about decisions that will need to be made later.[1]

After viability, aggressive management is the ethical standard of care. By aggressive management, we mean optimizing perinatal outcome by utilizing effective antepartum and intrapartum diagnostic and therapeutic modalities e.g. administering steroids for fetal lung maturity in preterm delivery.

There are, however, three important exceptions to aggressive management. The first exception is termination of pregnancy after fetal viability. This applies when there is certainty of diagnosis, and either certainty of death as an outcome of the anomaly diagnosed or, in some cases of short-term survival, certainty of the absence of cognitive developmental capacity as an outcome of the anomaly diagnosed.[1] Anencephaly is a classic example that satisfies these criteria. The second exception is non-aggressive management. This applies when there is a very high probability but sometimes less certainty about the diagnosis and, either a very high probability of death as an outcome of the anomaly diagnosed or survival with a very high probability of severe and irreversible deficit of cognitive developmental capacity as a result of the anomaly diagnosed.[2] When these two criteria apply, both aggressive and non-aggressive management can be justified, from which it follows that a choice between aggressive and non-aggressive management should be offered. Encephalocoele is a classic example that satisfies these criteria. The third important and ethically complex exception is cephalocentesis.[1]

This chapter will attempt to provide the best prognostic and probabilistic information regarding various outcomes, available to date, for obstetricians and prospective parents whose pregnancies are complicated by fetal brain anomalies. This information will be compiled, where possible, by the amalgamation of reports detailing the prognosis of antenatally diagnosed cases from the English world literature. In some instances, the antenatal prognosis will be compared with neurosurgical outcomes. The antenatal assessment and management of the most important anomalies will be discussed.

ANENCEPHALY

Anencephaly is an anomaly characterized by the absence of cerebral hemispheres and cranial vault. The crown of the head is covered by a vascular membrane which allows alphafetoprotein (αFP) to exude into the amniotic fluid, resulting in high maternal serum and amniotic fluid αFP levels. The incidence is 1 per 1000 births. The epidemiology of anencephaly is very similar to that of spina bifida, with considerable variation in the prevalence of the condition in different parts of the world.[3] The commonest associated malformations are: spina bifida in 17% of cases, cleft lip or palate in 2% and club foot in 1.7%. Omphalocoeles has also been described.[4] The recurrence risk is 4%, and as high as 10% if two previous pregnancies have been affected. The

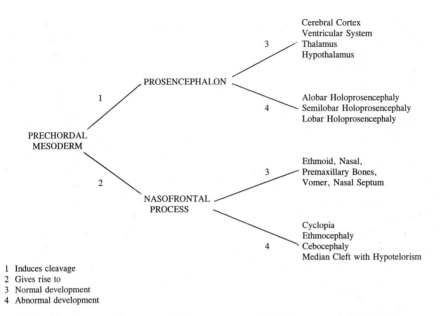

Fig.10.1 Embryology of holoprosencephaly and midline facial defects. (Reproduced with permission from Chervenak et al.[12])

antenatal diagnosis relies on the failure to demonstrate the cranial vault and other characteristic findings of a 'toad like' appearance; bulging eyes, large tongue and very short neck. The diagnosis can probably be made as early as the 12th week. In the third trimester, malpresentation may alert the clinician to the diagnosis. Polyhydramnios is frequently associated (40–50%) possibly owing to the failure to swallow, secondary to a brain stem lesion, excessive micturition or failure to reabsorb cerebrospinal fluid. There is also frequently increased fetal activity which may be caused by irritation of the exposed meninges.

The condition results in death usually in the first few hours or days of life and therefore termination of pregnancy is generally acceptable at any gestation.[5] Anencephalic infants are, however, a potential source of organs for transplantation.[6] Preconceptual maternal folate supplements should be given before future pregnancies.

HOLOPROSENCEPHALY

The term holoprosencephaly embraces a variety of cerebral abnormalities that result from a failure of cleavage of the primitive forebrain or prosencephalon. In holoprosencephaly, perhaps more than any other malformation, an understanding of the embryology can lead directly to ultrasound diagnosis (Fig. 10.1). The prosencephalon develops from the most rostral part of the

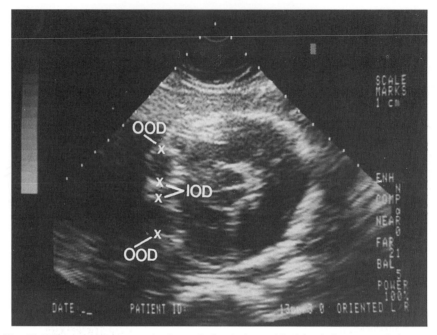

Fig. 10.2 Sonogram demonstrating hypotelorism in fetus with alobar holoprosencephaly.
OOD = outer orbital distance; IOD = inner orbital distance.

Defect in Central fusion

neural tube and gives rise to the cerebral hemispheres, thalamus and
hypothalamus. Failure of its sagittal division can result in a common ventricle, a fused thalamus, and cortex with neither lobes nor an interhemispheric
fissure.[7] Various midline facial anomalies are closely associated with this
entity.[8] A connective tissue mass, called the prechordal mesoderm, which is
situated between the oral cavity and the undersurface of the neural tube, is
thought to be the site of origin for both the development of the nasofrontal
process and the division of the prosencephalon. The nasofrontal process
gives rise to the ethmoid, nasal and premaxillary bones and the vomer and
nasal septum. Failure of these structures to develop normally can result in
the varying degrees of hypotelorism (diminished interorbital distance), cleft
lip and palate, and nasal malformation seen in this disorder (Figs 10.2 &
10.3).

Holoprosencephaly is divided into alobar, semilobar and lobar categories,
all based on the degree of separation of the cerebral hemispheres.[7] The alobar
variety is the most severe, with no evidence of division of the cerebral cortex.
The falx cerebri and interhemispheric fissure are absent.[9] The thalami are
fused and are seen to protrude into a large horseshoe-shaped monoventricular cavity[10] (Figs 10.4 & 10.5) and there is only a rudimentary corpus callosum, if one is present at all. When hypotelorism and the absence of midline
cerebral structures are observed the diagnosis is made with certainty.[11–18] The

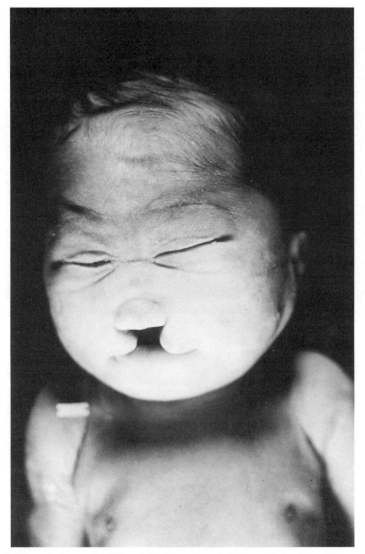

Fig. 10.3 Hypotelorism and midline cleft. (Reproduced with permission from Chervenak et al.[13])

semilobar and lobar varieties represent a higher degree of brain development, with semilobar having a partial separation of the hemispheres. There is much variability in the defects of the midline cerebral structures. Absent olfactory tracts and bulbs are usually associated with all of these conditions, thus the older term 'arrhinencephaly'.

In holoprosencephaly, certain facies predict the presence of the alobar type. Cyclopia, the presence of a single median bony orbit with a fleshy

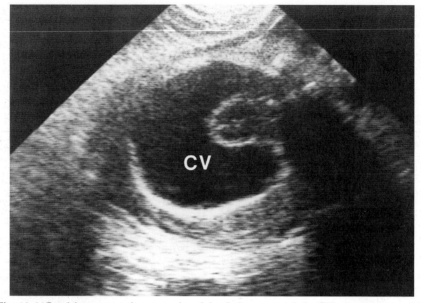

Fig. 10.4 Cranial sonogram demonstrating alobar holoprosencephaly. CV = common ventricle forming a large horseshoe-shaped monoventricular cavity.

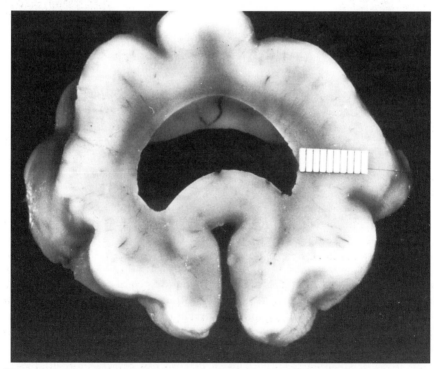

Fig. 10.5 An example of alobar holoprosencephaly with absent interhemispheric fissure and common ventricle. (Reproduced with permission from Chervenak et al.[13])

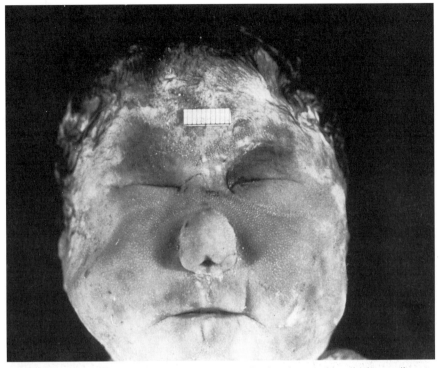

Fig. 10.6 Cebocephaly with hypotelorism and normally placed nose with a single nostril. (Reproduced with permission from Chervenak et al.[12])

proboscis above it, is the most severe of these malformations. Ethmocephaly, the least common, is characterized by two separate orbits with a proboscis in between. In cebocephaly, hypotelorism is associated with a normally placed nose with a single nostril (Fig. 10.6). Hypotelorism with a midline facial cleft also predicts the presence of alobar holoprosencephaly. Holoprosencephaly also may be associated with milder forms of midline facial dysplasia or normal facies.[7]

There are other anatomical aberrations, related to holoprosencephaly, that may be detected by antenatal ultrasound. Hydrocephalus is the most common of these. When seen in conjunction with macrocephaly, hydrocephalus is probably a result of obstruction to cerebrospinal fluid flow; when present with microcephaly, cerebral hypoplasia seems a more likely mechanism. Other associated structural defects detectable by ultrasound include midline facial cleft and polydactyly. Hydramnios also may be present, perhaps because of impaired fetal swallowing.[13] The incidence of holoprosencephaly has been reported to be between 1 in 5200 and 1 in 16 000 live births[19,20] but may affect as many as 0.4% of all conceptuses.[21] The aetiology of holoprosencephaly is heterogeneous and often not known for an individual case. There is a high incidence of chromosomal abnormalities (50–60%), mainly

Etiology ① Ch: abm: Trisomy 13, 8 ② Ionizing radiation ③ Diabetic mothers ④ Toxoplasmosis / Rubella ⑤ Heavy alcohol exposure ⑥ Familial

160   PROGRESS IN OBSTETRICS AND GYNAECOLOGY

trisomy 13[13,22] but also trisomy 18, triploidy, 13q-, and 18p.[23] Teratogenic agents including ionizing radiation[24] and certain alkaloids[25] have produced this malformation in experimental animals. However, no such agent has been clearly identified in man. A 200-fold increase in the incidence of holoprosencephaly has been reported in diabetic mothers.[26] It has also been associated with toxoplasmosis, amino-acid abnormalities, endocrine dysgenesis, intrauterine rubella or possible heavy alcohol exposure in early pregnancy.[27]

Familial occurrence has been documented in several cases. Autosomal recessive inheritance with variable expression has been suggested in some families and autosomal dominant inheritance with both incomplete penetrance and variable expression in others. The recessively inherited Meckel-Grüber syndrome (polydactyly, encephalocoele, polycystic kidney disease, microcephaly) also may include holoprosencephaly.[28]

The diagnosis of holoprosencephaly signals the need for a chromosomal determination to guide the management of future pregnancies. A chromosomal anomaly may predict either a low recurrence risk of less than 1%, if a trisomy is demonstrated, or a much higher risk if the aneuploidy involves a translocation and one of the parents is a carrier of the translocation chromosomes. In the absence of a chromosomal abnormality, an empirical recurrence of 6% has been calculated.[19] However, some families may be faced with the 25% recurrence risk associated with autosomal recessive inheritance.[29] It is usually impossible to designate these families, although consanguinity or a previously affected child may be suggestive. A further rare high-risk group includes adults with mild manifestations of dominantly inherited holoprosencephaly e.g. mild hypotelorism, hyposomia, mild midface hypoplasia or a single central maxillary incisor tooth.[30,31] Close examination of both parents is mandatory and sonographic examination of future pregnancies would be indicated.

The prognosis for alobar holoprosencephaly is uniformly poor with most dying either in utero or in the first year of life. The survivors usually have severe mental retardation.[7,8] Less is known about the prognosis in the lobar and semilobar varieties. Normal life span has been reported for some, but many are severely mentally retarded.[7,21,32] It is possible that individuals with subtle forms of lobar holoprosencephaly and very limited neurological abnormalities may exist.

The obstetrical management of holoprosencephaly is dependent upon the gestational age at the time of diagnosis, which is now even possible in the first trimester by early transvaginal ultrasound.[33,34] Pregnancy termination should be considered throughout gestation. Every attempt should be made to accomplish a vaginal delivery. If macrocephaly as a result of hydrocephalus is present, cephalocentesis – the decompression of the distended fetal ventricular system using transabdominal needle placement under ultrasound guidance – should be considered.[35] The potentially destructive nature of this procedure must be explained to the parents. Decision-making in lobar holoprosencephaly is difficult because data concerning outcome is not available.

HYDRANENCEPHALY

1.u infarction — Bilateral 1. caratid A occlusion sec: to Toxoplasmosis

Hydranencephaly is a destructive condition where most of the cerebral hemispheres are absent and replaced by cerebrospinal fluid (CSF). The cranial vault, meninges, cerebellum, midbrain, thalamus and basal ganglia are usually normal. The aetiology is thought to be either intrauterine infarction secondary to bilateral internal carotid artery occlusion[36] or secondary to toxoplasmosis infection.[37] The differential diagnosis is extreme ventriculomegaly and porencephaly (see below). Scanty data is available on the neurological performance of hydranencephalic infants. Most will have severe neurological abnormalities and die at birth. Chronic survival up to 3.5 years has been reported and seems to depend on an intact hypothalamus capable of thermoregulation.[38] Pregnancy termination should be considered throughout gestation.

TOP

INIENCEPHALY

Iniencephaly is an extremely rare complex developmental abnormality characterized by an exaggerated lordosis of the spine, usually associated with spina bifida and encephalocoele. Eighty-four per cent of iniencephalic infants have other associated anomalies such as anencephaly, hydrocephaly, cyclopia, cleft lip and palate, diaphragmatic hernia, single umbilical artery, omphalocoele, gastroschisis, situs inversus, polycystic kidneys, arthrogryposis and clubfoot.[39] The differential diagnosis includes anencephaly, the Klippel-Feil syndrome (shortness of the neck associated with fusion of the cervical vertebrae) and cervical myelomeningocoele. Some regard the Klippel-Feil syndrome and iniencephaly as different abnormalities of the same spectrum. Iniencephaly is virtually always fatal in the neonatal period.[39] Pregnancy termination should be considered throughout gestation. In the third trimester, iniencephaly can cause obstructed labour because of the hyperextended hydrocephalic head.[40,41] Cephalocentesis should be attempted and should this fail an embryotomy may be undertaken to avoid Caesarean section.

84'/.

TOP

MICROCEPHALY *1.6/1000*

Microcephaly is a clinical syndrome characterized by a head circumference of 3 standard deviations (SD) below the mean. However, the utility of head measurements alone and the comparison of biometric parameters e.g. head circumference; abdominal circumference ratio on serial scanning[42] and head circumference: femur length ratios[43] is limited as these can be markedly biased by factors such as incorrect dating or intrauterine growth retardation. As the most affected part in microcephaly is the forebrain, a potentially helpful diagnostic hint is possibly the ultrasound demonstration of a sloping forehead[44] or the assessment of the fetal frontal lobe.[45]

The incidence of microcephaly is estimated to be 1.6 per 1000 deliveries.

The aetiology is classified into two categories: with or without associated anomalies.[46] Some cases of microcephaly are associated with congenital infections (e.g. rubella, toxoplasmosis) but the majority are isolated defects and half of the latter are inherited as an autosomal recessive basis.[47] A recurrence risk of 1 in 8 is often quoted but microcephalic infants with no evidence of viral infection following consanguineous marriage can be regarded as recessive in aetiology. Microcephaly is associated with craniosynostosis (premature fusion of cranial sutures), Meckel-Grüber syndrome, chromosomal abnormalities including trisomies like 13 and 18, and radiation exposure. The prognosis for mental function is very poor as the impaired head growth is usually entirely secondary to poor brain growth. Avery et al[48] found the incidence of moderate to severe mental retardation of 33% and 62% in infants with head circumferences of 2–3 SD and < 3 SD, respectively, lower than the mean. Pryor and Thelander[49] found mean intelligence quotients (IQ) of 35 and 20 for infants with head circumferences of 4–7 SD and < 7 SD, respectively, lower than the mean.

Microcephaly is an untreatable condition and every attempt should be made to identify associated anomalies by both detailed ultrasound and amniocentesis for fetal karyotype. Pregnancy termination should be offered before viability.

PORENCEPHALY

Porencephaly is an extremely rare condition that describes an intracerebral CSF-containing cystic cavity which may or may not communicate with the ventricular system and the subarachnoid space. The condition is subdivided into true porencephaly and pseudoporencephaly. True porencephaly (schizencephaly) is a developmental anomaly caused by a failure in the migration of cells destined to form the cerebral cortex, resulting in a defect of both grey and white matter. In the absence of neural tissue, the subarachnoid space fills to form a cyst. Pseudoporencephaly, however, is a destructive condition that occurs as a result of vascular, infectious or traumatic cause that may happen in utero or at any time after birth.[50,51] As true porencephaly is characterized by cystic cavities of variable size usually localised around the Sylvian fissure, the diagnosis depends on the demonstration of intracranial cystic areas. A marked asymmetrical dilatation of the lateral ventricles with a shift of the midline is common and therefore porencephaly should always be considered whenever marked asymmetrical ventriculomegaly is found.[52]

The prognosis depends largely on the size of the lesion. As the basic defect of both true and pseudoporencephaly is localized absence of cerebral mass, the clinical course for both conditions is similar, where the outcome is extremely poor, with invariable, severe intellectual impairment and neurological sequelae.[51] Termination of pregnancy should be offered before viability. Cephalocentesis should be considered in cases of macrocephaly in order to avoid Caesarean section.

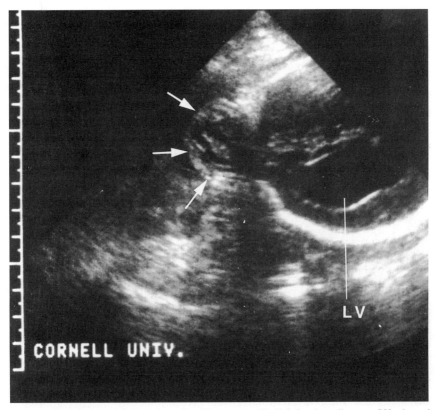

Fig. 10.7 Occipital encephalocoele outlined by arrows. Skull defect is easily seen. LV = lateral ventricle.

ENCEPHALOCOELE

An encephalocoele is an almost always midline defect of the cranial vault where brain tissue has herniated into a sac. It is usually situated in the occipital region (75%) but is occasionally frontal (13%), parietal (12%) or nasopharyngeal.[53] 'Cranial meningocoele' is the correct term where only meninges has herniated. The two conditions encompass the term cephalocoeles. The size of the defect varies from a few millimetres to a mass larger than the cranial vault. It may occur as a non-genetic sporadic syndrome e.g. amniotic band syndrome (predominantly non-midline, anterior, and multiple encephalocoeles, amputation of digits or limbs and bizarre oral clefts) or as part of an autosomal syndrome e.g. Meckel-Grüber, Chemke, Robert's, crytophtalmos syndromes.[54]

The prenatal diagnosis of encephalocoele relies on the demonstration of a paracranial mass[55–59] (Fig. 10.7). However, this criterion is insufficient to distinguish encephalocoeles from other non-neural masses, such as cystic hygromas, and soft tissue masses, such as scalp oedema/cephalohaematoma[60] and

D/D cystic Hygroma
Scalp oedema
Cephalohaematoma.
Haemangioma

haemangiomas.[61] For this reason, every effort should be made to identify the skull defect.[55] This may be difficult because the bony defect is usually smaller than the herniated mass.

A careful search of fetal anatomy is indicated as associated anomalies are frequently observed, such as hydrocephalus in 80% of occipital meningocoeles and 65% of occipital encephalocoeles[62] and spina bifida in 7–15% of all cephalocoeles.[55] Amniotic fluid αFP is usually elevated but not always.[55] The prognosis of encephalocoele depends largely on three factors:[63-67]

1. the most important discriminator is the presence of brain tissue in the herniated sac. Almost half of the infants with pure meningocoeles have normal development after surgery compared to less than 5% if brain tissue herniation has occurred.[65] There is little information on the correlation between amount of brain tissue herniation and handicap. Chervenak et al[55] reported two such children who are currently alive with moderate developmental delay

2. hydrocephalus – in the absence of brain tissue herniation and other associated anomalies this has a relatively favourable prognosis providing postnatal shunting is performed

3. microcephaly – the outlook is dismal in these cases.

Termination of pregnancy should be offered before viability and in cases associated with anomalies incompatible with life e.g. iniencephaly, Meckel-Grüber syndrome. After viability a choice between aggressive and non-aggressive management can be recommended.[1] Where no brain tissue has herniated, the outlook is much more favourable but parents should be advised that surgery will be necessary to repair the defect after delivery.

CHOROID PLEXUS CYSTS

The choroid plexus of the lateral ventricle is the first cerebral structure that can be identified in the fetus during the late first and early second trimester. This highly reflective echogenic structure is seen to occupy an unexpectedly large proportion of the cranial volume. It has a well defined smooth outline because of its interface with the cerebrospinal fluid, allowing it to be easily visualized in the axial, coronal or sagittal planes of the fetal head.

Choroid plexus (CP) cysts are found in approximately 50% of autopsy studies, occurring with about the same frequency in all age groups.[68] These cysts are believed to represent neuroepithelial folds that subsequently fill with cerebrospinal fluid and cellular debris.[68,69] On the other hand, symptomatic cysts (usually exceptionally large; 2–8 cm), although rare, have also been described in infants, young children and adults.[70]

The prenatal sonographic detection of CP cysts has stimulated considerable interest since the first report by Chudleigh et al,[71] suggesting their benign nature (Fig. 10.8). Since then there have been numerous conflicting reports raising the possibility of an association between CP cysts and

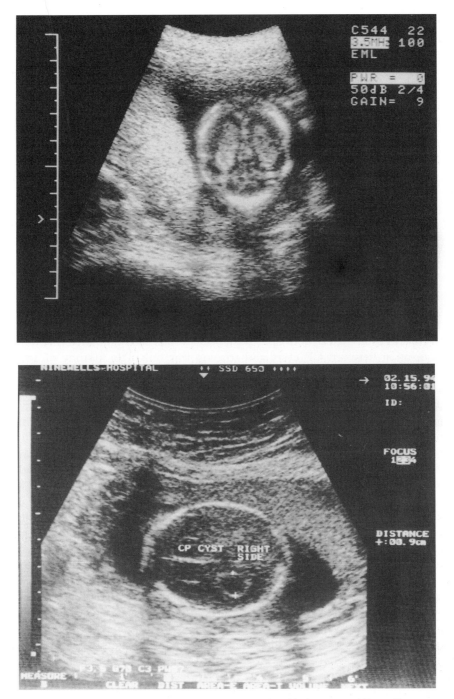

Fig. 10.8 Cranial sonogram demonstrating A. normal choroid plexuses; and B. small unilateral choroid plexus cyst.

[handwritten annotations at top: - age c̄ Trisomy 18, 21, Klinefelters Syndrome, Turner Syndrome, Validity - Isolated cyst → (N) out come]

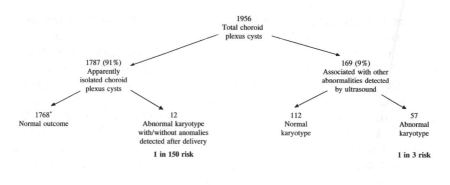

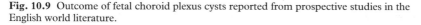

*7 cases lost to follow-up

For comprehensive tables of outcomes of all cases, see Gupta et al[73] and Gupta et al[82]

Fig. 10.9 Outcome of fetal choroid plexus cysts reported from prospective studies in the English world literature.

chromosomal abnormalities, particularly trisomy 18. In general, these studies have been case reports or retrospective studies with relatively small numbers. The prospective studies published suggest that the association is real, but not as great as estimated by retrospective reports. It has been estimated that if the association between CP cysts and trisomy was only 1%, a study of 1000 cases, i.e. 120 000 mid-trimester ultrasound scans, would be required to demonstrate a prevalence of this magnitude with 95% confidence limits of 0.5% and 1.5%.[72] The amalgamation of the world literature, concentrating on the prospective studies of unselected women, provides the best information on answering some of the questions. Comprehensive tables reporting the outcome of CP cysts from retrospective, prospective and case reports have been published previously.[73] There are 18 prospective studies in the world English literature reporting a total of 1956 CP cysts[74–91] (Fig. 10.9). The overall mean prevalence is 0.53%. Of the 1787 cases (91%) thought to be apparently isolated (i.e. not associated with other ultrasound detected anomalies), 12 (0.67% of 1787) were found to have an abnormal karyotype after delivery (8 trisomy 18, 3 trisomy 21 and 1 Klinefelter's (XXY)). The remaining majority (1768 cases), after excluding 7 cases that were lost to follow-up, were confirmed to be isolated cysts, and had a normal outcome with most of the cysts forming between 14–16 weeks and resolving by 26 weeks gestation. Just over one-third (57 cases) of the 169 cases associated with other abnormalities detected by ultrasound had an abnormal karyotype; 76% trisomy 18, 17% trisomy 21 and the remaining 7% comprising triploidy, mosaic Turner's syndrome and Klinefelter's syndrome. The prognosis is dismal in this group: follow-up not available in 24 cases, 26 terminations of pregnancy, 4 deaths and 3 live births (2 trisomy 18 and 1 trisomy 21, but the long-term outcome was not reported in these cases). Out of 112 cases where the karyotype was normal and associated with other ultrasound detected abnormalities, the outcome was available in 58 cases (52%): 9 terminations of pregnancy, 4 deaths and 45 (40%) with normal outcome or live births.[73,82]

The risk of aneuploidy is 1 in 150 (95% confidence intervals (CI), 1 in 95–1 in 341), if no other ultrasound anomalies, apart from CP cysts themselves, are detected. This risk is independent of diminishing cyst size as gestation progresses, complete cyst resolution (majority by 26 weeks), location of cysts (equally unilateral and bilateral) and small or large cyst size (60–80% <10 mm). The risk increases to 1 in 3 (95% CI, 1 in 2.5–1 in 3.8) if *any* other ultrasound abnormalities are detected. The risk of Down's syndrome in fetuses with apparently isolated CP cysts is lowered from 1 in 150 to 1 in 880 (17% of 1 in 150 risk).

Comment   *Incidence · 35% – 1%.*

The world literature reports an incidence of CP cysts that varies widely from 0.18%[80] to 3.6%.[77] The overall mean prevalence of 0.53% may not be a true reflection of the actual incidence as it is lowered by the single largest regional survey of a low-risk population, reporting 524 cases.[82] The authors of this study suspect that their low incidence of 0.35% was because of the failure of some districts to report all cases during the initial stages of the study, mainly owing to the lack of awareness and dilemma surrounding the significance of CP cysts. Overall, it could be assumed that CP cysts occur in approximately 1% of all pregnancies, if this series is removed from the analysis.

CP cysts are useful markers because they are easily seen in the standard biparietal view which is obtained for all routine anomaly scans. Alternative lesions detected by ultrasound screening that may have potentially higher sensitivities for chromosomal abnormalities are presently not easy to detect at a routine examination. For example, congenital heart disease abnormalities, such as ventricular septal defects, may be found in 90–99% of fetuses with trisomy 13 and 18 and in 50–80% of those with trisomy 21. However, these defects may be impossible to detect even by specialist echocardiographers in the second trimester.[92,93]

Management of fetal CP cysts

One disadvantage of screening a population for disease is that certain findings may be ambiguous and further, possibly invasive, tests would be required to determine whether disease is present. Amniocentesis and chorionic villus sampling are associated with a low, but significant, complication rate, and it is therefore desirable to define carefully the criteria for offering these tests to patients. With knowledge of the current available information on fetal CP cysts, we suggest that the scheme illustrated in Fig. 10.10 should be followed. We would regard CP cysts, maternal age of ≥ 37 years (or 'high risk' following Down's biochemical screening) and the sonographic detection of *any* other structural abnormalities as three important risk markers. If a

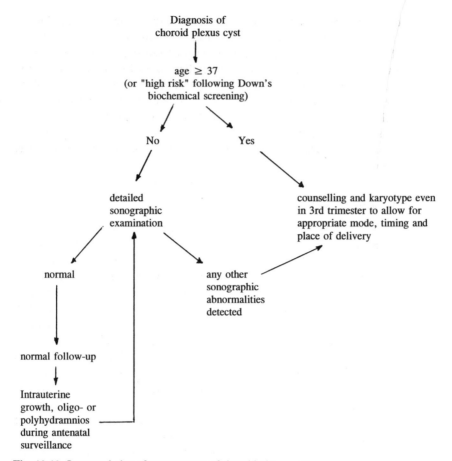

Fig. 10.10 Suggested plan of management of choroid plexus cysts.

combination of any two markers are found, then this is a clear indication for offering amniocentesis. As the majority of fetuses with trisomy 18 have detectable associated structural abnormalities, we suggest that careful attention is made to the hands, feet and face during the detailed sonographic examination. Subtle anomalies such as overlapping fingers, micrognathia and clubfoot are particularly important. The heart should be assessed with colour flow imaging to exclude small ventricular septal defects. If the fetus appears normal, we can reassure the parents. If any other abnormality is detected, including minor findings such as mild renal pelvis dilatation, then the parents should be offered karyotyping as the risk of aneuploidy is 1 in 3. Karyotyping is even of value in the third trimester, because knowledge that the fetus is chromosomally abnormal would give the parents and attending obstetrician a chance to reconsider the value of obstetric interventions, such as delivery by Caesarean section for fetal distress.

The dilemma arises when no other abnormalities are sonographically detected and CP cysts are the only finding. The risk of aneuploidy in this group is 1 in 150. Although representing only 12 reported cases, this worrying finding is confirmed by reports showing that 25% of fetuses with trisomy 18 have CP cysts as the only sonographic finding.[94-96] A further 24% of trisomy 18 fetuses have no sonographic anomalies detected by ultrasound i.e. not even CP cysts.[94,96,97] Therefore, although the sensitivity of CP cysts is relatively low even for trisomy 18, it compares favourably with the sensitivity of screening for chromosomal abnormalities on the basis for maternal age alone, which is approximately 25%.

Parental counselling

Parents should be advised that there is a distinct association between fetal CP cysts and chromosomal abnormality, most commonly trisomy 18, but also trisomy 21. The outcome of trisomy 18 cases is very poor with only 5% of babies surviving 1 year or more, almost all with severe mental handicap.[98] Many parents would regard this as a less serious condition than Down's syndrome, where life expectancy can be up to 55–60 years with the majority requiring long-term care because of a high incidence of Alzheimer's disease. As Down's syndrome will account for approximately 17% of all aneuploidic fetuses with CP cysts, the risk of this chromosomal abnormality, when CP cysts themselves and no other anomalies are detected antenatally, approximates to 1 in 880. We would, therefore, be unable to justify karyotyping all fetuses, if the parents were concerned mainly about Down's syndrome rather than trisomy 18, *unless* other sonographic abnormalities were detected. Conversely, the trade-off of performing amniocentesis on all cases of apparently isolated CP cysts is that almost equal cases of abnormal karyotype will be detected as losing normal fetuses from miscarriage as a direct result of amniocentesis.

AGENESIS OF THE CORPUS CALLOSUM

As the cerebral cortex develops, groups of fibres called commissures connect corresponding areas of the cerebral hemispheres with one another. The most important of these commissures cross in the lamina terminalis, situated in the rostral (anterior) portion of the forebrain. This lamina extends from the roof of the diencephalon (caudal or posterior part of the forebrain) to the optic chiasma. The first commissures to form, the anterior commissure (connecting the olfactory bulbs, olfactory centres and related brain areas) and the hippocampal commissure (connecting the hippocampal formations), are small fibre bundles that connect phylogenetically older parts of the brain. The largest cerebral commissure is the arched corpus callosum connecting neocortical areas. The rostral part of the corpus callosum forms first between the 12th and 20th week of gestation which then progresses caudally only after the 20th week. It is thought that complete agenesis of the corpus callosum

(ACC) is caused by a vascular or inflammatory lesion occurring before the 12th week. Later insults may lead to partial agenesis affecting the later developing posterior portion.[99] In ACC, commissural fibres do not cross the midline, forming instead thick bundles of intersecting fibres, called Probst bundles, which lie along the superomedial aspect of the lateral ventricles. These bundles indent and separate the anterior horns of the lateral ventricles, and the third ventricle may sometimes be displaced upward. In most cases, there is a stable, non-progressive dilatation of the caudal portion of the lateral ventricles.[100] The reason for this enlargement is not known; there is no evidence of obstruction along the cerebrospinal fluid pathways and intraventricular pressure is normal. As the corpus callosum is in close anatomical and embryological relationship with the underlying septum pellucidum, this latter structure is frequently absent in ACC.[101] The corpus callosum is phylogenetically a recent structure and its absence is not essential for life functions. Isolated ACC may be either a completely asymptomatic finding or revealed during the course of an examination of subtle neurological deficits – apocryphally Leonardo da Vinci had ACC. More efficient non-callosal connections, bilateral development of speech functions and the increased use of the ipsilateral somatic sensory pathways may compensate for the functions that the corpus callosum usually carries out.[99]

Four syndromes (e.g. acrocallosal, Aicardi, Andermann and Shapiro) are characterized by ACC, while others are only sporadically associated (e.g. fetal alcohol syndrome, Dandy-Walker syndrome, Leigh's syndrome, Arnold-Chiari II syndrome). There is a high incidence of ACC in abnormalities of chromosomes 8, 11, 13–15 and 18 suggesting their involvement in abnormal corpus callosum morphogenesis.[102] A further association with tuberous sclerosis, mucopolysaccharidosis, basal cell nevus syndrome, maternal toxoplasmosis and maternal rubella has also been reported.[43] A comprehensive table detailing syndromes and abnormalities associated with ACC has been published previously.[103]

Up to 85% of postmortem cases have other anomalies of the CNS and up to 62% have extra-CNS abnormalities.[104] Common abnormalities are mental retardation (85%), seizures (42%), ocular anomalies (42%), gyral abnormalities (32%), hydrocephalus (23%), other CNS lesions (29%) (e.g. holoprosencephaly, microcephaly, macrocephaly), costovertebral defects (24%)[102] and cardiovascular, gastrointestinal and genitourinary anomalies.[105] ACC is therefore usually an incidental discovery during investigation of the many associated anomalies. It is these associated anomalies which give rise to symptoms such as seizures, neurological problems and developmental delay and are not usually caused by ACC per se.[106]

There is a discrepancy in the reported incidence of ACC. In one autopsy study, the frequency was 1:19 (5.3%)[100] while a radiological series, based on 6450 pneumoencephalograms, found an incidence of 0.7%.[107] ACC is present in 2–3% of the mentally retarded.[108] Fetal ACC can be demonstrated using the following diagnostic features (Fig. 10.11):

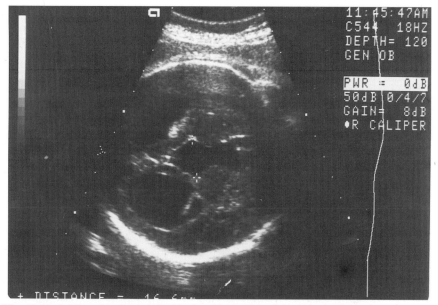

Fig. 10.11 Axial section through fetal brain with agenesis of the corpus callosum demonstrating dilated third ventricle (midline) and dilated occipital horns.

1. absence of the corpus callosum and septum pellucidum
2. increased separation of the lateral ventricles
3. marked separation of the slit-like anterior horns of the lateral ventricles and dilatation of the occipital horns creating the typical 'rabbit's ear' or 'tear drop' appearance, and
4. upward displacement of the third ventricle

Direct documentation of the absence of corpus callosum can be difficult with fetuses in vertex presentation but transvaginal sonography allows the diagnosis to be made with greater confidence and sometimes at early gestations.[109,110] The upward displacement of the third ventricle is regarded as a very specific sign[111] but this finding was only present in about one-half of the cases reported in two series.[43,110] The suspicion of partial or complete ACC should also be considered if lipoma of the corpus callosum is identified on antenatal sonography, which is easily visualized as a midline brightly echogenic mass. The chances of ACC in such cases is in the order of 50%, thought to be a result of the lipoma causing mechanical obstruction, thereby preventing normal development of the corpus callosum.[112]

The antenatal diagnosis of ACC has been reported in 70 cases from nine reports in the world English literature.[110,111,113–119] Detailed outcome of apparently isolated cases and cases where additional anomalies were detected on antenatal scans have been published previously.[103] There were 34 apparently isolated cases of which three were found to have other anomalies after

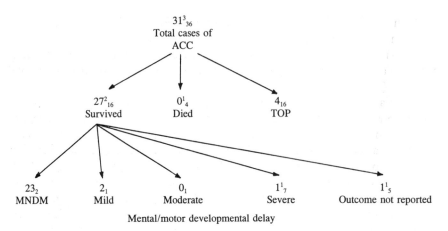

Fig. 10.12 Outcome of antenatally diagnosed cases of agenesis of corpus callosum reported in the English world literature. (Modified from Gupta and Lilford.[103])

delivery: one with severe developmental delay who had trisomy 8; one who died; and one in whom the outcome was not reported. Of the 31 confirmed isolated cases, there were four terminations of pregnancy and 27 survivors. Overall, 85% (23 of 27 cases) of the *apparently* isolated survivors (after excluding cases that died, had termination of pregnancy and where the outcome was not reported) are developing normally. Of the remaining four cases (15%), two have mild and two have severe mental/motor developmental delay; one of the latter group is associated with the fetal alcohol syndrome (Fig. 10.12). There were 36 cases (51%) where additional anomalies were detected during antenatal scans; almost half of the pregnancies were terminated and four died. Of the 16 survivors, only two (13%) are developing normally, nine (56%) have mental/motor developmental delay and the outcome was not reported in five (31%) (Fig. 12). In most cases the diagnosis of ACC was not made until the third trimester. This may be because the corpus callosum is not normally formed until 18 to 20 weeks gestation, thereby limiting early prenatal sonographic diagnosis. The mean duration of follow-up of all reported survivors was 29 months, but the range was wide: birth to 11 years.

Comment

Despite the limitations of early diagnosis, the value of an antenatal diagnosis of ACC is two-fold. First, as this condition is associated with a high incidence of other structural anomalies, a careful search of the entire fetal anatomy is required. The prognosis of cases with associated anomalies is very poor. Second, it is important to recognize that the sonographic appearance of ACC may be very similar to that of uncomplicated ventriculomegaly as the most striking finding is the enlargement of the occipital horns and atria resulting in the 'tear-drop' configuration.[110,119] Approximately 3% of all fetuses with ventriculomegaly[120] and almost 10% of those with mild ventriculomegaly[121] are noted to have ACC. The outcome in these cases is favourable; 59% of apparently isolated ventriculomegaly cases survive with a normal developmental quotient (see below).[122]

The diagnosis of *apparently* isolated fetal ACC (i.e. in the absence of other sonographically detectable anomalies) appears to carry an excellent prognosis, with an 85% chance of normal developmental outcome and 15% risk of handicap, after excluding cases that died, had termination of pregnancy or where the outcome was not reported. This is in keeping with the hypothesis that neurological impairment is not the consequence of ACC per se but rather of the many associated anomalies. However, fetal karyotyping may be indicated for all cases of ACC, independent of the presence of other sonographically detectable anomalies, as three of the four fetuses with trisomy 8 had ACC as the only sonographic finding; representing a 1 in 10 risk of aneuploidy (95% CI of 0.9–21.9%). Moreover, the diagnosis of ACC leads to concern regarding the possibility of an association with either genetic syndromes, inborn errors of metabolism or anatomic anomalies which cannot be tested by prenatal karyotyping. Other factors, which may aid the prognosis, have been reported. The upward displacement of the third ventricle and widened interhemispheric fissure are most frequently associated with neurological impairment, associated anomalies or both. Relative risks when these two findings are present are 2.2 (95% CI, 1.4–3) and 2.5 (95% CI, 1.6–3.4), respectively. Furthermore, there is a suggestion that fetuses with a good outcome tend to have larger cerebral ventricles than the ones with poor outcome.[110]

The precision of these estimations is low, but represent the best probabilistic information available to prospective parents at the current time. It is also possible that publication bias may reduce the accuracy of these estimates, but it is not possible to be certain how any such bias may work. Moreover, the duration of follow-up may be insufficient, and the results may therefore underestimate the incidence of minor neurological effects. Even in the presence of normal intelligence, ACC is associated with peculiar neurological findings and subtle cognitive deficits.[100,123–127] A possible relationship has also been hypothesized with psychotic disorders.[128]

DANDY-WALKER MALFORMATION

Dandy-Walker malformation (DWM) is characterized by the association of hydrocephalus of variable degree, a cyst in the posterior fossa and a defect in the cerebellar vermis through which the cyst communicates with the fourth ventricle[129] (Fig. 10.13). DWM is estimated to complicate approximately 1 in 25 000–35 000 pregnancies.[130]

The aetiology of DWM is unknown but it may occur as part of mendelian disorders such as Meckel-Grüber and Warburg syndromes. It has been found

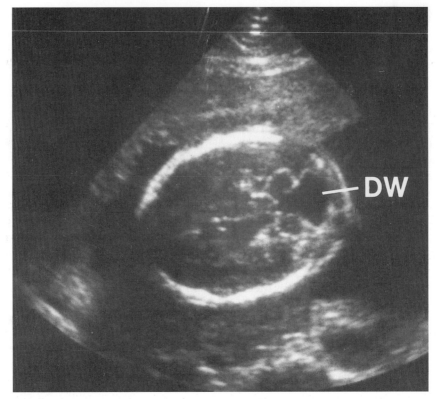

Fig. 10.13 Cranial sonogram demonstrating Dandy-Walker cyst (DW) with defect in the cerebellar vermis.

Recurrance 1-5%

in chromosomal aberrations e.g. trisomy 21, 18, and Turner's syndrome. Environmental factors such as viral infections, alcohol and diabetes have been suggested. When DWM is not associated with mendelian disorders, the recurrence risk has been quoted as 1–5%.[131] In rare cases, DWM is inherited as an autosomal recessive trait with a recurrence risk of 25%.[130] A similar anomaly to DWM, Joubert's syndrome (complete agenesis of the cerebellar vermis), is also inherited as an autosomal recessive trait, where the prognosis is universally poor.

The embryology of DWM is unclear. It was formally described by Dandy and Blackfan, at the beginning of the 20th century,[132,133] who postulated the condition to be secondary to congenital atresia of the foramina of Luschka and Magendie, leading to an enlargement of the ventricular system. Walker was the physician who described the first surgical treatment.[134] Benda[135] challenged the hypothesis suggested by these authors, but subsequently suggested the eponym, Dandy-Walker syndrome. The defect is now thought to represent a more complex developmental abnormality of the rhombo-encephalic structures.[135–137]

The differential diagnosis of DWM includes retrocerebellar arachnoid cyst and prominent fetal cisterna magna.[138–140] Unlike DWM, where the defect in the vermis is pathognomonic, the other two conditions are not associated with a vermian defect or other intrinsic cerebellar or cerebral abnormality.[138,141,142]

DWM is frequently associated with other CNS and extra-CNS abnormalities; necessitating a careful search of fetal anatomy in its entirety. A 50% incidence of CNS anomalies has been reported from clinical studies[143] and 68% from pathological studies.[137] ACC is particularly relevant because it is present in 7–17% of cases and carries a poor prognosis of intellectual outcome.[130, 143] Although hydrocephalus is usually described as a feature of DWM, it is present in an overall 60% (range 53–71%) of cases diagnosed in utero.[139, 144–146] Extracranial associated anomalies have been reported in 25–60% of cases.[137, 145] These include facial (e.g. dysmorphism, cleft palate haemangioma), heart (mainly ventriculoseptal defect, but also patent ductus arteriosus, pulmonary stenosis, coarctation of aorta, tetralogy of Fallot), skeletal (e.g. polydactyly, syndactyly), gastrointestinal (e.g. malrotation, Meckel's diverticulum) and genitourinary abnormalities (e.g. obstructive uropathy, urethral stenosis).[145]

The natural history of DWM is not well known. Enlargement of the posterior fossa cyst and worsening ventriculomegaly can be observed in utero,[139, 140, 145, 147] and because progressive changes are slow, conservative management is usually possible.[146] However, severe or rapidly progressing ventriculomegaly can necessitate aggressive intrauterine intervention[148] but its efficacy has yet to be proven. Of the cases not detected prenatally, 80–85% will present before 1 year of age with symptoms of hydrocephalus.[130,143]

The prognosis of DWM is difficult to determine because of ascertainment bias of the various antenatal and postnatal reports. The amalgamation of all the relevant reports gives the best available prognostic evidence.

The outcome of a total of 34 antenatally diagnosed cases of DWM have been reported in eight reports from the world English literature.[115,139,141,144–147,149] The overall mortality rate of the 26 survivors after excluding six cases of elective abortion and two cases of stillbirth, is 50%. Deaths were directly attributable to the associated congenital anomalies, mainly the extracranial malformations. Normal development was reported in only 15% of survivors but this is not a truly representative figure as the long-term outcome was not reported in 35% of cases. The analysis of postnatal neurosurgical series reports an overall mortality rate of 32% (42 cases out of 130).[130,143,150–152] Of the survivors, 53% (72 of 136 cases) have normal intelligence with an IQ greater than 80.[130,143,150–157] As with most other fetal brain abnormalities, the prognosis of in utero diagnosis of DWM appears to be worse than those reported postnatally, probably as the proportion of hopeless cases never come to surgery because of fetal or neonatal death. A less severe form of DWM, Dandy-Walker variant, has a much more favourable prognosis.[158] Seventeen cases have been reported from this series with 11 (65%)

survivors; 9 (82%) developing normally and the remaining 2 with severe developmental delay. Six of the 17 fetuses (35%) died in utero or during the neonatal period.

The obstetric management of DWM should include a detailed fetal sonographic examination, including fetal echocardiography, with an aim to identify additional cranial and extracranial anomalies. The presence of multiple congenital abnormalities adversely affects survival. If the diagnosis is made before viability, termination of pregnancy should be offered. If the parents choose to continue with the pregnancy, serial sonography should be performed for monitoring cyst size and ventriculomegaly. Fetal karyotyping is recommended.[131,139,144,145] Parents should be advised that there is a large probability that their child will eventually require neurosurgical shunting.

VENTRICULOMEGALY

Fetal ventriculomegaly, more commonly referred to as hydrocephalus, is defined as an increased intracranial content of CSF resulting in the enlargement of the ventricular system. CSF is formed mainly at the level of the choroid plexuses inside the ventricular system and flows slowly from the lateral ventricles via the third ventricle to the fourth ventricle. At this level, CSF passes through the foramina of Luschka and Magendie inside the subarachnoid space that externally bathes the cerebral structures. CSF is then absorbed by granulations distributed along the superior saggital sinus. Ventriculomegaly is the consequence of an obstruction along the normal pathway of the CSF.

The diagnosis of ventriculomegaly has traditionally relied on the demonstration of enlarged ventricles (Figs 10.14 & 10.15). Several nomograms have been developed where the lateral cerebral ventricular to hemispheric width (LVW : HW) ratio is abnormal for specific gestational ages.[159–161] However, the sensitivity of the LVW : HW ratio has been questioned in diagnosing early or mild ventricular dilatation.[160,162,163] Morphological, rather than pure biometrical, criteria have been suggested, including the simultaneous visualization of the medial and lateral ventricle,[163] the anterior displacement of the choroid plexus[164] and measurement of the atria of the lateral ventricle.[165]

Fetal ventriculomegaly is one of the most common congenital anomalies, reported to occur in approximately 0.5–2 per 1000 births.[166] The incidence of isolated neonatal hydrocephalus varies from 0.39–0.87 per 1000 births.[167] Several studies of isolated fetal ventriculomegaly give an incidence of 15–22% of all cases of antenatally diagnosed ventriculomegaly.[52,168,169] Many studies have demonstrated the frequency of concurrent anomalies associated with fetal ventriculomegaly – the incidence of associated intracranial and extracranial anomalies as 37% and 63%, respectively.[52] The single most common anomaly is spina bifida, with an incidence of 25–30%.[52,170,171] Other anomalies (cardiac, renal and gastrointestinal) range in frequency from 7–15%.[52] The

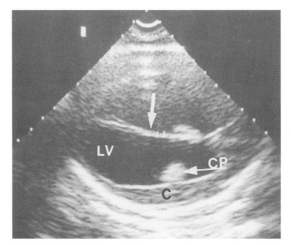

Fig. 10.14 Fetal ventriculomegaly. LV = dilated lateral ventricle; CP = dangling choroid plexus, arrow points to midline echo; C = compressed cerebral cortex.

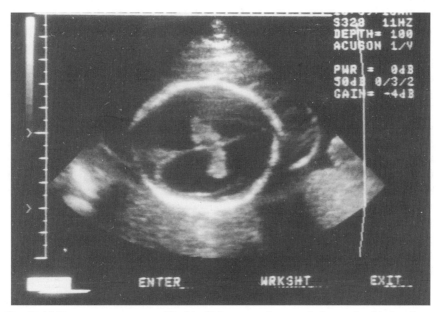

Fig. 10.15 Transverse sonogram of fetal head demonstrating ventriculomegaly with dangling choroid plexuses.

incidence of chromosomal abnormalities rises from 3%, with isolated ventriculomegaly, to 36% when additional anomalies are seen.[52,169,171]

Counselling is most difficult when none of these other features are detected because the prognosis is so uncertain (i.e. after excluding spina bifida, congenital infection (e.g. toxoplasmosis, cytomegalovirus, rubella),

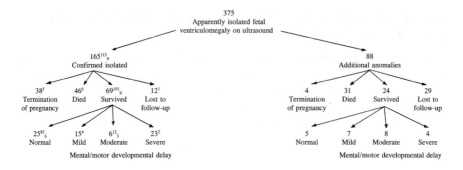

Numbers in superscript are cases with confirmed isolated borderline (mild) stable ventriculomegaly and cases with mild ventriculomegaly that resolved in utero

Numbers in subscript are those cases with progressive ventriculomegaly

For comprehensive tables of outcomes of all cases, see Gupta et al[191]

Fig. 10.16 Outcome of apparently isolated fetal ventriculomegaly reported in the English world literature.

chromosomal abnormalities and other structural anomalies). In mid-pregnancy, the most important decision is whether to continue or terminate the pregnancy. In late pregnancy the choice may be between cephalocentesis and vaginal delivery, with fetal sacrifice, versus Caesarean section. This information is very difficult to provide, especially as there is little or no correlation between the size of the ventricles and subsequent handicap.

A review of the world English literature on antenatal reports detailing the prognosis of apparently isolated ventriculomegaly is presented together with a summary of the current neurosurgical literature. A reference to the International Register of Fetal Surgery[172] and a separate analysis of reports of borderline (mild) isolated ventriculomegaly (e.g. Bromley et al[173]) and cases where ventriculomegaly resolved in utero (e.g. Mahony et al[174]) is included. The amalgamation of these reports gives prospective parents the best prognostic evidence available. Ventriculomegaly was graded in most reports on a scale from mild dilatation (cortex thickness >10 mm and normal biparietal diameter) to severe dilatation (cortex thickness <10 mm and an abnormally increased biparietal diameter).

There are 22 reports, covering 375 cases of apparently isolated ventriculomegaly.[168–170,172–190] Comprehensive tables detailing the outcomes have been published previously.[191] These include: 165 with confirmed isolated (non-borderline) ventriculomegaly, 113 with borderline (mild) ventriculomegaly, 9 with progressive ventriculomegaly and 88 with additional associated anomalies (Fig. 10.16). The mean duration of follow-up of all reported survivors was 19 months, but the range was wide; 1 to 66 months.

Prognosis for apparently isolated ventriculomegaly if additional anomalies were found after delivery

Nearly one-quarter of all cases of apparently isolated ventriculomegaly detected by ultrasound were shown to have additional associated structural anomalies after birth. The outcome for these cases is much worse than that for confirmed isolated ventriculomegaly (see below). Only 5 (21%) of the 24 survivors with additional anomalies where outcome is reported were found to be neurologically normal.

Prognosis of confirmed isolated ventriculomegaly

All cases out come / N mild, moderate, Severe handicap

Two hundred and eighty-seven cases were confirmed, at delivery, to have isolated ventriculomegaly. Forty-three pregnancies were terminated, 52 died, 13 were lost to follow-up and 179 survived: 114 (64%) with normal developmental quotient, and almost equal numbers were mildly (11%), moderately (12%) and severely (14%) handicapped. If the only cases included were those where follow-up was specifically reported to be over 18 months (*n* = 36), then 61% had normal developmental quotient, while 17%, 11% and 11% had mild, moderate and severe handicap, respectively. (Mild handicap, IQ 50–70; moderate handicap, IQ 35–49; severe handicap, IQ 20–34.)[192]

Borderline (mild) stable or resolving ventriculomegaly

A detailed breakdown of all 287 cases with confirmed isolated ventriculomegaly included 113 borderline cases; 101 of these had mild stable ventriculomegaly with 89 (88%) survivors of which 71 (80%) had a normal developmental quotient.[169,173,174,181,183,185,188] The remaining 12 cases of mild ventriculomegaly that resolved in utero had a normal developmental outcome.[173,174,185]

Progressive ventriculomegaly

Nine cases have been reported; six (67%) had a normal developmental quotient and three (33%) moderate developmental delay.[179,181,182,185,188] All required postnatal ventriculoperitoneal shunting.

Overall prognosis – apparently isolated ventriculomegaly

The overall prognosis for *apparently* isolated fetal ventriculomegaly (amalgamation of cases where additional anomalies were revealed at birth and similar cases confirmed to have isolated ventriculomegaly after birth) was available on a total of 286 infants (after excluding cases that underwent termination of pregnancy and those lost to follow-up), of whom 30% died, 29% survived with mental/motor developmental delay and 42% survived with normal developmental quotient. Similarly, if only cases where follow-up was specifically reported to be over 18 months ($n = 42$) are included, then 57% had a normal developmental quotient and 17%, 12% and 14% had mild, moderate and severe handicap, respectively.

Mode of delivery of isolated ventriculomegaly

The mode of delivery was detailed in 77 cases. Twenty-five cases were delivered by the vaginal route and 13 (52%) of these survived neurologically intact, three survived with developmental delay and nine (36%) died; five following intrapartum cephalocentesis. No cases had cephalocentesis and then survived. Of the 52 delivered by Caesarean section, 22 (42%) survived neurologically intact, 26 (50%) survived with developmental delay and four died. We accept, see below, that we might not be comparing like with like but can confirm that intrapartum cephalocentesis leads to death.

Prognosis and gestation at diagnosis

If the diagnosis of apparently isolated fetal ventriculomegaly was made by ultrasound in the second trimester ($n = 35$), 54% had a normal developmental outcome and 3% had mild or severe delay as opposed to 38%, 26% and 12%, respectively, where the diagnosis was made in the third trimester ($n = 66$). In 49 cases, the gestation when additional associated anomalies were missed, was reported. There is a three-fold increased risk of missing an additional anomaly if ultrasound is first performed in the third trimester rather than in the second trimester.

Fetal therapy

It would appear that fetal surgery has little to offer at the present time and may even be harmful; 27% deaths and 30% normal development compared to 5% deaths and 48% normal development in the in utero and postnatally treated cases, respectively.

Neurosurgical prognosis

The intellectual outcome of neurosurgical patients shows, by amalgamation of 19 reports covering a total of 1224 patients, that 74% survived at least 2 years and 53% of survivors have an IQ of 70 or above.[193-211] A comprehensive summary of these reports is given in Gupta et al.[191] The report from Laurence and Coates[200] is particularly interesting because, although 30 years old, it includes all cases, not just those deemed suitable for surgery. The prognostic figures in this series are worse than those reported in neurosurgical series and are in line with those reported for antenatally diagnosed cases.

There does not appear to be any method by which the prognosis of apparently isolated ventriculomegaly can be determined more accurately in the individual case. Some of the neurosurgical authors, for instance, find no relationship between prognosis and brain-mass-cortical thickness.[194,198,200,207] Others find a small correlation.[193,196,205,211,212] This distinction is not made in the antenatal cases.

Comment

Many abnormalities such as anencephaly, hydranencephaly, holoprosencephaly or microcephaly are either lethal or associated with severe handicap and a high mortality in infancy. The prognosis is uniformly bad and parents can be reliably advised of the expected outcome. Counselling is much more difficult when apparently isolated ventriculomegaly is discovered with no evidence of chromosomal abnormalities or intrauterine infection, because the prognosis is neither uniformly good nor overwhelmingly poor.

Parents should be warned that approximately one-quarter of cases of apparently isolated ventriculomegaly will subsequently be found to have other anomalies. Clearly, this figure will be higher in centres with the least experience and expertise and lower in those with the greatest skill.

There are, however, many biases in the prognostic figures given:

1. it could be argued that we have given an unduly pessimistic forecast by including cases from the International Register on in utero surgery,[172] because the outcome appears to be worse in this group. This could be the result of a harmful effect of the intervention and/or the bad prognosis of the cases referred for surgery (see below)
2. centres with a high termination of pregnancy rate among detected cases might have better prognosis among survivors, who might represent the milder cases. Against this, it is difficult to prognosticate because the cases with greatest dilatation might have only a slightly worse prognosis
3. centres whose patients tend to select a policy of intrapartum vaginal delivery might report a better prognosis through selective loss of the worst cases following cephalocentesis. Again, however, the cases requiring cephalocentesis might not, as mentioned above, have a much worse prognosis
4. centres with the longest follow-up might have the worst prognosis, because subtle neurological manifestations may be slow to appear
5. centres with unusually high or low follow-up rates might have better or worse prognosis; for example, families with severely affected children may be reluctant to move or may remain in contact with the hospital of birth
6. the threshold for reporting a case as positive may vary from centre to centre although, again, the potential for this form of bias is not great if we

are correct in our conclusion that the correlation between anatomical and functional severity is poor. In many series the proportion of cases needing postnatal shunting is low, suggesting that the degree of dilatation was mild in a large proportion of cases

7. centres with particularly good ultrasound, or reporting more recently, may record better outcomes for apparently isolated ventriculomegaly because they should detect a greater proportion of the associated anomalies on which the prognosis depends. Centres with a high invasive prenatal diagnosis rate should also bias results favourably by excluding chromosomal abnormalities

8. publication bias may influence the overall results although we cannot immediately see why particularly good or bad outcomes should be selectively reported

9. postnatally detected cases may have a better or worse prognosis. An improved prognosis might occur because other abnormalities are more easily detected and because some cases may have developed in late pregnancy. A worse prognosis would apply if some mild cases are not detected at all

10. the neurosurgical literature will inevitably be biased for survival from the perspective of parents who would like to think that Caesarean section is safer over vaginal delivery and cephalocentesis.

Is there any evidence that prenatal therapy, in the form of ultrasonically guided cephalocentesis or ventriculo-amniotic shunting, is of any positive benefit to the fetus? Experiments from animal studies[213] have shown encouraging results. In an effort to collate world experience of in utero treatment of fetal ventriculomegaly, the International Register of fetal surgery[172] includes the outcomes of these cases. This is obviously a potentially biased series but constitutes the best available evidence. However, the results of fetal surgery appear worse than those for postnatally operated cases.

There is little association between the degree of ventriculomegaly and intellect. This is because the aetiology of ventriculomegaly is more important than the degree. Ventriculomegaly commencing after the brain has formed (e.g. Arnold-Chiari) has little destructive effect because the brain is able to expand in the distensible fetal cranium. Ventriculomegaly caused by early obstruction (e.g. aqueductal stenosis) or brain shrinkage will, however, have a poor outlook which cannot be improved by fetal shunting. This said, our failure to find a clear relationship between severity (degree of dilatation) and prognosis might be influenced by intrapartum death in the most severe cases.

Ultrasonography is of limited help in distinguishing the underlying aetiology in cases of isolated hydrocephalus. Similarly, the size of the third ventricle or measurement of cerebrospinal fluid pressure are unlikely to provide good prognostic discrimination, but there is a possibility that nuclear resonance spectroscopy may be helpful in combination with electrophysiological measurements of brain function.[214]

Morbidity and mortality is associated not only with the underlying condition but also with the frequency of shunt infections, shunt obstruction and septicaemia, although these complications do not disturb intelligence.[193,196,204,206,207]

In conclusion, fetuses with ventriculomegaly, who on complete prenatal evaluation are otherwise normal, should be serially assessed by ultrasound (thereby excluding cases with progressive ventriculomegaly, which are uncommon). Delivery in these cases will depend upon the progressive increase in ventricular size, progressive cortical mantle thinning, abnormally rapid cranial growth and gestational age. The majority of remaining cases will either have borderline, non-progressive ventriculomegaly or ventriculomegaly that resolves in utero where a favourable outcome of normal mental development is expected. The outcome for antenatally diagnosed ventriculomegaly appears to be worse than that reported in the neurosurgical literature for children treated with congenital hydrocephalus. As most fetuses with ventriculomegaly will not have macrocrania, the method of delivery should be individualized as neither the vaginal route nor Caesarean section seems to have any advantage over the other. In utero shunting appears to offer no benefit and may even be harmful. Because of its destructive nature ultrasound-guided cephalocentesis should not be used on fetuses having hydrocephalus without severe anomalies. Postnatally, ventricular decompression with ventriculoperitoneal shunts should be performed using well established neurosurgical indications; this carries a favourable outcome. The outcome is much worse when other associated anomalies are present.

REFERENCES

1 McCullough L B, Chervenak F A. Obstetric ethics. New York: Oxford University Press, 1994
2 Beauchamp T L, Childress J F. Principles of biomedical ethics. 3rd ed. New York: Oxford University Press, 1989
3 Brocklehurst G. Spina bifida. In: Vinken P J, Bruyn G W, eds. Handbook of clinical neurology. Amsterdam: Elsevier/North Holland Biomedical Press, 1978; 32: pp 519–578
4 Giroud A. Anencephaly. In: Vinken P J, Bruyn G W, eds. Handbook of clinical neurology. Amsterdam: Elsevier/North Holland Biomedical Press, 1977; 30: pp 173–208
5 Chervenak F A, Farley M A, Walters L, Hobbins J C, Mahony M J. When is termination of pregnancy during the third trimester morally justifiable? N Engl J Med 1984; 310: 501–504
6 Holzgreve W, Beller F K, Buchholz B, Hansmann M, Köhler K. Kidney transplantation from anencephalic donors. N Engl J Med 1987; 316: 1069–1070
7 DeMyer W, Zeman W. Alobar holoprosencephaly (arhinencephaly) with median cleft lip and palate: Clinical, electroencephalographic and nosologic considerations. Confin Neurol 1963; 23: 1–36
8 DeMyer W. Holoprosencephaly (Cyclopia-arhinencephaly). In: Vinken P J, Bruyn G W, eds. Handbook of clinical neurology. Amsterdam: Elsevier/North Holland Biomedical Press, 1977; 30: pp 431–478
9 Pretorius D H, Russ P D, Rumack C M, Manco-Johnson M L. Diagnosis of brain neuropathology in utero. Neuroradiology 1986; 28: 386–397
10 Babcock D S. Sonography of congenital malformations of the brain. Neuroradiology 1986; 28: 428–439
11 Blackwell D E, Spinnato J A, Hirsch G, Giles H R, Sackler J. Antenatal ultrasound diagnosis of holoprosencephaly: A case report. Am J Obstet Gynecol 1982; 143: 848–849
12 Chervenak F A, Isaacson G, Mahoney M J, Tortora M, Mesologites T, Hobbins J C. The

obstetric significance of holoprosencephaly. Obstet Gynecol 1984; 63: 115–121
13 Chervenak F A, Isaacson G, Hobbins J C, Chitkara U, Tortora M, Berkowitz R L.
    Diagnosis and management of fetal holoprosencephaly. Obstet Gynecol 1985; 66: 322–326
14 Filly R A, Chinn D H, Callen P W. Alobar holoprosencephaly: Ultrasonographic prenatal
    diagnosis. Radiology 1984; 151: 455–459
15 Hill L M, Breckle C R, Bonebrake C R. Ultrasonic findings with holoprosencephaly. J
    Reprod Med 1982; 27: 172–175
16 Mok P M, Douglas-Jones A G. Prenatal diagnosis of holoprosencephaly by sonography.
    Aust Radiol 1983; 27: 5–7
17 Nyberg D A, Mack L A, Bronstein A, Hirsch J, Pagon R A. Holoprosencephaly: Prenatal
    sonographic diagnosis. Am J Roentgenol 1987; 149: 1051–1058
18 Pilu G, Romero R, Rizzo N, Jeanty P, Bovicelli L, Hobbins J C. Criteria for the prenatal
    diagnosis of holoprosencephaly. Am J Perinatol 1987; 4: 41–49
19 Roach E, DeMyer W, Conneally P M, Palmer C, Merritt A D. Holoprosencephaly: Birth
    data, genetic, and demographic analyses of 30 families. Birth Defects 1975; 11: 294–313
20 Saunders E S, Shortland D, Dunn P M. What is the incidence of holoprosencephaly? J Med
    Genet 1984; 21: 21–26
21 Matsunaga E, Shiota K. Holoprosencephaly in human embryos: Epidemiologic studies of
    150 cases. Teratology 1977; 16: 261–272
22 Berry S M, Gosden C, Snijders R J, Nicolaides K H. Fetal holoprosencephaly: associated
    malformations and chromosomal defects. Fetal Diag Ther 1990; 5: 92–99
23 Cohen M. An update of the holoprosencephalic disorders. J Pediatr 1982; 101: 865–869
24 Dekaban A S. Effects of X-radiation on mouse fetus during gestation: Emphasis on
    distribution of cerebral lesions. Part II. J Nucl Med 1969; 10: 68–77
25 Keeler R F. Teratogenic compounds of Veratrum Californicum (Durand) X. Cyclopia in
    rabbits produced by cyclopamine. Teratology 1970; 3: 175–180
26 Barr M, Hanson J W, Currey K et al. Holoprosencephaly in infants of diabetic mothers. J
    Pediatr 1983; 102: 565–568
27 Ronen G M, Andrews W L. Holoprosencephaly as a possible embryonic alcohol effect. Am
    J Med Genet 1991; 40: 151–154
28 Hsia Y E, Bratu M, Herbordt A. Genetics of the Meckal syndrome (dysencephalia
    splanchnocystica). Pediatrics 1971; 48: 237–247
29 Hennekam R C, van Noort G, de la Fuente A. Familial holoprosencephaly, heart defects,
    and polydactyly. Am J Med Genet 1991; 41: 258–262
30 Benke P J, Cohen M. Recurrence of holoprosencephaly in families with a positive history.
    Clin Genet 1983; 24: 324–328
31 Collins A L, Lunt P W, Garrett C, Dennis N R. Holoprosencephaly: a family showing
    dominant inheritance and variable expression. J Med Genet 1993; 30: 36–40
32 Manelfe C, Sevely A. Neuroradiological study of holoprosencephalies. J Neuroradiol 1982;
    9: 15–45
33 Bronshtein M, Wiener Z. Early transvaginal sonographic diagnosis of alobar
    holoprosencephaly. Prenat Diag 1991; 11: 459–462
34 Nelson L H, King M. Early diagnosis of holoprosencephaly. J Ultrasound Med 1992; 11:
    57–59
35 Chervenak F A, Romero R. Is there a role for fetal cephalocentesis in modern obstetrics?
    Am J Perinatol 1984; 1: 170–172
36 Myers R E. Brain pathology following fetal vascular occlusion: An experimental study.
    Invest Ophthalmol 1969; 8: 41–50
37 Altshuler G. Toxoplasmosis as a cause of hydranencephaly. Am J Dis Child 1973; 125:
    251–252
38 Halsey J H, Allen N, Chamberlin H R. Hydranencephaly. In: Vinken P J, Bruyn G W, eds.
    Handbook of clinical neurology. Amsterdam: Elsevier/North Holland Biomedical Press,
    1977; 30: pp 661–680
39 Nishimura H, Okamoto N. Iniencephaly. In: Vinken P J, Bruyn G W, eds. Handbook of
    clinical neurology. Amsterdam: Elsevier/North Holland Biomedical Press, 1977; 30: pp
    257–268
40 Bluett D. Iniencephaly causing obstructed labour. Proc Royal Soc Med 1968; 61:
    1281–1282
41 Cunningham I. Iniencephalus: A cause of dystocia. J Obstet Gynaecol Br Commonwealth
    1965; 72: 299–301

42 Chervenak F A, Rosenberg J, Brightman R C, Chitkara U, Jeanty P. A prospective study of the accuracy of ultrasound in predicting fetal microcephaly. Obstet Gynecol 1987; 69: 908–910

43 Romero R, Pilu G, Jeanty P, Ghidini A, Hobbins J C. The central nervous system. In: Prenatal diagnosis of congenital anomalies. Norwalk: Appleton & Lange, 1988: pp 1–79

44 Pearce J M, Little D, Campbell S. The diagnosis of abnormalities of the fetal central nervous system. In: Sanders R C, James E A, eds. The principles and practice of ultrasonography in obstetrics and gynecology. 3rd ed. Norwalk: Appleton-Century-Crofts, 1985: pp 243–256

45 Goldstein I, Reece E A, Pilu G, O'Connor T Z, Lockwood C J, Hobbins J C. Sonographic assessment of the fetal frontal lobe: A potential tool for prenatal diagnosis of microcephaly. Am J Obstet Gynecol 1988; 158: 1057–1062

46 Ross J J, Frias J L. Microcephaly. In: Vinken P J, Bruyn G W, eds. Handbook of clinical neurology. Amsterdam: Elsevier/North Holland Biomedical Press, 1977; 30: pp 507–524

47 Warkany J. Microcephaly. In: Congenital malformations. Chicago: Year Book, 1971: pp 237–244

48 Avery G B, Meneses L, Lodge A. The clinical significance of Measurement Microcephaly. Am J Dis Child 1972; 123: 214–217

49 Pryor H B, Thelander H. Abnormally small head size and intellect in children. J Pediatr 1968; 73: 593–598

50 Cantu R C, LeMay M. Porencephaly caused by intracerebral hemorrhage. Radiology 1967; 88: 526–530

51 Gross H, Simanyi M. Porencephaly. In: Vinken P J, Bruyn G W, eds. Handbook of clinical neurology. Amsterdam: Elsevier/North Holland Biomedical Press, 1977; 30: pp 681–692

52 Chervenak F A, Berkowitz R L, Romero R et al. The diagnosis of fetal hydrocephalus. Am J Obstet Gynecol 1983; 147: 703–716

53 Robinson H P, Hood V D, Adam A H, Gibson A, Ferguson-Smith M A. Diagnostic ultrasound: early detection of fetal neural tube defects. Obstet Gynecol 1980; 56: 705–710

54 Cohen M M, Lemire R J. Syndromes with cephaloceles. Teratology 1982; 25: 161–172

55 Chervenak F A, Issacson G, Mahoney M J, Berkowitz R L, Tortora M, Hobbins J C. Diagnosis and management of fetal cephalocele. Obstet Gynecol 1984; 64: 86–91

56 Fiske C E, Filly R A. Ultrasound evaluation of the normal and abnormal fetal neural axis. Radiol Clin N Am 1982; 20: 285–296

57 Graham D, Johnson T R, Winn K, Sanders R C. The role of sonography in the prenatal diagnosis and management of encephalocele. J Ultrasound Med 1982; 1: 111–115

58 Nicolini U, Ferrazzi E, Massa E, Minonzio M, Pardi G. Prenatal diagnosis of cranial masses by ultrasound: Report of five cases. J Clin Ultrasound 1983; 11: 170–174

59 Pilu G, Rizzo N, Orsini L F, Bovicelli L. Antenatal recognition of cerebral anomalies. Ultrasound Med Biol 1986; 12: 319–326

60 Winter T C, Mack L A, Cyr D R. Prenatal sonographic diagnosis of scalp/cephalohematoma mimicking an encephalocele. Am J Roentgenol 1993; 161: 1247–1248

61 Bronshtein M, Bar-Hava I, Blumenfeld Z. Early second-trimester sonographic appearance of occipital haemangioma simulating encephalocele. Prenat Diag 1992; 12: 695–698

62 Lorber J. The prognosis of occipital encephalocele. Dev Med Child Neurol Suppl 1967; 13: 75–86

63 Field B. Anencephalus, encephalocele and spinal meningomyelocele. Med J Aust 1974; 1: 889–890

64 Lipschitz R, Beck J M, Froman C. An assessment of the treatment of encephalomeningoceles. S Afr Med J 1969; 43: 609–610

65 Lorber J, Schofield J K. The prognosis of occipital encephalocele. Z Kinderchir 1979; 28: 347–351

66 McLaurin R L. Parietal cephaloceles. Neurology 1964; 14: 764–772

67 Mealey J, Ozenitis A J, Hockey A A. The prognosis of encephaloceles. J Neurosurg 1970; 32: 209–218

68 Shuangshoti S, Netsky M G. Neuroepithelial (colloid) cysts of the nervous system. Further observations on pathogenesis, location, incidence and histochemistry. Neurology 1966; 16: 887–903

69 Shuangshoti S, Roberts M P, Netsky M G. Neuroepithelial (colloid) cysts: Pathogenesis and relation to choroid plexus and ependyma. Arch Path (Chicago) 1965; 80: 214–224

70 Fakhry J, Schechter A, Tenner M S, Reale M. Cysts of the choroid plexus in neonates: Documentation and review of the literature. J Ultrasound Med 1985; 4: 561–563

71 Chudleigh P, Pearce J M, Campbell S. The prenatal diagnosis of transient cysts of the fetal choroid plexus. Prenat Diag 1984; 4: 135–137

72 Ostlere S J, Irving H C, Lilford R J. A prospective study of the incidence and significance of fetal choroid plexus cysts. Prenat Diag 1989; 9: 205–211

73 Gupta J K, Chervenak F A, Lilford R J. Assessment of other congenital abnormalities of the fetal brain. In: Levene M I, Lilford R J, Bennett M J, Punt J, eds. Fetal and neonatal neurology and neurosurgery. 2nd ed. Edinburgh: Churchill Livingstone, 1995; pp 231–248

74 Achiron R, Barkai G, Katznelson B, Mashiach S. Fetal lateral ventricle choroid plexus cysts: The dilemma of amniocentesis. Obstet Gynecol 1991; 78: 815–818

75 Camurri L, Ventura A. Prospective study on trisomy 18 and fetal choroid plexus cysts. Prenat Diag 1989; 9: 742

76 Chan L, Hixson J L, Laifer S A, Marchese S G, Martin J G, Hill L M. A sonographic and karyotypic study of second-trimester fetal choroid plexus cysts. Obstet Gynecol 1989; 73: 703–705

77 Chinn D H, Miller E I, Worthy L M, Towers C V. Sonographically detected fetal choroid plexus cysts. Frequency and association with aneuploidy. J Ultrasound Med 1991; 10: 255–258

78 Chitkara U, Cogswell C, Norton K, Wilkins I A, Mehalek K, Berkowitz R L. Choroid plexus cysts in the fetus: A benign anatomic variant or pathologic entity? Report of 41 cases and review of the literature. Obstet Gynecol 1988; 72: 185–189

79 Chitty L S, Chudleigh T. Choroid plexus cysts – when to karyotype? Br Med Ultrasound Soc Bull 1993; 1: 40–41

80 Clark S L, DeVore G R, Sabey P L. Prenatal diagnosis of cysts of the fetal choroid plexus. Obstet Gynecol 1988; 72: 585–587

81 Gabrielli S, Reece A, Pilu G et al. The clinical significance of prenatally diagnosed choroid plexus cysts. Am J Obstet Gynecol 1989; 160: 1207–1210

82 Gupta J K, Cave M, Lilford R J, Farrell T A, Irving H, Mason G, Hau C M. The clinical significance of choroid plexus cysts. Lancet 1995 (submitted)

83 Howard R J, Tuck S M, Long J, Thomas V A. The significance of choroid plexus cysts in fetuses at 18–20 weeks. An indication for amniocentesis? Prenat Diag 1992; 12: 685–688

84 Nadel A S, Bromley B S, Frigoletto F D, Estroff J A, Benacerraf B R. Isolated choroid plexus cysts in the second-trimester fetus: Is amniocentesis really indicated? Radiology 1992; 185: 545–548

85 Ostlere S J, Irving H C, Lilford R J. Choroid plexus cysts in the fetus. Lancet 1987; i: 1491

86 Ostlere S J, Irving H C, Lilford R J. Fetal choroid plexus cysts: A report of 100 cases. Radiology 1990; 175: 753–755

87 Platt L D, Carlson D E, Medearis A L, Walla C A. Fetal choroid plexus cysts in the second trimester of pregnancy: A cause for concern. Am J Obstet Gynecol 1991; 164: 1652–1656

88 Porto M, Murata Y, Warneke L A, Keegan K A. Fetal choroid plexus cysts: An independent risk factor for chromosomal anomalies. J Clin Ultrasound 1993; 21: 103–108

89 Twinning P, Zuccollo J, Clewes J, Swallow J. Fetal choroid plexus cysts: a prospective study and review of the literature. Br J Radiol 1991; 64: 98–102

90 Walkinshaw S, Pilling D, Spriggs A. Isolated choroid plexus cysts – the need for routine offer of karyotyping. Prenat Diag 1994; 14: 663–667

91 Zerres K, Schuler H, Gembruch U, Bald R, Hansmann M, Schwanitz G. Chromosomal findings in fetuses with prenatally diagnosed cysts of the choroid plexus. Hum Genet 1992; 89: 301

92 Allan L D, Crawford D C, Anderson R H, Tynan M J. Echocardiographic and anatomical correlations in fetal congenital heart disease. Br Heart J 1984; 52: 542–548

93 Copel J A, Pilu G, Kleinman C S. Congenital heart disease and extracardiac anomalies: Associations and indications for fetal echocardiography. Am J Obstet Gynecol 1986; 154: 1121–1132

94 Benacerraf B R, Harlow B, Frigoletto F D. Are choroid plexus cysts an indication for second-trimester amniocentesis? Am J Obstet Gynecol 1990; 162: 1001–1006

95 Fitzsimmons J, Wilson D, Pascoe-Mason J, Shaw C M, Cyr D R, Mack L A. Choroid plexus cysts in fetuses with trisomy 18. Obstet Gynecol 1989; 73: 257–260

96 Nyberg D A, Kramer D, Resta R G, Kapur R, Mahony B S, Luthy D A. Prenatal sonographic findings of trisomy 18: Review of 47 cases. J Ultrasound Med 1993; 12: 103–113

97 Benacerraf B R, Miller W A, Frigoletto F D. Sonographic detection of fetuses with trisomies 13 and 18: Accuracy and limitations. Am J Obstet Gynecol 1988; 158: 404–409
98 Root S, Carey J C. Survival in trisomy 18. Am J Med Genet 1994; 49: 170–174
99 Guibert-Tranier F, Piton J, Billerey J, Caille J M. Agenesis of the corpus callosum. J Neuroradiol 1982; 9: 135–160
100 Ettlinger G. Agenesis of the corpus callosum. In: Vinken P J, Bruyn G W, eds. Handbook of clinical neurology. Amsterdam: Elsevier/North Holland Biomedical Press, 1977; 30: pp 285–297
101 Leech R W, Shuman R M. Holoprosencephaly and related midline cerebral anomalies: a review. J Child Neurol 1986; 1: 3–17
102 Jeret J S, Serur D, Wisniewski K E, Lubin R A. Clinicopathological findings associated with agenesis of the corpus callosum. Brain Dev 1987; 9: 255–264
103 Gupta J K, Lilford R J. Assessment and management of fetal agenesis of the corpus callosum. Prenat Diag 1995 (in Press)
104 Parrish M, Roessman U, Levinsohn M. Agenesis of the corpus callosum: A study of the frequency of associated malformations. Ann Neurol 1979; 6: 349–352
105 Franco I, Kogan S, Fisher J et al. Genitourinary malformations associated with agenesis of the corpus callosum. J Urol 1993; 149: 1119–1121
106 Byrd S E, Harwood-Nash D C, Fitz C R. Absence of the corpus callosum. Computed tomographic evaluation in infants and children. J Can Assoc Radiol 1978; 29: 108–112
107 Grogono J L. Children with agenesis of the corpus callosum. Dev Med Child Neurol 1968; 10: 613–616
108 Jeret J S, Serur D, Wisniewski K E, Fisch C. Frequency of agenesis of the corpus callosum in the developmentally disabled population as determined by computerized tomography. Pediatr Neurosci 1985–1986; 12: 101–103
109 Hilpert P L, Kurtz A B. Prenatal diagnosis of agenesis of the corpus callosum using endovaginal ultrasound. J Ultrasound Med 1990; 9: 363–365
110 Pilu G, Sandri F, Perolo A et al. Sonography of fetal agenesis of corpus callosum: a survey of 35 cases. Ultrasound Obstet Gynecol 1993; 3: 318–329
111 Comstock C H, Culp D, Gonzalez J, Boal D B. Agenesis of the corpus callosum in the fetus. Its evolution and significance. J Ultrasound Med 1985; 4: 613–616
112 Mulligan G, Meier P. Lipoma and agenesis of the corpus callosum with associated choroid plexus lipomas – in utero diagnosis. J Ultrasound Med 1989; 8: 583–588
113 Bertino R E, Nyberg D A, Cyr D R, Mack L A. Prenatal diagnosis of agenesis of corpus callosum. J Ultrasound Med 1988; 7: 251–260
114 Blum A, André M, Droullé P, Husson S, Leheup B. Prenatal echographic diagnosis of corpus callosum agenesis. The Nancy experience 1982–1989. Genet Couns 1990; 1: 115–126
115 Bryce F C, Lilford R J, Rodeck C. Antenatal diagnosis of craniospinal defects. In: Lilford R J, ed. Prenatal diagnosis and prognosis. London: Butterworth, 1990; pp 5–29
116 Meizner I, Barki Y, Hertzanu Y. Prenatal sonographic diagnosis of agenesis of corpus callosum. J Clin Ultrasound 1987; 15: 262–264
117 Verco P W, LeQuesne G W. Agenesis of the corpus callosum in the fetus, neonate and infant. Australas Radiol 1987; 31: 129–135
118 Vergani P, Ghidini A, Mariani S, Greppi P, Negri R. Antenatal sonographic findings of agenesis of corpus callosum. Am J Perinatol 1988; 5: 105–108
119 Warren M E, Cook J V. Case report: Agenesis of the corpus callosum. Br J Radiol 1993; 66: 81–85
120 Filly R A, Cardoza J D, Goldstein R B, Barkovich A J. Detection of fetal central nervous system anomalies. A practical level of effort for routine sonogram. Radiology 1988; 172: 403–408
121 Goldstein R B, LaPidus A S, Filly R A, Cardoza J D. Mild lateral cerebral ventriculomegaly. Clinical course and outcome. Am J Obstet Gynecol 1990; 164: 863–867
122 Gupta J K, Bryce F, Lilford R J. Management of apparently isolated fetal ventriculomegaly. Obstet Gynecol Surv 1994; 49: 716–721
123 Fischer M, Ryan S B, Dobyns W B. Mechanisms of interhemispheric transfer and patterns of cognitive functions in acallosal patients of normal intelligence. Arch Neurol 1992; 49: 271–277
124 Jeeves M A. Stereoperception in callosal agenesis and partial callosotomy. Neuropsychologica 1991; 29: 19–34

125 Karnath H O, Schumacher M, Wallesch C W. Limitations of interhemispheric extracallosal transfer of visual information in callosal agenesis. Cortex 1991; 27: 345–350

126 Temple C M, Jeeves M A, Villaroya O. Ten pen men: Rhyming skills in two children with callosal agenesis. Brain Lang 1989; 37: 548–564

127 Temple C M, Jeeves M A, Villaroya O. Reading in callosal agenesis. Brain Lang 1990; 39: 235–253

128 Swayze V M, Andreasen N C, Ehrardt J C, Yuh W T, Allinger R J, Cohen G A. Developmental abnormalities of the corpus callosum in schizophrenia. Arch Neurol 1990; 47: 805–808

129 Brown J R. The Dandy-Walker syndrome. In: Vinken P J, Bruyn G W, eds. Handbook of clinical neurology. Amsterdam: Elsevier/North Holland Biomedical Press, 1977; 30: pp 623–646

130 Hirsch J F, Pierre-Kahn A, Renier D, Sainte-Rose C, Hoppe-Hirsch E. The Dandy-Walker malformation. A review of 40 cases. J Neurosurg 1984; 61: 515–522

131 Murray J C, Johnson J A, Bird T D. Dandy-Walker malformation: etiologic heterogeneity and empiric recurrence risks. Clin Genet 1985; 28: 272–283

132 Dandy W E, Blackfan K D. Internal hydrocephalus: An experimental, clinical and pathological study. Am J Dis Child 1914; 8: 406–482

133 Dandy W E. The diagnosis and treatment of hydrocephalus due to occlusions of the foramina of Magendie and Luschka. Surg Gynecol Obstet 1921; 32: 112–124

134 Taggart J K, Walker A E. Congenital atresia of foramens of Luschka and Magendie. Arch Neurol Psychiatr 1942; 48: 583–612

135 Benda C E. The Dandy-Walker syndrome or the so-called atresia of foramen Magendie. J Neuropathol Exp Neurol 1954; 13: 14–29

136 Gardner E, O'Rahilly R, Prolo D. The Dandy-Walker and Arnold-Chiari malformations: Clinical, developmental and teratological considerations. Arch Neurol 1975; 32: 393–407

137 Hart M N, Malamud N, Ellis W G. The Dandy-Walker syndrome: A clinicopathological study based on 28 cases. Neurology 1972; 22: 771–780

138 Mahony B S, Callen P W, Filly R A, Hoddick W K. The fetal cisterna magna. Radiology 1984; 153: 773–776

139 Pilu G, Romero R, DePalma L et al. Antenatal diagnosis and obstetrical management of Dandy-Walker syndrome. J Reprod Med 1986; 31: 1017–1022

140 Taylor G A, Sanders R C. Dandy-Walker syndrome: Recognition by sonography. Am J Neuroradiol 1983; 4: 1203–1206

141 Dempsey P J, Koch H J. In utero diagnosis of the Dandy-Walker syndrome: Differentiation from extra-axial posterior fossa cyst. J Clin Ultrasound 1981; 9: 403–405

142 Raybaud C. Cystic malformations of the posterior fossa: Abnormalities associated with the development of the roof of the fourth ventricle and adjacent meningeal structures. J Neuroradiol 1982; 9: 103–133

143 Sawaya R, McLaurin R L. Dandy-Walker syndrome. Clinical analysis of 23 cases. J Neurosurg 1981; 55: 89–98

144 Nyberg D A, Cyr D R, Mack L A, Fitzsimmons J, Hickok D, Mahony B S. The Dandy-Walker malformation: Prenatal sonographic diagnosis and its clinical significance. J Ultrasound Med 1988; 7: 65–71

145 Russ P D, Pretorius D H, Johnson M J. Dandy-Walker syndrome: A review of fifteen cases evaluated by prenatal sonography. Am J Obstet Gynecol 1989; 161: 401–406

146 Serlo W, Kirkinen P, Heikkinen E, Jouppila P. Ante- and postnatal evaluation of the Dandy-Walker syndrome. Childs Nerv Syst 1985; 1: 148–151

147 Hatjis C G, Horbar J D, Anderson G G. The in utero diagnosis of a posterior fossa intracranial cyst (Dandy-Walker cyst). Am J Obstet Gynecol 1981; 140: 473–475

148 Depp R, Sabbagha R E, Brown J T, Tamura R K, Reedy N J. Fetal surgery for hydrocephalus: Successful in utero ventriculoamniotic shunt for Dandy-Walker syndrome. Obstet Gynecol 1983; 61: 710–714

149 Newman G C, Buschi A I, Sugg N K, Kelly T E, Miller J Q. Dandy-Walker syndrome diagnosed in utero by ultrasonography. Neurology 1982; 32: 180–184

150 Carmel P W, Antunes J L, Hilal S K, Gold A P. Dandy-Walker syndrome: Clinico-pathological features and re-evaluation of modes of treatment. Surg Neurol 1977; 8: 132–138

151 Golden J A, Rorke L B, Bruce D A. Dandy-Walker syndrome and associated anomalies. Pediatr Neurosci 1987; 13: 38–44

152 Tal Y, Freigang B, Dunn H G, Durity F A, Moyes P D. Dandy-Walker Syndrome: Analysis of 21 cases. Dev Med Child Neurol 1980; 22: 189–201

153 Carteri A, Gerosa M, Gaini S M, Villani R. The dysraphic state of the posterior fossa. Clinical review of the Dandy-Walker syndrome and the so-called arachnoid cysts. J Neurosurg Sci 1979; 23: 53–59

154 Fischer E G. Dandy-Walker syndrome: An evaluation of surgical treatment. J Neurosurg 1973; 39: 615–621

155 James H E, Kaiser G, Schut L, Bruce D A. Problems of diagnosis and treatment in the Dandy-Walker syndrome. Childs Brain 1979; 5: 24–30

156 Maria B L, Zinreich S J, Carson B C, Rosenbaum A E, Freeman J M. Dandy-Walker syndrome revisited. Pediatr Neurosci 1987; 13: 45–51

157 Udvarhelyi G B, Epstein M H. The so-called Dandy-Walker syndrome: Analysis of 12 operated cases. Childs Brain 1975; 1: 158–182

158 Estroff J A, Scott M R, Benacerraf B R. Dandy-Walker variant: Prenatal sonographic features and clinical outcome. Radiology 1992; 185: 755–758

159 Denkhaus H, Winsberg F. Ultrasonic measurement of the fetal ventricular system. Radiology 1979; 131: 781–787

160 Jeanty P, Dramaix-Wilmet M, Delbeke D, Rodesch F, Struyven J. Ultrasonic evaluation of fetal ventricular growth. Neuroradiology 1981; 21: 127–131

161 Johnson M L, Dunne M G, Mack L A, Rashbaum C L. Evaluation of fetal intracranial anatomy by static and real-time ultrasound. J Clin Ultrasound 1980; 8: 311–318

162 Chervenak F A, Berkowitz R L, Tortora M, Chitkara U, Hobbins J C. Diagnosis of ventriculomegaly before fetal viability. Obstet Gynecol 1984; 64: 652–656

163 Fiske C E, Filly R A, Callen P W. Sonographic measurement of lateral ventricular width in early ventricular dilation. J Clin Ultrasound 1981; 9: 303–307

164 Chinn D H, Callen P W, Filly R A. The lateral cerebral ventricle in early second trimester. Radiology 1983; 148: 529–531

165 Campbell S, Pearce J M. Ultrasound visualization of congenital malformations. Br Med Bull 1983; 39: 322–331

166 Ferry P C, Pernoll M L. Rational management of perinatal hydrocephalus. Am J Obstet Gynecol 1976; 126: 151–152

167 Habib Z. Genetics and genetic counselling in neonatal hydrocephalus. Obstet Gynecol Surv 1981; 36: 529–534

168 Chervenak F A, Berkowitz R L, Tortora M, Hobbins J C. The management of fetal hydrocephalus. Am J Obstet Gynecol 1985; 151: 933–942

169 Nicolaides K H, Berry S, Snijders R J M, Thorpe-Beeston J G, Gosden C. Fetal lateral cerebral ventriculomegaly: Associated malformations and chromosomal defects. Fetal Diagn Ther 1990; 5: 5–14

170 Twinning P, Jaspan T, Zuccollo J. The outcome of fetal ventriculomegaly. Br J Radiol 1994; 67: 26–31

171 Vintzileos A M, Ingardia C J, Nochimson D J. Congenital hydrocephalus. A review and protocol for perinatal management. Obstet Gynecol 1983; 62: 539–548

172 Manning F A, Harrison M R, Rodeck C. Catheter shunts for fetal hydronephrosis and hydrocephalus. Report of the International Fetal Surgery Registry. N Eng J Med 1986; 315: 336–340

173 Bromley B, Frigoletto F D, Benacerraf B R. Mild fetal lateral cerebral ventriculomegaly: Clinical course and outcome. Am J Obstet Gynecol 1991; 164: 863–867

174 Mahony B S, Nyberg D A, Hirsch J H, Petty C N, Hendricks S K, Mack L A. Mild idiopathic lateral cerebral ventricular dilatation in utero: Sonographic evaluation. Radiology 1988; 169: 715–721

175 Amacher A L, Reid W D. Hydrocephalus diagnosed prenatally. Outcome of surgical therapy. Childs Brain 1984; 11: 119–125

176 Amato M, Huppi P, Durig P, Kaiser G, Schneider H. Fetal ventriculomegaly due to isolated brain malformations. Neuropediatrics 1990; 21: 130–132

177 Chervenak F A, Duncan C, Ment L R et al. Outcome of fetal ventriculomegaly. Lancet 1984; ii: 179–181

178 Clewell W H, Meier P R, Manchester D K, Manco-Johnson M L, Pretorius D H, Hendee R W. Ventriculomegaly: evaluation and management. Semin Perinatol 1985; 9: 98–102

179 Cochrane D D, Myles S T. Management of intrauterine hydrocephalus. J Neurosurg 1982; 57: 590–596

180 Cochrane D D, Myles S T, Nimrod C, Still D K, Sugarman R G, Wittmann B K. Intrauterine hydrocephalus and ventriculomegaly: associated anomalies and fetal outcome. Can J Neurol Sci 1985; 12: 51–59

181 Drugan A, Krause B, Canady A, Zador I E, Sachs A J, Evans M I. The natural history of prenatally diagnosed cerebral ventriculomegaly. JAMA 1989; 261: 1785–1788

182 Glick P L, Harrison M R, Nakayama D K et al. Management of ventriculomegaly in the fetus. J Pediatr 1984; 105: 97–105

183 Goldstein R B, La Pidus A S, Filly R A, Cardoza J. Mild lateral cerebral ventricular dilatation in utero: Clinical significance and prognosis. Radiology 1990; 176: 237–242

184 Harrod M J E, Friedman J M, Santos-Ramos R, Rutledge J, Weinburg A. Etiologic heterogeneity of fetal hydrocephalus diagnosed by ultrasound. Am J Obstet Gynecol 1984; 150: 38–40

185 Hudgins R J, Edwards M S B, Goldstein R et al. Natural history of fetal ventriculomegaly. Pediatrics 1988; 82: 692–697

186 Oi S, Yamada H, Kimura M et al. Factors affecting prognosis of intrauterine hydrocephalus diagnosed in the third trimester – computerized data analysis on controversies in fetal surgery. Neurol Med Chir (Tokyo) 1990; 30: 456–461

187 Pober B R, Greene M F, Holmes L B. Complexities of intraventricular abnormalities. J Pediatr 1986; 108: 545–551

188 Serlo W, Kirkinen P, Jouppila P, Herva R. Prognostic signs in fetal hydrocephalus. Childs Nerv Syst 1986; 2: 93–97

189 Vintzileos A M, Campbell W A, Weinbaum P J, Nochimson D J. Perinatal management and outcome of fetal ventriculomegaly. Obstet Gynecol 1987; 69: 5–11

190 Williamson R A, Schauberger C W, Varner M W, Aschenbrener C A. Heterogeneity of prenatal onset hydrocephalus: Management and counseling implications. Am J Med Genet 1984; 17: 497–508

191 Gupta J K, Bryce F, Lilford R J. Assessment and management of fetal ventriculomegaly and other associated congenital anomalies. In: Levene M I, Lilford R J, Bennett M J, Punt J, eds. Fetal and neonatal neurology and neurosurgery. 2nd ed. Edinburgh: Churchill Livingstone, 1995; pp 215–230

192 American Psychiatric Association DSM III. Diagnostic and statistical manual of mental disorders, 3rd ed. 1980

193 Amacher A L, Wellington J. Infantile hydrocephalus: Long-term results of surgical therapy. Childs Brain 1984; 11: 217–229

194 Billard C, Santini J J, Gillet P, Nargeot M C, Adrien J L. Long-term intellectual prognosis of hydrocephalus with reference to 77 children. Pediatr Neurosci 1985–1986; 12: 219–225

195 Fernell E, Hagberg B, Hagberg G, von Wendt L. Epidemiology of infantile hydrocephalus in Sweden. II. Origin in infants born at term. Acta Paediatr Scand 1987; 76: 411–417

196 Foltz E L, Shurtleff D B. Five-year comparative study of hydrocephalus in children with and without operation (113 cases). J Neurosurg 1963; 20: 1064–1079

197 Guthkelch A N, Riley N A. Influence of aetiology on prognosis in surgically treated infantile hydrocephalus. Arch Dis Child 1969; 44: 29–35

198 Jansen J, Gloerfelt-Tarp B, Pederson H, Zilstorff K. Prognosis in infantile hydrocephalus. Follow-up in adult patients, born 1946–1955. Acta Neurol Scand 1982; 65: 81–93

199 Jones R F C. Long-term results in various treatments of hydrocephalus. J Neurosurg 1967; 26: 313–315

200 Laurence K M, Coates S. The natural history of hydrocephalus. Detailed analysis of 182 unoperated cases. Arch Dis Child 1962; 37: 345–362

201 Lorber J. The results of early treatment of extreme hydrocephalus. Dev Med Child Neurol Suppl 1968; 16: 21–28

202 Lorber J, Zachary R B. Primary congenital hydrocephalus. Long-term results of controlled therapeutic trial. Arch Dis Child 1968; 43: 516–527

203 McCullough D C, Balzer-Martin L A. Current prognosis in overt neonatal hydrocephalus. J Neurosurg 1982; 57: 378–383

204 Mealey J, Gilmor R L, Bubb M P. The prognosis of hydrocephalus overt at birth. J Neurosurg 1973; 39: 348–355

205 Oberbauer R W. The significance of morphological details for developmental outcome in infantile hydrocephalus. Childs Nerv Syst 1985; 1: 329–336

206 Overton M C, Snodgrass S R. Ventriculo-venous shunts for infantile hydrocephalus. A review of five years' experience with this method. J Neurosurg 1965; 23: 517–521

207 Renier D, Sainte-Rose C, Pierre-Kahn A, Hirsch J F. Prenatal hydrocephalus: Outcome and prognosis. Childs Nerv Syst 1988; 4: 213–222

208 Rosseau G L, McCullough D C, Joseph A L. Current prognosis in fetal ventriculomegaly. J Neurosurg 1992; 77: 551–555

209 Shurtleff D B, Foltz E L, Loeser J D. Hydrocephalus. A definition of its progression and relationship to intellectual function, diagnosis and complications. Am J Dis Child 1973; 125: 688–693

210 Shurtleff D B, Kronmal R, Foltz E L. Follow-up comparison of hydrocephalus with and without myelomeningocele. J Neurosurg 1975; 42: 61–68

211 Young H F, Nulsen F E, Weiss M H, Thomas P. The relationship of intelligence and cerebral mantle in treated infantile hydrocephalus (IQ potential in hydrocephalic children). Pediatrics 1973; 52: 38–44

212 Hanigan W C, Morgan A, Shaaban A, Bradle P. Surgical treatment and long-term neurodevelopmental outcome for infants with idiopathic aqueductal stenosis. Childs Nerv Syst 1991; 7: 386–390

213 Nakayama D K, Harrison M R, Berger M S, Chinn D H, Halks-Miller M, Edwards M S. Correction of congenital hydrocephalus in utero. I. The model: intracisternal kaolin produces hydrocephalus in fetal lambs and rhesus monkeys. J Pediatr Surg 1983; 18: 331–338

214 Blum T, Saling E, Bauer R. First magnetoencephalographic recordings of the brain activity of a human fetus. Br J Obstet Gynaecol 1985; 92: 1224–1229

11 Intrapartum stillbirths and deaths in infancy: The first CESDI report

R. Neale

Obstetricians have always been at the forefront of clinical audit. The General Registry Office first started collecting childbirth statistics in 1837. It was succeeded by the Office of Population Censuses and Surveys in 1973. The history of the setting up of the Confidential Enquiry into Maternal Deaths is now well known.[1] The National Perinatal Epidemiology Unit (NPEU) was set up in 1978, and has published numerous reports. The Cochrane database which arose from the NPEU has meant that obstetricians have also been at the forefront of evidence-based medicine. Finally, the Royal College of Obstetricians and Gynaecologists collects annual statistical returns from all UK hospitals.

Despite this wealth of outcome data there are some perceived gaps. Drife in 1995[3] indentified a lack of rigour in the collection of national statistics, with deteriorating quality nationwide. Furthermore, trusts have not been part of the culture which attaches so much importance to the accurate accumulation of data from which so many important lessons can be learned. The NPEU has suggested[4] ways in which new information about pregnancy care might be collected.

Another perceived gap was the dearth of information on some types of stillbirth. The perinatal mortality rate has fallen from 32.8 in 1960 to 7.6 in 1993. Despite this the cause of most stillbirths remains an enigma. A recent study looking for obstetric antecedents of unexplained stillbirths failed to produce any real answers.[5] Thus, while it has always been recognized that many stillbirths, occurring as in-utero deaths in late pregnancy, are unpredictable and unpreventable, there is a smaller subset of stillbirths, a little over 10%, which occur in labour, wherein the death is, as it were, under the 'very noses' of the midwives and obstetricians. This perception, together with the logarithmic rise in the expectations of parents-to-be, led to the formation of CESDI whose National Advisory Body (NAB) is chaired by Lady Littler. CESDI is a unique initiative worldwide.[6] The first full report published in 1995 analyses data from the first study year, which was 1993. CESDI is

---

Note. All statistical information is taken from the Confidential Enquiry into Stillbirths and Infant Deaths (CESDI) annual report for 1993[2] (CESDI 1993) unless otherwise quoted.

Table 11.1 Evidence of suboptimal care. CESDI definitions

0	No suboptimal care
I	Suboptimal care, but different management would have made **NO** difference to the outcome
II	Suboptimal care – different management **MIGHT** have made a difference – an avoidable factor of uncertain clarity or influence on the outcome
III	Different management **WOULD REASONABLY BE EXPECTED** to have made a difference to the outcome – a clearly avoidable factor implying that an adverse outcome could have been prevented

organized on a regional basis, and the author has been privileged to analyse over 60 cases from two regions (Northern and Yorkshire).

The numbers are relatively small. In the UK (Scotland excepted) in 1993 the rate of early fetal loss (defined as babies born between 20 weeks and 23 weeks and 6 days, or babies who had a birth weight of over 500 g) was 2.1 per 1000 total births. The corresponding stillbirth rate was 5.3, and the neonatal mortality rate 3.9. The perinatal mortality rate for the nation in the middle part of the decade is approximately 7–8 per 1000 total births.

METHODS USED IN CESDI

Rapid reporting

A nominated person in each maternity unit was made responsible for completing a rapid reporting form after every late fetal loss, stillbirth or early or late neonatal death. Any deaths following late terminations under the Abortion act were excluded from CESDI. The aim was that the report should be dispatched to the regional CESDI office within 1 week, and from thence to the national office within 1 month. As this was the first year of full reporting, performance predictably improved as time passed, with 76% of reports reaching London on time in the last quarter of the year. The rapid reporting form contains 30 items of data, mostly of a demographic nature but including the all-important extended Wigglesworth classification of death.[7,8] Late terminations of pregnancy were excluded. There were 9221 reported deaths from all four groups. This included a total of 3726 stillbirths, and of these only 433 occurred in labour (11.6%). These deaths formed the subject of the report.

Confidential enquiries

A number of stillbirths (506) were initially deemed to fit the criteria by the regional offices. These were the subject of a confidential enquiry. The criteria were:

1. Deaths of babies during labour and early neonatal deaths possibly related to labour.
2. Birth weight of 2.5 kg or more; no gross or life-threatening abnormality.

Thus it will be seen that although all women were deemed to be in labour, some deaths occurred in the home rather than at hospital. In 1993 there were just 10 home deliveries of which 2 were planned.

Of the 506 cases submitted 73 were eventually judged not to fit the criteria; of the remaining 433 cases, 45 were submitted too late for analysis; this left 388 cases which were analysed. These were the subject of a confidential enquiry held on a regional basis. The notes of each case were collated and anonymized by a research midwife, a summary of the case prepared and the papers forwarded to the members of the panel. Each panel usually considers 4–7 cases at a sitting taking up to 1 hour to discuss each case. The panel consists of one or more members from the following professional groups: obstetricians (usually at least two), midwives, neonatal nurses, paediatricians, health visitors, public health physicians and perinatal pathologists. Additional members of the panel such as anaesthetists or general practitioners can be co-opted if the subject matter of the case under discussion suggests that would be advantageous. The regional co-ordinator ensures that no member of the panel comes from a hospital involved with any of the cases. A special assessment form, which reflects the views of the panel, is completed by the chairman.

The first task is to identify evidence of suboptimal care. There may be several well defined episodes of care in any individual case which may be so categorized (Table 11.1). Panels were encouraged to err on the side of being critical in their analysis as this would assist in the educational nature of the exercise. On the other hand, some panels did not hesitate to offer praise if it was felt that the tragedy had arisen despite a high level of care. The views recorded on each case are recognized as being subjective and probably non-reproducible representing as they do consensus and, on occasions, compromise. Nevertheless, panels quickly develop a chemistry of their own and all members frequently have expressed the educational value for their own personal practice.

For each episode of suboptimal care the panel is required to make two further judgements, first to categorize the type and the chronology of the failing, and second to identify the persons contributing to the failing (Tables 11.2, 11.3 and 11.4).

The panel is required to fix the overall grade of suboptimal care. This will normally be the highest grade accorded to an individual episode of suboptimal care, although three episodes of grade II care might be judged to be grade III overall.

Panels are required to comment on any documentation thought to be missing. Regional co-ordinators have experienced some difficulty and delay in collating hospital notes when the perinatal death was the subject of a coroner's enquiry or when the case was already the subject of litigation. Panels are also asked to comment on the quality of record keeping and any tests or investigations which were not performed that should have been.

The panel is then required, with the help of its perinatal pathologist

Table 11.2 Type of failure

Clinical practice
Failure to recognize a problem
Failure to act appropriately
Poor communication
Patient and/or family
Lack of human Resource
Lack or failure of equipment

Table 11.3 Timing of failure

Antepartum
Intrapartum
Postpartum
Post death

Table 11.4 Persons contributing to suboptimal care

General practitioner	Community midwife
Hospital midwife	Obstetrician
Paediatrician	Anaesthetist
Pathologist	Parent/family
The organization	Other

---

member, to comment on the adequacy of the pathological investigation. If a postmortem was not performed the hospital must indicate on the rapid reporting form whether this was because permission had been refused or because the parents were not asked.

Lastly, panels were required to categorize the death using the extended Wigglesworth, Obstetric (Aberdeen),[9] and Fetal and Neonatal Classifications.[10] See Tables 11.5, 11.6 and 11.7.

MAIN RESULTS

Obstetric parameters

Of 388 deaths analysed 54% of the babies were boys and exactly 50% were nulliparous at booking. There were 21 home births of which 9 were planned and 12 unplanned. The latter group included 8 concealed pregnancies. There were 13 cases (3%) of multiple pregnancy; all except one were twins. Among the twins the first twin was the subject of the enquiry in three cases, the second twin in nine.

The gestational age ranged from 30 to 44 weeks, but only a small number (7%) were preterm (< 37 weeks). The mean birthweight was 3.4 kg; 3% of babies were > 4 kg.

Table 11.5 Extended Wigglesworth classification

1. Severe/lethal congenital malformations*
2. Unexplained antepartum fetal death*
3. Death from intrapartum 'asphyxia', 'anoxia', or trauma
4. Immaturity
5. Infection
6. Specific causes (e.g. *fetal* – hydrops or twin-to-twin transfusion, *neonatal* – haemorrhagic shock from vasa praevia, pulmonary haemorrhage)
7. Owing to accident or other forms of (non-obstetric) trauma including non-accidental injury
8. Sudden infant death – cause unknown
9. Unclassifiable – the reason for this choice must be stated. To be used only as a last resort

*These two categories would not normally appear on CESDI forms as they fall outside the definition for inclusion in a CESDI enquiry.

Table 11.6 Obstetric (Aberdeen) classification

Congenital anomaly
1. Neural tube defects
2. Other anomalies

Isoimmunization
3. Owing to Rh (D) antigen
4. Owing to other antigens

Pre-eclampsia (true)
5. Without APH
6. Complicated by APH

Antepartum haemorrhage (APH)
7. Placenta praevia
8. Abruption
9. Of uncertain origin

Mechanical
10. Cord prolapse
11. Cephalic malpresentations
12. Breech presentation
13. Abnormal lie, uterine rupture, etc.

Maternal disorder
14. Hypertension
15. Other maternal disease
16. Maternal infection

Miscellaneous
17. Neonatal infection
18. Other neonatal condition
19. Specific fetal conditions

Unexplained
20. > 2.5 kg
21. < 2.5 kg
22. *Unclassifiable*

The lowest numbered category that fits should be chosen. Definitions and explanations of each category are given to CESDI panels for guidance.

Table 11.7 Fetal and neonatal classification

Congenital anomaly
1. Chromosome defect
2. Inborn error of metabolism
3. Neural tube defect
4. Congenital heart defect
5. Renal anomaly
6. Other malformation
7. *Isoimmunization*

Asphyxia before birth
8. Antepartum asphyxia
9. Intrapartum asphyxia
10. *Birth trauma*
11. *Severe pulmonary immaturity*

Hyaline membrane disease (HMD)
12. HMD alone
13. HMD with IVH
14. HMD with infection

Intracranial haemorrhage
15. Intraventricular bleed
16. Other intracranial bleed

Infection
17. Necrotizing enterocolitis
18. Antepartum infection
19. Intrapartum infection
20. Postpartum infection
21. *Miscellaneous*

Unclassifiable/unknown
22. Cot death
23. Unattended delivery
24. Other undocumented death

The lowest numbered category that fits should be chosen. Definitions and explanations of each category are given to CESDI panels for guidance.

Induction of labour was a feature of 23% of cases and augmentation of 40%.

The assisted delivery rate was very high – 55% overall – see Table 11.8.

All 388 deaths were classified according to the extended Wigglesworth classification. The results in Table 11.9 gave no surprises, with an overwhelming predominance of intrapartum related death.

Approximately 30% of the babies in the series were born at the weekend with Saturday being the peak day for both birth and death; 17% of deaths occurred on this day against the expected 14%. Among the stillbirths there was a slight increase in the numbers of births occurring in the late evening and early hours of the morning with a peak at 22.00 hours. Of course, the precise time of death of the fetus in utero is often unknown.

Table 11.8 Mode of delivery

	%
Unassisted vaginal	45
Unplanned Caesarean*	35
Forceps	11
Ventouse	8

*There were no elective Caesarean sections.

Table 11.9 Wigglesworth classification of deaths

%		
Unexplained antepartum*	0.5	
Intrapartum related death	79.1	
Immaturity	0.5	
Infection 5.4		
Other specific causes	9.8	
Accident/trauma	0.3	
Sudden unexplained infant death		2.8
Unclassifiable	1.5	

*In theory these should not appear in a study of *intrapartum* deaths.

Analysis of grade of care

This is the most noteworthy part of the report. In only 17% of cases was there no suboptimal care (Grade 0). In almost one-half of the cases was the suboptimal care graded as III where different management *would reasonably be expected to have made a difference* to the outcome (Table 11.10).

Therefore, there was a mean of 3.2 episodes of substandard care per death. These figures, coupled with virtually 80% of the deaths being classified as intrapartum-related according to extended Wigglesworth demonstrates that his audit leaves little room for complacency so far as maternity services are concerned.

Grade III suboptimal care was more likely to be seen with primigravidae (52%) than with multipara (37%). Clearly, in any one individual case some of the comments about episodes of suboptimal care may relate to events occurring at different times: ante, intra and postpartum; 51% of episodes deserving adverse comment occurred in the intrapartum phase and 39% of intrapartum stillbirths were associated with Grade III suboptimal care compared with 44% of early neonatal deaths.

The grading is, of course, purely subjective and therefore some variation between regions was expected. This proved to be the case. This variation was all the more likely as 1993 was the first year of study. Thus Mersey and Trent region found an overall level of grade III substandard care in 59% of cases, with Wessex coming to the same conclusion in just 11%. The mean was 42%. The NAB is addressing this regional variation by inviting representatives

Table 11.10 Overall grade of care and graded comments concerning episodes of substandard care

Grade	%	No. of comments ($n = 1278$)	%
0	17.3	80	6.3
1	12.1	388	30.4
2	28.1	465	36.4
3	42.3	345	27.0

Table 11.11 Type of event

Failure to act appropriately	34%
Failure to recognize problem	29%
Communication failure	17%
Failure to follow/accept advice	5%
Human resource (staffing problems)	5%
Equipment failure	2%
Miscellaneous	7%

from each region to participate in national panels as an educational and discussive exercise.

Slightly more than one-third of adverse events represented a *failure to act appropriately* when faced with a certain clinical situation, whereas a little under one-third referred to a *failure to recognize the problem* in the first place (Table 11.11).

As would perhaps be expected, both hospital midwives and obstetricians perform badly when the type of personnel contributing to suboptimal care are examined; they are the personnel who look after mothers in labour (Table 11.12).

The problem with interpreting these data is that there are no denominator data available for comparison. Nevertheless some comment is possible. Given that some 75–80% of women are delivered by midwives without medical intervention, obstetricians, who are the most frequently mentioned group and feature in 47% of cases, must accept much of the blame for suboptimal care in the labour ward. As perhaps expected, midwives were more likely to be guilty of failing to recognize the nature of the problem, while obstetricians were more likely to be guilty of failing to act appropriately. Failure to communicate involved all professional groups in equal proportions. Similarly, it was the registrar, the person most frequently involved in difficult deliveries, who was most frequently implicated compared to other grades of staff. The absence of consultant involvement in many of these tragedies was a notable feature (Table 11.13). Again, denominator data on staffing levels is not available.

Clinical scenarios

The previous section has demonstrated that in many intrapartum-related stillbirths and neonatal deaths there is an unacceptable level of care among

Table 11.12 Personnel implicated

No. of mentions	On own	With others	Total
Obstetrician	33	213	246
Hospital midwife	19	185	204
Paediatrician	10	93	103
Patient and/or family	12	58	70
Organization	0	52	52
General practitioner	3	38	41
Community midwife	3	37	40
Anaesthetist	0	27	27

Table 11.13 Seniority of obstetrician involved

Consultant only	48
Registrar only	149
SHO only	34
Consultant and registrar	56
Consultant and SHO	17
Registrar and SHO	67
Consultant, registrar and SHO	20

obstetricians and hospital midwives. If matters are to improve – closing the audit circle – it is important to look carefully at the clinical scenarios within which these deaths occurred so that an educational process may begin to improve the quality of care in these areas.

The main clinical problems recorded in the 388 deaths analysed are recorded in Table 11.14.

OXYTOCICS

The overwhelming feature which stands out from this table is the use of oxytocics, syntocinon or prostaglandin (PgE_2), to stimulate the uterus. Their use was by far and away the most frequently recorded – 36% of the recorded factors.

Oxytocin or prostaglandin were used to induce 23% of the labours in the series and 40% were augmented. In the group where syntocinon was used the operative delivery rate was 66% (half Caesarean and half Ventouse or forceps) compared with the operative delivery rate of 55% in the whole group (see Table 11.8). Prostaglandin use was associated with an increased risk of uterine rupture; the overall incidence of this complication was 3% whereas 6% of the mothers in whom prostaglandin had been used suffered a ruptured uterus.

The following aspects of oxytocic stimulation were identified by CESDI review panels:

- Delay in inducing or augmenting labour when clear indications were present.

Table 11.14 Clinical factors recorded for intrapartum related deaths

	Stillbirths	Neonatal deaths	Total
Maternal factors			
Pregnancy-induced hypertension including true pre-eclampsia	35	33	68
Chronic hypertension	10	3	13
Asthma	8	14	22
Diabetes	10	12	22
Infection	35	40	75
Smoking	32	37	69
Obesity	16	11	27
Haemorrhage			
APH (unspecified)	19	33	52
Abruption	16	11	27
Difficult delivery			
Ruptured uterus	5	7	12
Shoulder dystocia	17	12	29
Birth weight > 4 kg	22	34	56
Nuchal cord	34	38	72
Cord prolapse	4	8	12
Compound presentation	1	3	4
Home delivery			
Planned	2	7	9
Unplanned	8	4	12
Other factors			
Induction of labour	33	57	90
Augmentation of labour	72	83	155
Breech	4	11	15
			672*

*388 deaths analysed.

- Dubious indications for induction including poor documentation for so-called 'social' reasons.
- Overdosage with prostaglandins – often a third dose of vaginal prostin would be administered when there were no clear indications for induction and without reference to senior staff.
- Uterine hypertonus, usually resulting from high-dosage oxytocin infusion regimens.
- Failure to recognize hypertonus when it occurred.
- Failure to slow down or stop an oxytocin infusion when there was clear cardiotocographic (CTG) evidence of a compromised fetus.
- Delay in starting induction (the usual excuse being that the labour ward was busy) such that a high-risk patient would be in the active phase of labour in the middle of the night.
- Inappropriate management of 'failed' induction.

- Failure to conduct adequate fetal surveillance when oxytocics were being used.
- Lack of supervision by senior staff.
- Poor communications between midwives and medical staff.
- Failure to respect the mother's wishes.

This is a sorry catalogue of criticisms but all were recorded. The most common problem appeared to be starting inductions late in the day.

It is, of course, recognized that many of the deaths associated with the use of oxytocic agents may reflect the underlying problem that caused these drugs to be used in the first place. Nevertheless, these drugs are not without risk and it appears that problems associated with their use are not uncommon, at least as evidenced by the CESDI survey.

Part of the problem may arise from poor understanding of the nature of the dysfunction in labour. 'Failure to progress' is a catch-all phrase and is frequently cited as the indication for Caesarean section. In the great majority of labour wards the clinician does not know, having excluded disproportion, whether the slow rate of cervical dilatation is caused by decreased cervical compliance or poor myometrial function leading to a failure to generate adequate intrauterine pressures or to a combination of both. If it is a combination of both factors it is not known which is the major contibutor.[11] While intrauterine pressure monitoring is routinely used in the USA it is infrequently used in the UK outside tertiary units (PJ Steer, personal communication). A generation of obstetricians have been brought up on the safety of oxytocin infusions following the pioneering work of Kieran O'Driscoll.[12] It was his claim that in his institution uterine hypertonus did not occur. However, the model described by Gee,[11] wherein there is a non-compliant cervix which does not modulate uterine wall tension and so generates high intrauterine pressures and poor placental perfusion, is in contrast with the bland assurances from Dublin, and this group of patients would appear to be particularly vulnerable to oxytocin. The syntocinon data sheet[13] provided by the company lists 'hypertonic uterine inertia' (i.e. failure of the cervix to dilate despite strong contractions) as an absolute contraindication to the use of oxytocin. This may not be observed in routine clinical practice/Failure to respond to the presence of hypertonus when it was clearly demonstrable by tocography and failure to reduce or stop the oxytocin infusion in the presence of an abnormal CTG were two of the most common problems recorded by CESDI review panels. There is much to be said for more widespread use of intrauterine pressure monitoring during oxytocin infusions.

Another problem revolves around the absence of a standard protocol in the UK. Although the American College of Obstetricians and Gynaecologists issued a guideline document as long ago as 1987,[14] no such guideline has appeared in the UK. The need for such was identified by Thornton and his Newcastle colleagues in 1993[15] who surveyed the Northern Region and found a five-fold variation in the volume of solute administered. The maximum infusion rate varied between 25 and 64 mU/min. They recommended a protocol which started with an infusion rate of 1 mU/min, increasing at 30 minute intervals to a maximum of 12 mU/min. This is in agreement with the studies of Seitchik and Castillo,[16] who found that the great majority of patients achieved effective cervical dilatation at infusion rates of 4 mU/min, and those of Bidgood and Steer,[17] who found that there was a lower rate of hyperstimulation with a lower starting infusion rate. Steer, reviewing several papers reported hyperstimulation rates of 30–40% when infusion rates of up to 40 mU/min were employed.[18] Lastly, it is also known that plasma oxytocin levels are markedly higher during augmentation than they are during natural labour when the levels remain low.[19]

For all these reasons there is now a cogent argument for the production of national guidelines on the use of oxytocic agents to induce and augment labour and on the care of the fetus while these procedures are underway.

FETAL SURVEILLANCE

Fetal surveillance in labour was one of the most important issues to arise from the CESDI report. In some 8% of the 388 cases analysed there was no recorded form of fetal monitoring of any sort. Of the rest, electronic fetal monitoring (EFM) using an external transducer was easily the most favoured method, being recorded in 73% of cases.

The principal problems associated with cardiotocography (CTG) were either a failure to recognize the severity of the problem indicated by the CTG trace or the failure to take appropriate action. In 221 cases (57%) the reaction to the CTG was specifically cited as 'poor' by review panels.

Other than this there were technical problems with the equipment coupled with an unwillingness to 'listen through' a contraction when the electronic pick up was poor.

Another problem concerned fetal blood sampling (FBS). Although the worth of this has recently been discussed by Steer[20] it appears that less than half the maternity units in the UK were using the technique in Wheble's 1989 survey.[21] This trend is reflected in the CESDI report where FBS was also infrequently used. There were also instances of unnecessary delay caused by performing a scalp sample when the CTG appearances were severe enough to demand urgent delivery. Clearly, good judgement is not always in evidence.

Another frequently voiced concern was a failure of senior staff to become involved both in questions of interpretation and in decision making.

These results surely imply a failure of training of junior medical staff. Despite a number of papers by Neilson and others[22,23] attesting to the failure of electronic fetal monitoring when applied to whole obstetric populations to improve fetal outcome, and other papers attesting to the poor specificity of the technique and poor predictive value,[24] the use of the technique appears to be inexorably increasing. While accepting this at an intellectual level, many obstetricians appear unwilling to reverse the trend towards ever more liberal use of the technique, perhaps because of medico-legal concerns.[25] Equally, the admission test appears to be well established in routine labour ward practice despite a lack of evidence from randomized trials.[26] In view of this widespread use of EFM, evidence-based or not, the profession has a clear duty to provide the best possible training for those who are responsible for interpretation and decision making. Ennis[27] in 1991 identified the fact that half of the Senior House Officers in his survey had received no formal training in CTG interpretation during the whole of their 6 month rotation on the labour ward.

There is additional evidence that serious changes on CTGs are being missed. Murphy and others reviewed the CTG traces of 38 severely asphyxiated infants and found gross changes, with slow response times in 87%.[27a] In terms of appropriate action Niswander and others[28] consider that a failure to take action within 90 minutes after the onset of late decelerations represented suboptimal care. In medico-legal terms this interval might now seem too long.

Under these circumstances there is a clear need for structured training in fetal surveillance for junior medical staff and midwives. The British Royal College of Obstetricians and Gynaecologists, unlike its Australian counterpart, has no module for such education in the MRCOG diploma. Despite the efforts of Gibb and Arulkumaran, whose enterprise, Fetal Monitoring Education, has instructed over 10 000 persons in the past decade, there is no *requirement* for trainee obstetricians to attend such instruction. The considerable majority of persons attending Gibb's courses are midwives and not junior obstetricians. (Donald Gibb – personal communication)

Part of the reason for this educational failure may lie in the complexity of classification schemes for CTG patterns.[29,30] There may be some merit in a more simplified scheme as used in the Dublin trial.[31] Teaching methods need to be researched so that optimum results for time spent in teaching may be achieved.

Another reason may be the difficulty in appreciating trends in CTGs over time; Chard[32] identified the difficulty in making an adequate visual assessment in changes in dip area, and yet computer analysis, which solves this problem, is not used widely.

From the perspective of future CESDI reports, it might well be useful to apply quantitative, as opposed to subjective, criteria to CTG analysis and the utilization of FBS to the analysis of future CESDI confidential enquiries.

Until the following objectives are achieved, the first being adequate training in the principles and practice of fetal surveillance for junior medical staff and senior midwives, and the second to ensure the availability of senior medical staff when difficult questions of judgement need to be addressed, there would seem to be little prospect of making inroads into the intrapartum stillbirth rate or the labour ward litigation problem.

SHOULDER DYSTOCIA

Among the 388 cases identified by CESDI there were 29 cases of shoulder dystocia. Of these, 17 (59%) were stillborn and the rest were neonatal deaths. Nineteen (65%) weighed in excess of 4 kg at birth. Shoulder dystocia was associated with 33% of the pregnancies affected by diabetes in the series, and 34% of all the babies whose birth weight exceeded 4 kg. This triad of large baby, diabetes and shoulder dystocia still seems to go unrecognized. In the past shoulder dystocia has been regarded as unpredictable and unpreventable but recent reviews by Roberts[33] and Gibb[40] in 1994 would suggest that this concept is no longer tenable and that there are many mothers in whom a high index of suspicion should exist. In such cases labour ward staff should be notified of the possibility of shoulder dystocia and rehearsed in their duties should it arise.

In the author's experience of the confidential enquiries two features of deficient management stood out. The first was delay in seeking senior help and the second was organizational confusion. Nobody would be in charge and nobody would have a clear idea of priorities.

Analysis of the reports suggests that the all important McRoberts manoeuvre described by Gonik and others[35] in 1983 is infrequently employed.

There is a clear and compelling need for an agreed guideline document jointly published by the Royal College of Obstetricians and the Royal College of Midwives, together with high quality posters for labour ward staff rest rooms and SHO's on-call bedrooms. Deaths from shoulder dystocia should largely be preventable and the responsibility must fall heavily on the shoulders of midwives because of the time factor. Similarly, Erb's palsy litigation is in the ascendancy, which is a further reason for urgent action by responsible bodies.

RUPTURED UTERUS

There were 12 cases of ruptured uterus in the series, of whom 9 had a previous Caesarean section. Five were stillborn, the rest early neonatal deaths. Two clinical features stood out:

1. Delay in making the diagnosis. Fetal distress was invariably present but no action was taken.
2. The use of prostaglandins to induce labour. In some cases multiple doses of Prostin were used in the face of an unripe cervix which had not been 'tested' in a previous labour – the usual scenario being a mother who had been delivered by elective Caesarean in her first pregnancy for a breech presentation without going into labour. It would not be unusual to find somewhat spurious indications for induction.

McKenzie and his colleagues[36] in Oxford studied 439 women who had an induction of labour using vaginal PgE$_2$ in the presence of a lower uterine segment scar. In five patients the scar gave way; four cases of dehiscence were found at repeat Caesarean and one case of overt rupture. In all five patients oxytocin augmentation had been used compared with 62% in the whole group.

PROLAPSED UMBILICAL CORD

This emergency occurred in 12 cases. The most common criticism voiced by review panels was a failure on the part of staff present to have a routine, a knowledge of what to do to try and preserve the fetus' life.

CESDI, RISK MANAGEMENT AND MEDICAL NEGLIGENCE

The CESDI team at the Department of Health, chaired by Lady Littler, have always gone out of their way to emphasize the confidential nature of the exercise in order that the worth and trustworthiness of the study may come to be recognized by the profession in the same way that the Confidential Enquiry into Maternal Deaths has become over nearly a half century. As with that well established enquiry the CESDI report makes for sober reading. It is clear that there can be no room for complacency on the part of those whose duty it is to determine labour ward policies and working patterns in their own unit. The high level of incidence of obstetricians being implicated indicate that there is still much to be done in terms of making UK labour wards safer places for women and the babies they are delivering.

In medical negligence terms the claims continue to spiral. Obstetrics remains the most vulnerable speciality. Brian Capstick[37] has recently analysed the outstanding claims that have been registered against Trusts in south-west London. He calculates that in a trust with a turnover of £10 million a year there will be an average of one birth-asphyxiated baby per annum – the range in his survey was 0–3. He also calculates that a trust of that size will have up to 16 such cases 'on its books', and that if none could be defended it would mean a liability of some £11 million. These are scary figures for any trust Financial Director. The new Clinical Negligence Special Trust, chaired by Sir Brian Martin QC and under the day-to-day management of the Medical Protection Society will lose no time in establishing a database of claims, and the premiums that trusts will be required to subscribe will be based upon a trust's claims history.

It therefore behoves a trust to have an active risk management policy, and no part of a hospital is more fundamental to this than the Maternity Unit. One of the most important aspects of Risk Management is incident reporting and analysis of 'near misses'. In this context a stillbirth that occurs in labour should be regarded as a 'near miss'. In litigation terms a stillbirth is very cheap, a brain damaged baby is horrifically expensive. Both may arise from the same sort of clinical management mistakes.

All maternity units should have regular perinatal meetings. There is

Table 11.15 Incident reporting

Apgar scores of < 7 at delivery
Scalp trauma (fracture, sub-galeal haemorrhage or cephalhaematoma)
All cases of shoulder dystocia
Facial nerve palsy following forceps delivery
Erb's palsy
Mid-cavity rotational forceps delivery*
Delay of > 40 minutes in the performance of an urgent CS
Documented cases of staff communication difficulty
Unexpected admissions to SCBU
Third degree tears
Post-partum haemorrhages requiring transfusion
Failure to summon a paediatrician to attend a delivery in cases of a compromised fetus
Intrapartum stillbirths and neonatal deaths

---

*As an exercise in decision analysis.

evidence that in some hospitals little importance is attached to them, attendance by all is poor, especially at consultant level and the level of debate and analysis regrettable. Nothing could be more important. The recent onset of CME points may serve to improve consultant attendance, but junior staff must be in no doubt that their presentations are of the highest order, rather than something hastily prepared 5 minutes before the meeting. A written summary should be provided, which includes a brief survey of the relevant literature. Senior midwives should be encouraged to take their turn with presentations and that the fact that they may outperform their medical colleagues acts as a good-natured spur to improve. Careful records should be kept of these meetings together with interval reports on paediatric follow-up of babies born in poor condition.

One registrar or senior registrar should be put in charge of an incident reporting system, ideally backed up by a computer programme and an audit assistant. Table 11.15 lists some of the events that should be reported.

Such a list is not meant to be exhaustive but should serve as a stimulus for debate. Cases should be presented in a non-adversarial and anonymized manner so that the ensuing discussion can be educational rather than recriminatory.

Regular teaching sessions for new medical and midwifery staff should be undertaken, together with an annual review of the labour ward policy manual. Posters in midwive's staffrooms and junior medical staff on-call rooms on topics such as simplified CTG analysis (e.g. MacDonald 1985)[31] and first aid procedures for shoulder dystocia and cord prolapse will pay dividends, as will such ventures as lunchtime quizzes (with prizes), debates with one consultant pitted against another, videotapes and other audio-visual material provided by commerical companies.

Most important of all is to inculcate an atmosphere of joint trust, respect, responsibility and accountability on the part of all who work in the labour ward. Fostering such a beneficial atmosphere is a test of true leadership qualities among consultants, heads of midwifery and managers. Discord and poor working conditions on the labour ward is fertile ground for mistakes, and mistakes are extraordinarily expensive in both humanitarian and financial terms.

Lastly, one of the regular features recorded by the author in the 100 or so cases he has analysed at Confidential Enquiry meetings is a dearth of consultant input at critical moments in the conduct of a high-risk labour. There may be any number of reasons for this, many of which have to do with unsociable hours of the day. However, the profession, our managers and, in particular, the Royal College of Obstetricians and Gynaecologists is going to have to grasp the nettle of increased consultant input into the labour ward if the vicious circle of spiralling litigation costs is to be broken.

SUMMARY

CESDI is arguably the most important audit exercise in this speciality in our generation. It has the same capacity to save life, this time babies, as the maternal mortality reports, begun nearly 50 years ago, did for mothers. If this possibility is to be turned into a reality then the audit loop must be closed by those regulatory authorities whose responsibility it is to govern the twin professions of obstetrics and midwifery by appropriate educational programmes.

One problem which the NAB itself will have to address is the lack of denominator data for many of the figures quoted. While this does not negate the value of the study it does prevent meaningful statistical analysis much of the time and good quality denominator data would undoubtedly enhance the worth of the project.

The NAB made eight recommendations in the 1993 report published in 1995, most of which were of an administrative nature. However, a plea was also made for better communication between all grades of staff and for better record keeping. This may act as a spur towards the development of a national maternity record. On intrapartum care the NAB has this to say:

Relevant professional and statutory bodies should ensure that training for intrapartum care emphasises risk recognition and management, in particular for induction of labour, management of labour in the presence of a uterine scar; rehearsal of procedures required in rare emergencies such as uterine rupture, haemorrhage, cord prolapse and shoulder dystocia; and the interpretation of the CTG.

It is hoped that this recommendation will be heeded.

REFERENCES

1 Godber G. The origin and inception of the confidential enquiry into maternal deaths. Br J Obstet Gynaecol 1994; 101: 946–947
2 Confidential enquiry into stillbirths and deaths in infancy. Annual report for 1993, Parts 1 & 2. London Department of Health, 1995
3 Drife J O. Assessing the consequences of changing childbirth. Br Med J 1995; 310: 144

4 Macfarlane A. Perinatal mortality surveys. Br Med J 1984; 289: 1473–1474
5 Mathias G, Morgan G. Unexplained stillbirths; antenatal characteristics. J Obstet Gynaecol 1995; 15: 299–300
6 Department of Health. Press release H91/304, 1991
7 Wigglesworth J S. Monitoring perinatal mortality: a pathophysiological approach. Lancet 1980; ii: 684–686
8 CESDI coordinators introductory pack. NAB, 1992
9 Cole S K, Hey E N, Thomson A M. Classifying perinatal death: an obstetric approach. Br J Obstet Gynaecol 1986; 93: 1204–1212
10 Hey E N, Lloyd D J, Wigglesworth J S. Classifying perinatal death: fetal and neonatal factors. Br J Obstet Gynaecol 1986; 93: 1213–1223
11 Gee H, Olah K S. Failure to progress in labour. In: Studd J, ed. Progress in obstetrics and gynaecology. Vol 10. Edinburgh: Churchill Livingstone 1993: pp 159–181
12 O'Driscoll K, Meagher D. Active management of labour. London: WB Saunders, 1980: pp 42–43
13 ABPI Data sheet compendium. London: Datapharm Publications, 1995/6: pp 1539–1540
14 American College of Obstetricians and Gynaecologists. Induction and augmentation of labour. Technical Bulletin 1987; 110
15 Irons D W, Thornton S, Davison J M, Baylis P H. Oxytocin infusion regimens: time for standardisation? Br J Obstet Gynaecol 1993; 100: 786–787
16 Seitchik J, Castillo M. Oxytocin augmentation of dysfunctional labour. 1. Clinical data. Am J Obstet Gynecol 1983; 144: 899–905
17 Bidgood K A, Steer P J. A randomised controlled study of oxytocin augmentation of labour. 1. Obstetric outcome. Br J Obstet Gynaecol 1987; 94: 512–517
18 Steer P J. Intrapartum care including the detection and management of fetal dysfunction. In: Clements R V, ed. Safe practice in obstetrics and gynaecology. Edinburgh: Churchill Livingstone, 1994: 195–197
19 Thornton S, Davison J M, Baylis P H. Plasma oxytocin during the first and second stages of spontaneous human labour. Acta Endocrinol 1992; 126: 425–429
20 Steer P J. Fetal scalp blood analysis: current practice. In: Spencer J A D, Ward R H T, eds. Intrapartum fetal surveillance. London: RCOG press, 1993; pp 127–137
21 Wheble A M, Gillmes M D G, Spencer J A D, Sykes G S. Changes in fetal monitoring practice in the UK 1977–1984. Br J Obstet Gynaecol 1989; 96: 1140–1147
22 Neilson J, Grant A M. The randomized trials of electronic fetal heart rate monitoring. In: Spencer J A D, Ward R H T, eds. Intrapartum fetal surveillance. London: RCOG press, 1993: pp 77–93
23 Neilson J. Cardiotocography during labour. Br Med J 1993; 306: 347–348
24 Mires G J, Patel N. Advances in the diagnosis and management of fetal distress in labour. In: Bonnar J ed. Recent advances in obstetrics and gynaecology. No 18. Edinburgh: Churchill Livingstone, 1994: pp 79–90
25 Smith J H. Is continuous intrapartum fetal monitoring necessary? In: Chard T, Richards M P M, eds. Obstetrics in the 1990s: Current controversies. Oxford: Blackwell Scientific, 1992: pp 192–201
26 Ingemarsson I. EFM as a screening test. In: Spencer J A D, Ward R H T, eds. Intrapartum fetal surveillance. London: RCOG press, 1993: pp 45–52
27 Ennis M. Training and supervision of obstetric senior house officers. Br Med J 1991; 303: 1442–1443
27a Murphy K W, Johnson P, Moorcroft J, Pattinson R, Russell V, Turnbull A. Birth asphyxia and the intrapartum cardiotocograph. Br J Obstet Gynaecol 1990; 97: 470–479
28 Niswander K, Hanson G, Elbourne D et al. Adverse outcome of pregnancy and the quality of obstetric care. Lancet 1984; ii: 827–831
29 Steer P J, Danielian P J. Fetal distress in labour. In: James D K, Steer P J, Wiener C P, Gonik B, eds. High risk pregnancy. London: WB Saunders, 1994,: p 1083
30 FIGO news. Int J Gynecol Obstet 1987; 25: 159–167
31 MacDonald J D, Grant A M, Sheridan-Pereira M, Boylan P, Chalmers I. The Dublin randomized trial of intrapartum fetal heart rate monitoring. Am J Obstet Gynecol 1985; 152: 524–539
32 Chard T. The role of computers in obstetrics. In: Chard T, Richards M P M, eds. Obstetrics in the 1990s: Current controversies. Oxford: Blackwell Scientific, 1992: pp 202–211

33 Roberts L. Shoulder dystocia. In: Studd J, ed. Progress in obstetrics and gynaecology. Vol 11. Edinburgh: Churchill Livingstone, 1994: pp 201–216
34 Gibb D. Operative delivery. In: Clements R V, ed. Safe practice in obstetrics and gynaecology. Edinburgh: Churchill Livingstone, 1994: pp 233–234
35 Gonik B, Stringer C, Held B. An alternative maneuver for management of shoulder dystocia. Am J Obstet Gynecol 1983; 145: 882–884
36 McKenzie I Z. The therapeutic roles of prostaglandins in obstetrics. In: Studd J, ed. Progress in obstetrics and gynaecology. Vol 8. Edinburgh: Churchill Livingstone, 1990: 149–174
37 Capstick B. Incident reporting and claims analysis. Clin Risk 1995; 1: 165–167

PART TWO

Gynaecology

12 Adolescent gynaecology

O. Sheil   M. Turner

Adolescence is described as that period of life when the carefree child becomes the responsible adult. Developmental changes rather than age limits or physical milestones are probably the best markers. There is no statutory legal age limit of when adolescence begins and ends. In general, the age range we are talking about is 13 to 18 years, but the physical and psychological changes which occur may begin before and continue after this age span. At this time, there is a marked acceleration of physical and emotional development to which the adolescent must adjust. To date, little attention has been paid to the health problems of teenagers. When one considers that 10% of our population is in this age group, this lack of attention to their health is unsatisfactory. Fortunately, this situation is now changing as health professionals realize that arguments exist for a separate specialty for adolescents.[1] Adolescent gynaecology is not a new subject: adolescents have always suffered from genital tract disorders; however, awareness of this subject is new.[2] Hence, as gynaecologists, we must now address this issue and strive to protect the health of our female teenagers.

The gynaecological problems of teenagers can pose difficulties in management, not just from the physical nature of the problem, but from associated emotional and psychological factors. These girls are often shy and embarrassed to discuss the more personal aspects of their lives. Hence, they often do not know where to turn for help. Added to this is a lack of knowledge and understanding as to what is happening to their bodies at this time. This may lead to fear. They may be fearful that they are abnormal compared to their sisters and friends; they may be afraid to confide and afraid to seek advice. How the medical profession deals with these girls is important. One study reported what teenagers expect from doctors when they attend: understanding, friendliness and personality.[3]

It is important that we address this need whether it is at general practitioner or hospital level. Teenage girls with gynaecological problems must be dealt with sensitively if we are to encourage them to come forward and communicate their anxieties and problems, and ultimately protect their health. One way to do this is to establish adolescent gynaecology clinics. The aim of such a service should be to provide an environment that is friendly, not intimidating, and private. Ideally, it should take place away from the often

215

frenetic general outpatients department, which can be terrifying to a multi-parous 50 year old, never mind an inhibited 15 year old girl. The girl must be able to feel she is being treated with respect and confidentiality. We have developed such a service, which has been in operation for two years and which has been favourably received by teenage girls and family doctors.

This chapter will now discuss the management of adolescents with gynaecological problems and address the following areas: history and examination, normal and delayed puberty, common gynaecological disorders in this age group (menstruation disorders, abdominal pain, vaginal discharge), neoplasia and, finally, contraception in teenagers. The aim is to provide a practical, problem-orientated approach.

HISTORY AND EXAMINATION

The approach to history taking and examination of the adolescent must differ from that of the adult. As suggested, privacy and comfort are essential. We believe it best to interview the girl alone as this allows a rapport to be established and confidentiality to be maintained. At the end of the interview, the problem and any additional information necessary can be discussed with the girl's parent or guardian. In our experience, the girl herself appreciates this sort of approach and confidential information may be revealed, which might not have otherwise been obtained. Interestingly, often the mother also finds this approach helpful as it allows her daughter to feel she is being treated as an adult. It also minimizes any unwelcome effects of a dominant mother. In our clinic, neither medical students nor nurses are present, and the girls are interviewed on a one-to-one basis. Occasionally, this is not possible, as in the very young girl or those with mental handicap – in this situation, the mother's presence is essential. It is best to begin by asking general questions, for example, about her position in the family, schooling and interests, rather than moving directly to the presenting problem. This allows her to relax and gain confidence. Regarding the gynaecological problem, direct questioning is often necessary to obtain a clear picture of the situation. Accurate details of any previous medical problems are essential and often the mother is a more reliable historian in this regard. This information, however, can be obtained at the end of the interview. Most teenagers will give an honest answer to questions about sexual activity once they realize that confidentiality is guaranteed. It is important not to avoid this question or presume it is irrelevant in a particular girl as her management may well differ if she is sexually active. We found it less easy to obtain information regarding sexual abuse at the initial unit but when confidence has been obtained it may be that this information is given. It has become obvious in our clinic that the problem presented may simply be caused by ignorance of what is normal, for example, menstrual cycle disturbances or a vaginal discharge.

Once the history has been completed, a physical examination should be performed. This must include a general examination with appraisal of sec-

Table 12.1 Physical changes during puberty

Physical feature	Age (years)
Breast growth	9–13
Pubic hair growth	9–13
Axillary hair growth	10–14
Growth in height	10–14
Menstruation	11–15

ondary sexual development, congenital anomalies, height and weight. A gynaecological examination can be performed in those who are sexually active and should include speculum examination and cervical smear. A limited digital vaginal examination is possible without distress in girls using vaginal tampons; however, we do not routinely perform speculum examinations in this group. Where this is not possible, ultrasound examination of the pelvis provides more valuable information than a rectal examination, which may cause distress. Examination under anaesthesia is rarely required. In general, the gynaecological examination of the adolescent can be performed simply and sensitively. Patience, awareness of the patient's need to be treated with respect and honesty and some modification of the adult technique will allow a helpful examination in almost all cases.

On completion of the examination, the nature of the problem and its management should be discussed in detail with the girl. At the end of this, her mother can be brought in and the situation explained in the girl's presence. In this way, the patient will appreciate that confidentiality has been maintained. There is an inevitable conflict between the patient's right to confidentiality and the parent's wish to be fully informed of all matters relevant to her daughter. In general, however, it is in the patient's best interest to respect her confidences, regardless of her age, unless of course she is being exploited and in need of protection.

NORMAL PUBERTY

Puberty has been defined as the state of being functionally capable of procreation. This term is generally used in a more comprehensive sense, however, to refer to the whole period of time during which secondary sexual characteristics develop, menstruation begins and the psychosexual outlook of the patient changes. There are five main physical features of puberty: breast growth, pubic hair growth, axillary hair growth, growth in height, and menstruation. The average age range at which these changes occur is shown in Table 12.1. The order of appearance of these changes is not strict. Approximately 50% of girls begin with breast development and growth in height, followed by pubic and axillary hair growth, and then by the onset of menstruation. However, in the remaining 50%, these events occur in a different pattern, for example, pubic hair growth before breast growth, menstruation

Table 12.2 Delayed puberty: causes

Symptom	Cause
Normal development but amenorrhoea	Anatomical cause
	Resistant ovary syndrome
Poor or absent development	Constitutional delay
	Gonadal dysgenesis
	Hypothalamic or pituitary failure of rhythmic FSH/LH production
Heterosexual development	XY female
	Congenital adrenal hyperplasia
	Adrenal tumour
	Masculinizing ovarian tumours
	Cushing's Syndrome

before axillary hair growth. It is important to note this variability. The changes vary in the age of onset, time of full development and order of their appearance. It is a mistake to expect any two girls to be the same. What is reasonably constant, however, is that menstruation usually commences after the maximum growth rate (which can be as much as 6–11 cm per year). Also, there is a relationship between skeletal maturity and the onset of menstruation. At the menarche, the majority of girls have a bone age of 13 to 14 years. It is unusual for menstruation to begin before a bone age of 12.5 years or after 14.5 years. This feature is useful in the assessment of pubertal delay (see below). Although menstruation may have begun, regular menstrual cycles may not become established for a further 1–2 years.

DELAYED PUBERTY

The first question to be addressed here is: when is delayed puberty abnormal? This must be considered in terms of the complete development of the patient, and not just restricted to the onset of menstruation. Therefore, one must consider both the secondary sexual development and menstrual status of.the girl. It is not possible to state an exact age at which puberty should take place. This is evident from the range of ages shown in Table 12.1 at which the various physical features of puberty develop. In general, however, if secondary sexual development has not begun by the age of 15 years, investigations should be instigated. Regarding the menarche, if in the process of normal secondary sexual development this has not occurred by 16 years of age, then assessment of possible reasons for the delay is advisable.

The approach to management of these girls can be based on their secondary sexual development. As shown in Table 12.2, the causes of delayed puberty can be divided into three groups according to the degree of sexual development: normal development but amenorrhoea; poor or absent development; heterosexual development. The assessment of these girls should include the following facts: age; height; weight; the degree of secondary sexual development, including the presence of any heterosexual development or associated abnormal physical features (such as neck webbing in gonadal dysgenesis); the presence of cyclical abnormal pain; examination for an abdominal or pelvic swelling and inspection and examination of the vulva and introitus for abnormalities. The investigations will depend on the clinical assessment. The management of these patients is summarized in Table 12.3.

Normal development with amenorrhoea

The commonest cause of primary amenorrhoea in a girl with normal secondary sexual development is the presence of an imperforate hymen. Menstrual blood accumulates in the vagina causing haematocolpos. She may describe intermittent abdominal pain, which may be cyclical. On examination an abdominal and/or pelvic mass is present, and inspection of the introitus reveals a tense bulging bluish membrane. Treatment is simple with incision of the imperforate hymen to release retained menstrual fluid. Occasionally the situation is more complex with either the presence of a transverse vaginal septum or congenital absence of the vagina. In these cases, complete assessment of the degree of vaginal development is essential before surgery is performed. The presence of co-existing urinary tract anomalies should be sought and hence intravenous pyelography performed. The surgery for those patients with a low vaginal septum involves excision of the septum and anastomosis of the upper and lower vagina. Where the vaginal septum is high, more extensive surgery is required, for example, an abdominoperineal approach and reconstruction of the vagina over a solid mould to allow epithelialization. A detailed description of these procedures is outside the scope of this chapter.[4,5] For patients with congenital absence of the vagina, the uterus is usually absent or at least rudimentary. Hence, their management must include appropriate psychological support. Initial therapy should be non-surgical using the Frank technique of indentation.[6] Surgery should be reserved for those patients not responding to this method. The surgery involves vaginoplasty – either that described by Williams[7] or in more recent years, the use of skin or amnion to line the new vaginal space.[8,9] Our experience using amnion vaginoplasty is that the procedure is not difficult and that, provided the patient complies with dilator use postoperatively, functional and anatomical success is achieved.

The resistant ovary syndrome is rare. It is characterized by primary amenorrhoea in the presence of secondary sexual development with elevated gonadotrophins and normal ovarian structure.[10] It is important not to misdiagnose this syndrome as premature ovulation failure as the ovaries contain ova and, hence, although reduced, fertility is possible with ovarian stimulation. If the oestrogen levels are low, then hormone replacement therapy is advisable to protect against osteoporosis. If not, however, treatment is not necessary until ovulation induction is requested.

Table12. 3 Management of delayed puberty

Cause		Investigations	Treatment
Normal development but amenorrhoea			
Anatomical	Imperforate hymen	Clinical examination	Surgery
	Vaginal septum	Clinical examination	
	Vaginal absence	EUA	
		IVP	
		Pelvic ultrasound	Psychological support
Resistant ovary syndrome		FSH ↑	Hormone replacement
		LH ↑	if oestrogen low
		Oestrogen may be low	Ovulation induction
		Laparoscopy and ovarian biopsy	
Poor or absent development			
Constitutional delay		History	Wait
		Bone age	
Gonadal dysgenesis		Chromosomal analysis	Hormonal
		FSH ↑	Ethinyloestradiol
		LH ↑	followed by
		Streak ovaries at	progestogen
		laparoscopy	Anabolic steroids
			Growth hormone
			Gonadectomy if Y
			chromosome present
			Psychological support
Hypothalamic/pituitary failure of FSH/LH production		FSH ↓ LH ↓	Hormonal as in b
		Skull X-ray	Ovulation induction
		CT scan	
		LHRH stimulation test	
		TFTs	
		Laparoscopy + ovarian biopsy	
Heterosexual development			
XY female		Chromosomal analysis	Hormone replacement
		Testosterone ↓ or ↑	Gonadectomy
		FSH ↑	External genitalia
		LH↑	reconstruction
		Laparotomy +	Psychological support
		gonadal biopsy	
Congenital adrenal hyperplasia		Chromosome analysis	Steroids
		Urinary oxosteroids	External genitalia
		Serum 17-hydroxy	reconstruction
		progesterone	
		ACTH stimulation test	
Adrenal tumours		Androstenedione, dehydroepiandrosterone test	Surgery
Malignant ovarian tumours		Radiological and ultrasound evaluation	Surgery
Cushing's Syndrome		Cortisol assay	Medical management
		ACTH assay suppression test	

TFTS = thyroid function tests

Poor or absent development

Constitutional delayed puberty is usually diagnosed from the history and examination. There may be a history of significant medical conditions which can retard development at puberty. Often there is a familial tendency to this problem. Clinical examination will often show that pubertal development has begun and the growth spurt has started. Investigations can be limited to the radiological assessment of bone age – if this is less than the chronological age, it is reasonable to wait and allow development to progress. One other feature worth consideration is anorexia nervosa. There is a loose association between weight and the onset of menstruation in that most girls will not menstruate until a weight of 47 kg is achieved. In patients where secondary sexual development has not started and the girl is underweight, anorexia nervosa should be considered.

The commonest form of gonadal dysgenesis is Turner's Syndrome, where an X chromosome is missing giving a 45X karyotype. Other chromosomal anomalies exist such as mosaic patterns – 45X/46XX, 45X/46XY – or structural abnormalities with deletion of part of the chromosome ($46XX_q$–$46XX_p$).[11] In these situations, the clinical features will vary from the classical features of Turner's Syndrome. Discussion here will concentrate on the commonest form except to state that, where mosaic patterns exist and a Y chromosome is present, the management should include gonadectomy because of the risk of subsequent malignancy.

The clinical features of Turner's Syndrome include short stature, absent secondary sexual development, wide carrying angle of the arms, webbed neck, widely spaced nipples and primary amenorrhoea. Associated features include short metatarsals and coarctation of the aorta. There are streak gonads without ova, but normal uterus, tubes, vagina and vulva. Investigations must include chromosome analysis and determination of follicle-stimulating hormone (FSH) and luteinizing hormone (LH) levels which will be markedly elevated. Laparoscopy and ovarian biopsy are only necessary where the chromosomal pattern is other than 45X. The treatment is based on hormonal replacement therapy and psychological support. Care must be taken when hormone therapy is commenced because excess oestrogen administration will restrict skeletal growth by causing epiphysial fusion. Treatment should begin with low doses such as ethinyloestradiol 1–2 µg/day. This can then be increased gradually over 2 years to 20–30 µg/day. The aim of this treatment is to mimic natural puberty. Progestogens should be added for 5 days every 4 weeks to prevent the problems of unopposed oestrogen on the uterus. This treatment approach allows secondary sexual development and menstruation. The adult dose of 20–30 µg ethinyloestradiol should only be used when secondary sexual development has occurred. Other treatment options for growth promotion in these patients include anabolic steroids, such as oxandrolone, and growth hormone. Growth hormone has been shown to be effective even in those girls without a deficiency of growth hormone.[12,13] Obviously these patients require considerable psychological and social support. They are infertile but perhaps ovum donation may be an option in the future. Many countries now have groups which provide useful psychological support.

The presence of hypothalamic or pituitary lesions can result in delayed sexual maturation and primary amenorrhoea. Detailed investigation is required to diagnose the nature of the problem. There may be associated conditions such as Kallman's syndrome or Laurence-Moon-Biredl syndrome. Central nervous system lesions such as craniopharyngioma, gliomas and pituitary neoplasms may be present. Others have a functional disorder in the hypothalamic–pituitary axis. Clinical assessment must include identification of any associated signs. Radiological examination of the hypothalamus and pituitary with skull X-ray, CT scans and/or Magnetic Resonance Imaging should be performed. Endocrine tests should include gonadotrophin levels, thyroid function tests and, if anatomic lesion is excluded, the LHRH test to determine whether the problem lies in the hypothalamus or pituitary. For a functional disorder of gonadotrophin production the treatment involves hormonal treatment as for gonadal dysgenesis. These patients are not infertile and can respond to ovulation induction regimens.

Heterosexual development

Patients who present with amenorrhoea and are found to have heterosexual features on examination are rare. The most distressing problem here is the diagnosis of the XY female. Detailed descriptions are available elsewhere.[14] Briefly, the condition results from one of three main causes: failure of the testes to produce androgens; androgen insensitivity; true hermaphrodite. Where there is an anatomical failure of the testes to produce androgens, there is also a failure to produce Mullerian inhibitor and hence these patients have a uterus, fallopian tubes and vagina. Where the problem is caused by an enzymatic failure in androgen production, however, Mullerian inhibitor is produced and therefore there is no uterus, fallopian tubes or vagina. The management of either of these conditions, however, is the same with hormone replacement therapy as in gonadal dysgenesis except that those without a uterus do not require progestogens. Gonadectomy is essential because of the risk of malignancy caused by the presence of the Y chromosome. In some cases of enzymatic failure, surgery of the external genitalia will be required, for example creation of a neovagina. Once again psychological support is required and patients should continue to be reared as females. These patients usually present as tall girls without secondary sexual development and with amenorrhoea; they may have some secondary feminization depending on the production of oestrogens and androstenedione.

The patient with androgen insensitivity has normal testes and hence normal testosterone and mullerian inhibitor production. The uterus, tubes and upper vagina are absent but there may be some lower vaginal development from the urogenital signs. The classical picture is a patient presenting with primary amenorrhoea from oestrogen conversion of androtenedione. Pubic and axillary hair will be sparse or absent; the vulva will look normal, testosterone levels will be normal but FSH and LH levels elevated. The management involves gonadectomy and oestrogen replacement to prevent menopausal symptoms. Surgical elongation of the short vagina is rarely necessary.

The condition of true hermaphroditism has usually been diagnosed in the neonatal period when an infant has ambiguous genitalia and the other causes of masculinization of a female infant (such as congenital adrenal hyperplasia masculinizing tumours, exogenous maternal hormone administration) have been excluded. Rarely, the condition may present in adolescence with the development of heterosexual features. The same approach to its diagnosis in infancy is required with laparotomy and gonadal biopsy for confirmation. Surgical reconstruction of the genitalia, such as clitoral reduction and division of labial adhesions, may be required; gonadectomy will necessitate appropriate hormonal replacement therapy.

The other causes of masculinization of a female at adolescence are congenital adrenal hyperplasia (CAH), adrenal tumours, masculinizing ovarian tumours and, rarely, Cushing's syndrome. Chromosomal abnormalities must be excluded and the management of these patients then depends on the underlying condition, for example appropriate steroid regimens in CAH and excision of adrenal or ovarian neoplasms. Some reconstruction of the external genitalia may be required.

The problem of precocious puberty has not been addressed in this discussion of normal and delayed puberty as this is not a condition of adolescence and usually rather presents in childhood.

COMMON GYNAECOLOGICAL DISORDERS IN ADOLESCENCE

Menstrual disorders

Disturbances of menstruation, either actual or perceived, are the commonest presenting complaint in our Adolescent Gynaecology Clinic (75% of new patients). There are three main complaints: dysmenorrhoea, irregular menses and excessive menstrual bleeding. It is important to remember that the onset of menstruation does not mean that ovulation has occurred. Forty-five per cent of girls do not have ovulatory menstrual cycles for 2 years after the menarche. The first menses are usually anovulatory. This is of importance in relation to the problems of irregular and excessive menses. Table 12.4 outlines the management approach for menstrual disorders.

DYSMENORRHOEA

Of the adolescent girls with menstrual disorders attending our clinic the most frequent complaint was dysmenorrhoea. It is classified as primary or

Table 12.4 Menstrual disorders in adolescence

Type	Investigation	Treatment
Dysmenorrhoea		
Primary	History	PGSI
	Examination	COCP
Secondary	History	PGSI
	Examination	COCP
	Pelvic ultrasound	Treat underlying condition if present
	Laparoscopy	
	Hysteroscopy	
Irregular menses		
Polymenorrhoea	History	Progestogens in luteal phase
	Examination	COCP
Oligomenorrhoea	Prolactin	Bromocriptine
	TFTs	
	FSH LH (PCOS)	Oestrogen progesterone preparation ±
	Androgens	
	Oestradiol	Cyproterone acetate
Excessive Menstrual Bleeding	FBC	PGSI
	Coagulation studies	Progestogens
	TFTs	COCP
	Pelvic ultrasound	
	Hysteroscopy	

PGSI, prostaglandin synthetase inhibitor; COCP, combined oral contraceptive pill; FBC, full blood count; FSH, follicle-stimulating hormone; LH, luteinizing hormone; PCOS, polycystic ovarian syndrome.

secondary. Primary dysmenorrhoea starts on the first day of menstruation and usually lasts for 12 to 24 hours. It only occurs in ovulatory cycles and so usually does not present until ovulation has been established. It does not indicate underlying pathology. Secondary dysmenorrhoea usually begins before menstruation and lasts for the duration of the bleeding. It may be predictive of uterine or pelvic pathology such as endometriosis, uterine anomalies or pelvic adhesions. In adolescents, primary dysmenorrhoea is the commonest type. Its aetiology is thought to be caused by increased prostaglandin synthesis, mainly PGE_2 and PGF_2.[15] While as many as one-half of all women at some stage in their lives complain of dysmenorrhoea, it tends to be most severe in young nulliparous women. In adolescence it can be severe and cause as many as 5–10% to miss school, college or work. The problem may be compounded by fear, especially where the young girl has seen her mother suffer from the same problem on a regular basis. This fact has been reported as long as 20 years ago and in our experience still persists today.[16] More than 20% of our patients with dysmenorrhoea report that their mothers or sisters also had similar problems.

The management of these girls begins with a complete history, paying particular attention to the disruption to her life at the time of menstruation. An attempt should be made to differentiate primary from secondary dysmenorrhoea. A past history of renal problems in childhood should raise the question of an associated uterine anomaly. A general physical examination should be performed. As discussed earlier it is often easy to perform a gentle vaginal examination. Pelvic ultrasound is useful if a uterine anomaly is suspected. A hysteroscopy or laparoscopy is rarely required. In our practice we treat first and then only proceed to these investigations if the treatment is unsuccessful, unless of course the history is suggestive of endometriosis. Diagnostic curettage is now regarded as unnecessary and unhelpful in these patients and so should no longer be routinely performed.[17] The management of these girls begins with an explanation of the reason for the dysmenorrhoea and a reassurance that treatment is available. One study has reported that there is substantial ignorance and misinformation among female adolescents regarding the causes and treatment of dysmenorrhoea.[18]

The pharmacological treatment of dysmenorrhoea in adolescence is with either prostaglandin synthatase inhibitors or combined oestrogen progesterone preparations. Where contraception is not required, drugs such as mefenamic acid or naproxen sodium, ideally starting premenstrually, provides symptomatic relief in up to 70% of patients. In girls who need contraception or in those not responding to analgesics, the combined oral contraceptive pill provides effective relief.[19] Another study has shown that adolescents who improve symptomatically with oral contraceptives are eight times more likely to continue treatment.[20] This has benefits in terms of contraception compliance in this age group.

Some patients will not report any improvement and these require further evaluation. Pelvic ultrasound, hysteroscopy and/or laparoscopy should be performed. The commonest pathological finding in this group is endometriosis. One of the most important factors in the treatment of these girls, however, is the support they receive in attending for help. Hence, it is important that they should be reviewed to monitor whatever treatment has been prescribed.

IRREGULAR MENSTRUAL CYCLES

Normal menstrual cycles are generally defined as 28 days long (range 21–35 days) with bleeding for 4 days (range 2–7 days). This regular cycle depends on the presence of ovulation. Forty-five per cent of adolescents do not ovulate for 1 to 2 years after menarche. Hence it is not surprising that irregular or infrequent cycles is a common occurrence in this age group. Furthermore, the lack of regular menstruation seem to be a considerable cause for concern amongst many girls and their mothers. Much less common is the complaint of polymenorrhoea. In our experience this complaint arises more from a lack of understanding of how to estimate the duration of the menstrual cycle, and of the range of normal, than from an actual true increased frequency of menses.

When a patient presents with oligomenorrhoea, however, it is important to determine whether this is significant. For example, in the first year after the menarche the occurrence of infrequent menses, with delays of several months in between, is normal. Reassurance that this is a self-limiting problem is generally all that is required. The girl who presents, however, with infrequent menses following a previously regular cycle warrants further assessment. The most common reason is suppression of hyothalamic or pituitary function caused by emotional stress. Acute weight loss and excessive exercise are another possibility and it is always worthwhile considering the possibility of anorexia nervosa. Some patients may have just recently stopped the oral contraceptive pill. Rarely, patients will be found to have prolactin-producing pituitary adenomas, and appropriate radiological evaluation is necessary. Thyroid function should also be assessed. Others may have ovarian or adrenal lesions. Polycystic ovarian syndrome can cause oligomenorrhoea. It is often associated with obesity and hirsutism. Measurement of the LH/FSH ratio and androgen levels together with the classical ovarian ultrasound picture will confirm this diagnosis. Laparoscopy is no longer necessary to confirm this condition. Occasionally a patient will be found to have an ovarian tumour which produces androgens but in this situation virilizing changes are usually also present. Even more rare are adrenal tumours or lesions, such as congenital adrenal hyperplasia or Cushing's syndrome. The current consensus that diagnostic curettage is of little value in this age group makes the diagnosis of Asherman's syndrome unlikely.

Patients presenting with secondary amenorrhoea may have any of the possible causes discussed above. One must always consider pregnancy, although, the history may not be forthcoming.

Therefore, the clinical assessment and investigation approach to these patients depends on the most likely underlying problem – only a thorough history and examination can direct the gynaecologist in this regard. Where there is hypothalamic or pituitary suppression from emotional or physical factors, such as weight loss, it is best to address these issues, and pharmacological manipulation of the cycle is unnecessary. Hyperprolactinaemia is easily treated with bromocriptine with a rapid return of the menses. However, some patients will require neurosurgical treatment. Whether polycystic ovarian syndrome requires treatment in this age group is unclear and depends on the severity of the symptoms. Cycle regularity can be restored with combined oestrogen-progestogen preparations. In the presence of hirsutism the addition of cyproterone acetate is helpful but it is important the patient realises that significant cosmetic improvements will not be evident for 6 months. What is important for these patients is that they understand that the presence of infrequent menses in their teens does not predict subsequent infertility. In many the problem is self-limiting; in others, where the problem persists and they wish to become pregnant, ovulation induction is generally successful.

In adolescence, polymenorrhoea is usually caused by luteal phase dysfunction. These patients respond well to either progestogen treatment in the luteal phase or combined oestrogen-progesterone preparations, usually of the monophasic type.

EXCESSIVE MENSTRUAL BLEEDING

The young girl who has just started menstruating may find that she experiences excess menstrual loss both in amount and duration. Occasionally this bleeding can continue for several weeks. This may be frightening not only for her but also for her mother and family doctor. Once again the problem of anovulation is the likely cause and therefore this problem occurs much more commonly in the younger teenager. As ovulation has not occurred the endometrium continues to be stimulated by unopposed oestrogen; when menstruation eventually occurs the bleeding tends to be excessive and prolonged. This can be a recurrent problem until the cycle becomes regular, and each episode is usually separated by several weeks of amenorrhoea. Occasionally anaemia results with haemoglobin levels as low as 6 or 7 g/dl. The history of such a patient must also include an assessment of any coagulation disorder or blood dyscrasia. Physical examination is therefore important to detect anaemia, bruising and abdominal or pelvic swellings. Occasionally a complaint of prolonged menses is the presenting feature of genital tract neoplasia. Pelvic examination in these young girls may, however, not be possible and the ultrasound examination is often helpful. Other investigations should include full blood count and coagulation profiles, but endocrine investigations are unnecessary.

The management begins with explanation of the nature of the problem and reassurance that it will resolve over the ensuing months. In many patients no further therapy is required. Hormonal treatment is worthwhile where the girl is anaemic or where the problem is recurrent and restricts her activities. Progestogens alone are generally effective but can be used in combination with oestrogens where breakthrough bleeding occurs. High-dose oestrogen alone is not advisable as it will stimulate endometrial proliferation further. The advantage of progestogen therapy alone is that it can prevent the development of endometrial hyperplasia. Prolonged hormonal therapy, particularly if combined oestrogen-progesterone preparations are used, is not necessary. It may also lead to hypothalamic suppression with subsequent amenorrhoea. The occasional patient will not respond to hormonal therapy and in these patients diagnostic curettage may be warranted. Its main purpose is to assess whether endometrial hyperplasia has developed. If so, cyclical progestogen therapy is necessary and should be continued for up to 12 months. Repeat curettage should then be performed to examine the endometrium. The other aspect of management of patients who have become anaemic is to correct this and, where the bleeding is recurrent, regular haematological checks should be performed.

ABDOMINAL PAIN

Teenagers presenting with abdominal pain, regardless of its nature, are frequently concerned about the presence of ovarian cysts. This concern is often fuelled by maternal anxiety, especially where the girl's mother herself has required surgery for ovarian neoplasms. In our experience, many of the girls presenting have already had a pelvic ultrasound examination for recurrent abdominal pain and the incidental finding of physiological follicular or luteal cysts is the reason for referral to the specialized adolescent gynaecology clinic. However, significant ovarian cysts in adolescence are uncommon. A recent study in Michigan showed 88 ovarian neoplasms, over a 25 year period, in children and adolescents attending a tertiary referral centre.[21] The majority of ovarian neoplasms are benign. Nevertheless the quoted incidence of malignancy varies from 9.8%[22] to 35%.[23] Hence, appropriate evaluation and treatment is essential. Once again a detailed history is the most important starting point. Pathological ovarian neoplasms in adolescence usually present with an episode of acute abdominal pain and often with the presence of an abdominal or pelvic swelling. In our own experience, the chronic recurrent abdominal pain, which is the most common presenting complaint, rarely reveals ovarian pathology and is more likely to be caused by conditions such as irritable bowel syndrome, or in other cases may reflect psycho-social stresses.

Ultrasound examination of the ovaries is valuable and can help differentiate these cysts which can be managed conservatively, by laparoscopy and those which require laparotomy and ovarian cystectomy or oophorectomy. Where possible it is always important to try and conserve the affected ovary and contralateral ovary if oophorectomy is required. In our practice a simple unilocular cyst of less than 5 cm in diameter is managed conservatively, initially, with serial ultrasound examination at 4-weekly intervals. If the cyst persists or enlarges then laparoscopic aspiration is attempted provided the laparoscopic findings confirm a benign appearance, and cytology is performed on the aspirated fluid. Where a multilocular or mixed solid/cystic neoplasm is present then laparotomy is performed. Ovarian cystectomy is performed if, macroscopically, the neoplasm is benign. This is particularly important where dermoid cysts are present as 10% of these are bilateral. Oophorectomy is performed where malignancy is suspected, but again only if the tumour is unilateral. The contralateral ovary is conserved. Germ cell tumours are the commonest malignant ovarian neoplasm in this age group.[21] Adjunctive combination chemotherapy is successful in these patients where necessary.[24]

VAGINAL DISCHARGE

Adolescents are often concerned about vaginal discharge because its occurrence is associated with infection. However, they are often ignorant about physiological vaginal discharge and unaware that this varies with the menstrual cycle. Hence a clear history of the nature, quantity, colour and odour of the discharge, together with the presence of any associated symptoms such as pruritus, is essential. Questions about sexual activity and sexual abuse must be asked.

Details of any previous treatments such as antimicrobials, local douches, disinfectants, etc., must be elicited. Attention to hygiene and clothing is also important. If the discharge is persistent, foul smelling, discoloured and associated with pruritus then vaginal infection should be suspected. Examination of the vulva and lower vagina is easily performed without speculum examination. Obviously, if the patient is sexually active or is using vaginal tampons for menstruation then a speculum examination should be performed. High vaginal and/or endocervical swabs should be obtained for culture and sensitivity. This is also an opportunity to perform a cervical smear. A blood-stained discharge should alert the gynaecologist to the possibility of vaginal neoplasia or trauma. In our service a mullerian adenofibroma of the cervix presented as a profuse bloodstained discharge in a 14 year old. Although she was not sexually active a limited vaginal examination was possible in the outpatient department, and the tumour was diagnosed. She was then admitted for further evaluation and treatment.

The management depends on the type of discharge. In physiological discharge, explanation and reassurance, with hygiene advice including avoidance of local chemical treatments, is all that is required. If a specific infection is diagnosed then an antimicrobial therapy is appropriate. For those girls who are sexually active, the question of sexually transmitted disease (STD) is important. The clinical presentation of STD in adolescents is the same as in adults. However, adolescents are at an increased risk of STD as they are less likely to anticipate the consequences of their actions.[25] Adolescents account for 25–50% of all cases of gonorrhoea in the USA. However, chlamydia infection is more common than gonorrhoea, occurring in 8% to 27% of adolescent girls.[25] Human papilloma virus and herpes simplex virus infections are also common. Therefore, gynaecologists should have a high index of suspicion for STD in this age group. A discussion of STD prevention through delaying sexual activity, the use of barrier methods of contraception and limiting the number of sexual partners should be part of routine care for adolescents.

GYNAECOLOGICAL MALIGNANCY IN ADOLESCENTS

A detailed discussion of all the potential gynaecological malignancies in adolescents is outside the scope of this chapter. However, the management of three particular malignancies will be briefly described – vulvovaginal rhabdomyosarcoma, clear cell adenocarcinoma of the vagina and ovarian germ cell tumours – mainly because of the recent advances in their treatment.

Vulvovaginal rhabodomyosarcoma

This mixed mesodermal tumour is the most common malignancy of the lower genital tract in young girls. More commonly known as sarcoma botryoides, its site of origin can be the vulva, vagina, cervix or uterus, with cervical or uterine lesions occurring more frequently in the adolescent age group. The patient can present with vulval, perineal or vaginal lesions, or with a polypoid mass resembling a bunch of grapes protruding through the introitus. Histologically there is a continuous condensed band of tumour cells below the surface epithelium with smaller pleiomorphic tumour cells, some of which have rhabdomyoblastic differentiation embedded in a myxoid stroma. In the 1970s multimodality therapy with radical surgery, radiotherapy and combination chemotherapy was the main treatment.[26] More recently, however, local excision with or without chemotherapy, has been shown to be effective,[27–29] thus preserving fertility.

Clear cell adenocarcinoma of the vagina

The first report of the association between intrauterine exposure to diethylstilbestrol (DES) and the development of adenocarcinoma of the vagina was in 1971.[30] The most recent report from the Registry for Research on Hormonal Transplacental Carcinogenesis reveals 547 cases of clear adenocarcinoma of the vagina and cervix in the USA.[31] Initially, treatment for this condition was either radical pelvic surgery (radical hysterectomy, pelvic lymphadenectomy, total vaginectomy and replacement of the vagina with split-thickness skin graft) or whole pelvic radiation and vaginal radiation. In 1987, however, the combination of wide local excision (with preservation of vaginal function and fertility) with retroperitoneal pelvic lymphadenectomy, to exclude lymph node metastasis, followed by local radiation was reported as an effective treatment for lesions less than 2 cm in diameter.[32] Theoretically, effective chemotherapy would allow for even less localized therapy but this modality has yet to be developed.

Ovarian germ cell tumours

Germ cell tumours of the ovary are another gynaecological malignancy that, owing to the development of newer chemotherapeutic agents, has seen major improvements in survival with more conservative therapy; at the same time future fertility has been preserved. From the treatment point of view these tumours can be divided into (a) pure dysgerminoma and (b) nondysgerminoma including endodermal sinus tumour embryonal carcinoma, immature teratoma, choriocarcinoma and mixed germ cell tumours.

Dysgerminomas

These are the most common germ cell tumours of the ovary and account for 3% to 51% of all ovarian malignancies. They are bilateral in 15% of patients and are associated with early pelvic and para-aortic lymph node metastases. They are extremely radiosensitive. Conservative surgery with unilateral salpino-oophorectomy followed by ipsilateral hemipelvic and para-aortic lymph node radiation, while shielding the contralateral ovary and uterus, has been reported with good results.[33] More recently, reports using cisplatin-based combination chemotherapy following conservative surgery suggest that such chemotherapy will replace radiotherapy in these patients.[34]

Nondysgerminomas

This group of tumours differs from the dysgerminoma group in that less than 1% are bilateral. However, with the change to cisplatin-based chemotherapeutic regimens a similar approach of unilateral salpingoophorectomy followed by combination chemotherapy provides effective treatment with higher cure rates. Therefore, this once-lethal disease of young girls can now be cured with retention of future fertility.

TEENAGE CONTRACEPTION

Sexual activity in teenagers is increasing. A recent publication shows that 54% of 15–16 year olds are sexually active.[35] This compares with a figure of 15% for 15–19 year olds in the UK in 1965.[36] Mellanby et al[35] reported that those who had sex before the age of 16 were almost twice as likely to have had sex at some time without using contraception, were twice as likely to have had sex within a short relationship, and were three times more likely to know a close friend with a sexually transmitted disease. The medical problems associated with teenage sexual activity, including teenage pregnancies and complications from sexually transmitted disease, are increasing, despite the efforts of schools and parents, the availability of family planning clinics, and advertising. The problem of preventing unwanted pregnancies in teenagers remains, and needs to be urgently addressed.[37] Methods of contraception that are effective among older women are not necessarily ones that work for adolescents. The most effective contraceptive method for adolescents is the oral contraceptive pill; compliance, however, remains a problem, particularly in the younger patient. Provided there are no absolute contraindications it has few, if any, significant side effects and some benefits, such as a reduction in dysmenorrhoea. As adolescents do not usually plan sexual encounters, barrier methods are not as effective in this population. Other patients may be better advised to use injectable contraception, such as medroxyprogesterone acetate; however, its association with menstrual irregularity and amenorrhoea make it unacceptable to some. Whatever the method chosen all doctors looking after adolescents have an obligation to provide appropriate education and advice to this vulnerable group.

CONCLUSIONS

Teenagers with gynaecological problems need to be sensitively dealt with. The majority of their problems can be dealt with simply. Nevertheless, adolescent gynaecology remains an area to which greater attention should be given if we are to protect and promote the health of our teenagers. This can perhaps best be done in specialized adolescent gynaecology clinics.

REFERENCES

1 Malus M. Towards a separate adolescent medicine. Br Med J 1992; 305: 789
2 Dewhurst J. Practical paediatric and adoloescent gynaecology. 2nd edn. Edwards K, ed. London: Butterworths, 1989
3 Sternlieb J J, Munan L. A survey of health problems, practices and needs of youth. Paediatrics 1972; 49: 177–186
4 Sheares B H. Congenital atresia of the vagiana: a new technique for funnelling the space between bladder and rectum and construction of the new vagina by a modified Wharton technique. J Obstet Gynaecol Br Emp 1960; 67: 24–31
5 Rock J A, Zacur M A, Dlugi A M, Jones H W, TeLinde R W. Pregnancy success following surgical correction of imperforate hymen and complete transverse vaginal septum. Obstet Gynaecol 1982; 59: 448–451
6 Frank R T. The formation of an artificial vagina without operation. Am J Obstet Gynecol 1938; 35: 1053–1057
7 Williams E A. Congenital absence of the vagina: a simple operation for its relief. J Obstet Gynaecol Br Commonwealth 1964; 71: 511–512
8 Counsellor V S, Flor F S. Congenital absence of the vagina. Surg Clin N Am 1957; 37: 1107
9 Morton K E, Dewhurst C J. Human amnion in the treatment of vaginal malformations. Br J Obstet Gynaecol 1986; 93: 50–54
10 Jones G S, De Moraes-Ruehesen M. A new syndrome of amenorrhoea in association with hypergonadotropism and apparently normal ovarian follicular apparatus. Am J Obstet Gynecol 1969; 104: 597–600
11 Dewhurst C J. Chromosome abnormalities and the gynaecologist. J Obstet Gynaecol Br Commonwealth 1971; 78: 1058–1076
12 Rosenfeld R G, Hintz R L, Johansen A J et al. Three year results of a randomized prospective trial of methionyl human growth hormone and oxandrolone in Turner syndrome. J Paediatr 1988; 113: 393–400
13 Rengen-Westerlaker C, Fokker M M, Wit J M et al. Two year results of treatment with methionyl human growth hormone in children with Turner syndrome. Acta Paediatr Scand 1990; 79: 658–663
14 Dewhurst C J, Spence J E H. The XY Female. Br J Hosp Med 1977; 17: 498–506
15 Rees M C P, Anderson A B M, Demens L M, Turnbull A C. Prostaglandins in menstrual fluid in menorrhagia and dysmenorrhoea. Br J Obstet Gynaecol 1984; 91: 673–680
16 Dickens A. Excessive menstrual bleeding and dysmenorrhoea. Clin Obstet Gynaecol 1974; 17: 655–659
17 Sheil O, Turner M J. Diagnostic dilatation and curettage. Br Med J 1993; 306: 719
18 Johnson J. Level of knowledge among adolescent girls regarding effective treatment for dysmenorrhoea. J Adolesc Health Care 1988; 9: 398–402
19 Milsom I, Sundell G, Andresch B. The influence of different combined oral contraceptives in the prevalence and severity of dysmenorrhoea. Contraception 1990; 42: 497–506
20 Robinson J C, Plichta S, Weismen C S, Nathasan C A, Ensminger M. Dysmenorrhoea and use of oral contraceptives in adolescent women attending a family planning clinic. Am J Obstet Gynecol 1992; 166: 578–583
21 Haefner H K, Roberts J A, Schmidt R W. The university experience of clinical and pathological findings of ovarian neoplasia in children and adolescents. Adolesc Pediatr Gynecol 1992; 5: 182–187
22 Diamond M P, Baxtor J W, Peerman G, Burnett L S. Occurence of ovarian malignancy in childhood and adolescence – A community wide evaluation. Obstet Gynecol 1988; 71: 858–860
23 Breen J C, Maxon W S. Ovarian tumours in children and adolescents. Clin Obstet Gynecol 1977; 20: 607–623
24 Schwartz P E, Chambers S K, Chambers J T, Kohorn E, McIntosh S. Ovarian germ cell

malignancies – the Yale University experience. Gynecol Oncol 1992; 45: 26–31

25 Berry P L, Schubiner H, Giblin P T. Issues in adolescent gynaecological care. Obstet Gynecol Clin N Am 1990; 17(4): 837–849

26 La Vecchia C, Draper G J, Fransceshi S. Childhood non ovarian genital tract cancer in Britain 1962–1978. Cancer 1984; 54: 188–192

27 Hays D M, Schimada H, Reney R B, Teffft M, Newton W, Crist W M, Lawrence W, Regab A, Beltangady M, Maurer H M. Clinical staging and treatment results in Rhabo myosarcoma of the female genital tract among children and adolescents. Cancer 1988; 61: 1893–1903

28 Daya D, Scully R E. Sarcoma boryoides of the uterine cervix in young women: A clinicopathological study of 13 cases. Gynecol Oncol 1988; 29: 290–304

29 Gordon A N, Montag T W. Sarcoma Botroides of the cervix: Excision followed by adjuvant chemotherapy for preservation of reproductive function. Gynecol Oncol 1990; 36: 119–124

30 Herbst A L, Ulefelder H, Poskanzer D C. Adenocarcinoma of the vagina of maternal stilbestrol therapy with tumor appearance in young women. N Eng J Med 1971; 284: 878–881

31 Herbst A L, Anderson D. Clear cell adenocarcinoma of the vagina and cervix secondary to intrauterine exposure to diethylboestrol. Semin Surg Oncol 1990; 6: 343–346

32 Serekjian E K, Frey K W, Anderson D et al. Local therapy in stage I clear cell adenocarcinoma of the vagina. Cancer 1987; 60: 1319–1324

33 De Palo G, Lattuada A, Kenda R et al. Germ cell tumour of the ovary: The experience of the National Cancer Institute of Milan. Dysgerminoma Inst J Radiat Oncol Biol Phy 1987; 13: 853–860

34 Gershensar D M, Morris M, Canger A et al. Treatment of malignant germ cell tumours of the ovary with Bleomycin, etoposide and cisplatin. J Clin Oncol 1990; 8: 715–720

35 Mellanby A, Phelps F, Tripp J H. Teenagers, sex and risk taking. Br Med J 1993; 307: 25

36 Schofield M. The sexual behaviour of young people. London: Longhams, 1965

37 Smith T. Influence of socio economic factors on attaining targets for reducing teenage pregnancies. Br Med J 1993; 306: 1232–1235.

13 Anatomy of female continence

M. J. Quinn

The pathoanatomy of urinary stress incontinence (USI) was originally described as 'posterior and inferior rotation of the bladder neck with an increase in intra-abdominal pressure'. [1-4] 'Anatomic' stress incontinence (ASI) described the *loss of anatomical support* of the urethrovesical junction, although the indirect nature of bead-chain cystourethrography ensured that it could not be differentiated from continent patients with genital prolapse. Real time imaging of the bladder neck using X-rays[5] or ultrasound[6] has enabled urinary loss concurrent with a cough (pathophysiology) to be demonstrated *with* the loss of anatomical support (pathoanatomy). Between ASI and its recent description with real-time imaging techniques, traditional urodynamic theory has developed 'genuine' stress incontinence (Table 13.1) and the 'pressure transmission theory' of female continence[7] although it is remarkable that its validity was questioned by the author shortly after its original description. Some of the premises associated with the traditional urodynamic theory will be contrasted with contemporary anatomical views of female continence and illustrated with magnetic resonance (MR) imaging techniques.

Table 13.1 Definitions of stress incontinence based on clinical, radiological and urodynamic observations.

'Urinary' stress incontinence	The patient's complaint of an involuntary loss of urine with an increase in intra-abdominal pressure
'Demonstrable' stress incontinence	The demonstration of urine loss concurrent with a cough, usually with the patient in the erect position
'Anatomic' stress incontinence	Posterior and inferior rotation of the urethrovesical junction with an increase in intra-abdominal pressure demonstrated by fluoroscopy in a patient with urinary incontinence
'Genuine' stress incontinence	An involuntary loss of urine occurring, when in the absence of a detrusor contraction, the intravesical pressure exceeds the maximum urethral pressure demonstrated by twin-channel, subtraction cystometry with, or without, fluoroscopy

235

THEORIES OF FEMALE CONTINENCE

The 'pressure transmission' hypothesis of female continence depends upon the female urethra being divided into 'intra-abdominal' and 'extra-abdominal' portions by the pelvic floor (Fig. 13.1). Any increase in intra-abdominal pressure is transmitted concurrently to the bladder and the proximal urethra to prevent urinary leakage.[7] Similarly, genuine stress incontinence is portrayed in terms of changes in intravesical pressure to differentiate it from detrusor incontinence (Table 13.1), however, the definition does not describe the pathoanatomy of USI and may not be exclusive to the condition that is successfully treated by suprapubic surgery. In the testing situation where a series of coughs is used to provoke urinary leakage, genuine stress incontinence is associated with passive, concurrent, urinary loss and associated with posterior and inferior rotation of the vesical neck (Fig. 13.9) whereas detrusor incontinence may vary in both the nature and timing of urinary loss relative to the cough (Fig. 13.10) and may not be associated with anatomical displacement of the vesical neck.[6] The primary objection to the pressure transmission hypothesis is the absence of an anatomical feature that separates the intra-abdominal from the extra-abdominal urethra; pubococcygeus, and other components of the levator ani, have no direct relationship with the urethra.

The hammock hypothesis is an alternative theory of female continence that re-emphasises anatomical principles.[8] Continence is maintained by - compression of the urethrovesical junction against the hammock of the anterior vaginal wall and the pubocervical fascia during an increase in

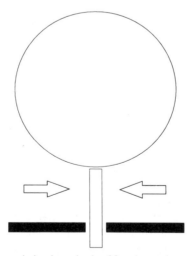

Fig. 13.1 The pressure transmission hypothesis of female continence depends on the transmission of any increase in intra-abdominal pressure to the intra-abdominal proximal urethra to maintain continence. There is no anatomical feature that separates the intra-abdominal urethra from the extra-abdominal urethra (see Figs 13.5 & 13.6).

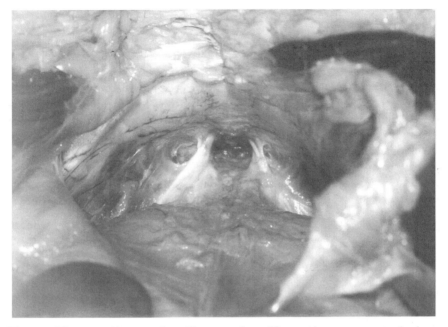

Fig. 13.2 The retropubic space of a nulliparous cadaver. The anterior suspensory mechanism of the vesical neck is clearly demonstrated and connects the posterior surface of the pubis, the anterior surface of the vesical neck, the urethra and the pubococcygeus. The pubovesical component (white ligamentous structures) inserts into the anterior surface of the bladder and extends posteriorly to the ischial spines as the arcus tendineus fasciae pelvis, otherwise known as the white line over the obturator internus.

intra-abdominal pressure. The anterior vaginal wall is stabilized by its attachments:

1. laterally, to the pelvic side wall by its insertions into the arcus tendineus fasciae pelvis via the pubocervical fascia (Fig. 13.2)
2. anteriorly, to the pubis via the anterior suspensory mechanism of the vesical neck (Fig. 13.2)
3. posteriorly, to the uterine cervix and the uterosacral-cardinal ligament complex via the pericervical connective tissue

Damage to the integrity of this layer at vaginal delivery contributes to both genital prolapse and urinary stress incontinence,[9–12] and explains why the two conditions frequently co-exist. Disruption, or attentuation, of other anatomical supporting structures may also contribute to loss of anatomical support and the potential for 'subsequent development of genital prolapse or USI.[13–16] The relative merits of these two hypotheses of female continence will be discussed by examining some urodynamic aphorisms before considering the detailed anatomy of the lower urinary tract as demonstrated with advanced imaging techniques.

'. . . Symptoms (and signs) are unreliable in the evaluation of bladder function'

Many studies have demonstrated the lack of a relationship between patient's symptoms and urodynamic diagnoses.[17,18] Mundy[19] has questioned the significance of non-weighted comparisons between symptoms and urodynamic diagnoses, many of which do not take into account the demonstration of USI on physical examination or the validity of urodynamic observations. Urodynamic studies have been extensively standardized,[20-24] although none have been validated.[25] Early urodynamic definitions have been arbitrarily defined and recent ambulatory studies have described unstable detrusor activity in 40% of asymptomatic continent subjects calling into question the relationship between abnormal urodynamic findings, particularly phasic increases in intravesical pressure, and clinical symptoms.[26]

'The problem here is one of definition. There is no problem with defining detrusor instability in urodynamic terms, as long as it is recognised that this definition has no real clinical meaning. That, unfortunately, is not the case, and the ICS has suggested that "urge incontinence" be divided into two separate categories: **motor urge**, in which the incontinence is shown to be related to a detrusor contraction by cystometry, and **sensory urge**, where the cystometry does not show a detrusor contraction. The ICS goes on to state then that "sensory urgency incontinence" is incontinence not caused by detrusor contraction. That simply is not proven and not provable.

In addition there is now substantial evidence that detrusor instability which occurs during the course of a cystometrogram may be entirely asymptomatic. Thus the cystometric study is plagued by false negative and false positive results, and it cannot be used as a definitive test of anything except bladder compliance.'

Edward McQuire, 1988[26A]

One view of urodynamic investigation is that it should seek to reproduce the patient's symptoms in the testing situation; failure to do so leaves open the question as to their precise aetiology, and the significance of changes in intravesical pressure conjectural.[27]

'. . . The primary objective of suprapubic surgery is elevation of the bladder neck

According to the pressure transmission theory, the primary objective of suprapubic surgery for primary stress incontinence is elevation of the bladder neck into an intra-abdominal pressure zone. Although this objective secures high rates of continence (80%) and may be appropriate for some subgroups of patients,[28] there is a significant rate of postoperative complications including high rates of irritative symptoms, voiding difficulties and recurrent entercoele.[29-32] Postoperative, pressure transmission ratios of more than 100% are regularly recorded, indicating that alternative mechanisms may be important in restoring female continence.[33] Successful suprapubic surgery restores continence by creating an alternative hammock using a vaginal shelf,[10,34] needle suspension operations[35,36] or an autologous sling, to prevent downward displacement of the urethrovesical junction with an increase in intra-abdominal pressure. In surgical terms this translates into not seeking tissue apposition of the supporting sutures at colposuspension and providing a hammock for the urethrovesical junction either using conventional or laparoscopic techniques to deliver the supporting sutures.[37] Objective evaluation of tissue apposition versus absence of tissue apposition in selected groups of patients has not yet been addressed; however, many surgeons have adopted the latter approach on clinical grounds alone. Creation of a supporting hammock rather than over-elevation of the vaginal fornices may explain some of the differences in the rates of postoperative complications following suprapubic surgery.

'. . . *Detrusor instability is made worse by suprapubic surgery.*'

Objective studies of retropubic surgery for GSI demonstrate that detrusor instability (DI) is caused or cured in equal proportions by colposuspension and that these results persist over medium and long-term follow-up (Table 13.2).[29,38-42] Another expression of these findings is that the cystometrogram (CMG) has a sensitivity of 32% and a specificity of 36% in the prediction of postoperative, symptomatic DI.[25] These observations raise the question as to whether there is there any merit in demonstrating the presence of detrusor instability prior to suprapubic surgery for genuine stress incontinence. Systolic or high pressure DI has been suggested as an important prognostic finding prior to surgery; however, its precise definition is unclear and limited evidence has been advanced to support this proposal.

Part of the explanation of this view is the significance attributed to the

Table 13.2 Relative risk of the predictive value of preoperative detection of detrusor instability (DI) in the postoperative development of DI following colposuspension. Of 396 patients undergoing colposuspension in six series, 68/396 (17%) developed de novo DI postoperatively[43]

Author	No. of patients	Preoperative UDS DI	No DI	Postoperative UDS DI	No DI	De novo DI	Relative risk
Cardozo (1979)[29]	92	0/92	92/92	17/92	75/92	17/92	-
Sand (1988)[44]	66	20/66	46/66	14/66	52/66	5/66	5.9 (2.3–15.7)
Langer (1988)[40]	62	30/62	32/62	29/62	33/62	17/62	1.5 (0.8–2.7)
Milani (1985)[45]	65	20/65	45/65	21/65	44/65	4/65	13.2 (2.2–7.7)
Jorgensen (1988)[46]	56	19/56	37/56	26/56	30/56	11/56	4.0 (2.2–7.7)
Eriksen (1990)[39]	55	21/55	34/55	21/55	34/55	14/55	1.3 (0.6–2.7)

analogy between bladder outflow obstruction secondary to benign prostatic hypertrophy and its association with DI in the high pressure male system and the postoperative finding of DI following primary colposuspension for female urinary stress incontinence in a low pressure outflow unit. No obstructive effect has been consistently described with colposuspension and no urodynamic evidence of obstruction has been demonstrated in a studies of continent postoperative patients with persistent irritative symptoms.[47] The aetiology of DI following suprapubic surgery remains unclear and may result from the over sensitivity of cystometric techniques, inaccurate surgery or putative obstructive effects. Postoperative, symptomatic DI is persistent in the medium term and suggests a persistent aetiology following suprapubic surgery[48] that may be determined by the accuracy of suprapubic surgery.[49] Inaccurate placement of sutures (too high on the vaginal wall) with apposition of the vaginal fornices to the iliopectineal ligaments may result in the trigone being placed under sustained tension and explain persistent irritative symptoms.

'. . . Evidence-based urodynamic investigations'

Most urodynamic definitions and investigations have been standardized although none have been validated in appropriate randomized studies. Literature review with appropriate analysis has produced some controversial conclusions regarding the standard of contemporary urodynamic investigations.[25]

1. no evidence to support the routine, non-investigational use of simple uroflowmetry in the evaluation or management of stress urinary incontinence
2. no evidence that the resting urethral pressure profile can yet separate clearly continent women from those with stress incontinence secondary to urethral dysfunction
3. a routine cystometrogram used to make the diagnosis of DI is a blunt instrument: if negative it does not rule out the condition; if positive: it does not mean stress incontinence is not also present, nor does it necessarily suggest a bad operative result.

Aagard, 1991[25]

Uncontested indications for cystometry may include patients with neurological symptoms, voiding difficulties, etc., however, they are not universal and comprise a minority of urodynamic referrals.[50] Urinary stress incontinence may be defined by clinical history and physical examination supported by appropriate imaging techniques to describe the pathoanatomy and pathophysiology of the condition e.g. fluoroscopy or ultrasound.[51,52] Combining cystometry and fluoroscopy in the investigation of synchronous videocystourethrography (VCU) may be the investigation with the optimal chance of defining both GSI and DI because they are performed concurrently. Concomitant DI in a patient with GSI appears to have little prognostic value and begs the question as to whether intravesical pressure measurements are necessary in a patient with anatomical evidence of GSI. At present the safest interpretation of urodynamic studies, particularly retrograde filling cysto-metry, may be that they present the opportunity to reproduce a patient's symptoms in the testing situation, though even this limited proposition has not been evaluated.

THE ANATOMY OF THE LOWER URINARY TRACT

Much misunderstanding of the anatomy of the lower urinary tract has been attributable to variations in nomenclature and absence of appropriate imag-ing techniques. DeLancey's studies[8,27,53-56] of serial histological sections of (largely) parous cadavers have provided detailed and considered nomencla-ture of the anatomy of the lower urinary tract that will be used throughout this discussion. Aspects of terminology relating to macroscopic anatomy have been a persistent problem in this subject and have been clarified recently:

1. the anatomy of the endopelvic fasciae and their contribution to the female pelvic floor
2. the internal (smooth) and external (striated, rhabdosphincter) urinary sphincters.

The endopelvic fasciae is the term applied collectively to the connective tissue associated with the lower pelvis; its organized components include the pubourethral ligaments of the vesical neck, the arcus tendinei fasciae pelvis, the pubocervical fascia, the transverse cervical ligaments and the uterosacral ligaments (Figs 13.2 & 13.3A,B). Many clinicians are unfamiliar with the precise anatomy of some of these features although they readily appreciate the difference between surgical procedures in a nulliparous subject when all these structures are intact, and those in a parous subject where many of these supporting structures may have been attenuated or disrupted.

The retropubic space of a nulliparous cadaver illustrates the complex of supporting structures that comprise the anterior suspensory mechanism of the vesical neck (Fig. 13.3A,B). This complex of structures includes a pubo-urethral component (sometimes termed the pubourethral ligaments), a pubovesical component (sometimes termed the pubovesical ligaments) and its continuation as the arcus tendineus fasciae pelvis (white line over the obturator fascia). The precise function of the anterior suspensory mechanism (ASM) remains unclear although it is a substantial feature in all nulliparae and is appropriately placed to prevent downward displacement of the ure-throvesical junction during an increase in intra-abdominal pressure. There have been few opportunities to study the retropubic space in continent nulli-parous subjects and it is rare to see significant remnants of the ASM at retropubic urethropexy because they have been disrupted or attenuated at vaginal delivery. Disruption of the ASM following traumatic vaginal delivery is associated with excessive mobility of the entire urethra and early onset of urinary stress incontinence in the puerperium though both lateral and sub-urethral supports may also be disrupted in such circumstances.[6]

DeLancey (1992) has defined three levels of vaginal support that corre-spond with selected MRI sections of the pelvis (levels I–III). The vagina is successively suspended, attached and fused with adjacent supporting struc-tures. The upper third of the vagina is *suspended* by the uterosacral-lateral cervical ligament complex (level I), the middle third is *attached* to the arcus tendineus on the lateral pelvic side wall via the pubocervical fascia (level II) and the lower third is *fused* to adjacent structures including the perineal membrane in its distal 3 cm.[8] The perineal membrane provides a platform for the insertion of the distal fibres of pubococcygeus and disruption of the per-ineal membrane may be one of the features associated with loss of control of bowel functions.

The arcus tendineus (or white line over the obturator internus) is a thicken-ing in the fascia over the obturator internus that provides for attachment of the pubocervical fasciae; the latter is a definite layer of connective tissue that is a continuation of the cardinal ligaments. The layer may best be considered as a triangular sheet with its apex at the symphysis pubis, lateral attachments to the arcus tendinei and its free posterior limit as the transverse cervical ligaments. The lateral attachments of the anterior vaginal wall to the arcus tendinei by the pubocervical fasciae constitute a hammock that prevents downward displace-ment of the urethrovesical junction with an increase in intra-abdominal pres-sure (Fig. 13.8). Defects in this layer of support contribute to the development of different sites of cystocoele with accompanying urinary symptoms that are predictable by the anatomical features of the cystocoele.[9]

The perineal body is not a prominent feature of the lower pelvis and refers to those structures between the vagina and the anus (Fig. 13.5). It is largely composed of circular striated muscle fibres of the external anal sphincter that are connected via the anococcygeal raphe to the coccyx; however it is not a significant feature of pelvic support (Fig. 13.5). Absence of the perineal body through neglected obstetric trauma is not associated with significant degrees of genital prolapse. The perineal membrane and the pubococcygeus may be more significant in this context with the perineal membrane provid-ing a platform for the external genitalia and the pubococcygeus providing a closure mechanism for the pelvic outlet. Continuous resting tone of the pub-ococcygeus may have a significant role in the support of the pelvic viscera although complete denervation is not necessarily associated with significant prolapse (Fig. 13.7). The pelvic floor may refer to both the pubococcygeus and the elements of endopelvic fasciae that collectively prevent displacement of the pelvic viscera.

The external striated sphincter is the term applied to the striated muscle associated with the urethra and includes: the external, circular layer of striated muscle of the urethra; the compressor urethrae; and the urethrovagi-nal sphincter (Figs 13.6 & 13.8). The compressor urethrae and urethrovagi-nal sphincter are minor striated components associated with the distal urethra proximal to the perineal membrane whose function is unclear although may be concerned with voluntary interruption of flow, emptying the distal urethra, or, in some circumstances where continence is threatened. The internal urinary sphincter refers to the two extensions of detrusor smooth muscle that pass around the vesical neck and are not under voluntary control.[27]

MRI ANATOMY OF THE LOWER URINARY TRACT

Normal anatomy of the lower urinary tract has been defined in vivo using advanced MRI techniques in a series of asymptomatic nulliparous women (Figs 13.4–9). Previous studies have described some features of the pathoanatomy of urinary stress incontinence; however, controlled studies of the anatomical effects of vaginal delivery are awaited.[57-61] Serial axial and sagittal images of 4 mm thickness demonstrate the urethra and its adjacent, soft tissue, supporting structures in nulliparous subjects (imaging with a pelvic surface coil and a parent unit; General Electric Signa, 1.5T, using fast spin echo techniques with T2 weighting of the imaging sequences). Three important axial sections of the lower pelvis have been defined at the levels of the ischial spines, the proximal urethra and the perineal membrane, and correspond to the levels of vaginal support described by DeLancey.

The ischial spines define an important axial plane that includes the uterine cervix and the lateral cervical ligaments (Level I). The second axial plane associated with the proximal urethra is identified by the increased ratio of longitudinal smooth muscle to circular striated muscle (Level II) (Fig. 13.4A,B). The prominent soft tissue landmark associated with the distal urethra is the perineal membrane that provides a platform for the external genitalia and serves as the distal anchor for the midline viscera (Level III) (Fig. 13.5). The prominent anatomical feature of the lower female pelvis is the characteristic, H-shape of the nulliparous vagina that is formed by the anterior attachments to the medial border of pubococcygeus and the posterior attachments to the rectum via the rectovaginal pillars (Figs 13.4, 13.6 & 13.8). Primary supports of the vagina include the cardinal and uterosacral ligaments at the level of the cervix at its upper extent and the perineal membrane at its lower extent. Between these attachments it is connected to the arcus tendinei by the pubocervical fasciae. These lateral attachments, together with the vaginolevator attachment, stabilize the anterior vaginal wall and pubocervical fascia against which the urethra may be compressed by an increase in intra-abdominal pressure.

Magnetic resonance techniques provide reliable and consistent imaging of the components of the levator ani at different levels of the pelvis with the sling of pubococcygeus prominent in all sections of the lower pelvis (Figs 13.6 & 13.8). Relaxation of the pubococcygeus prior to voiding may cause opening of the vesical neck and proximal urethra because of the direct connection

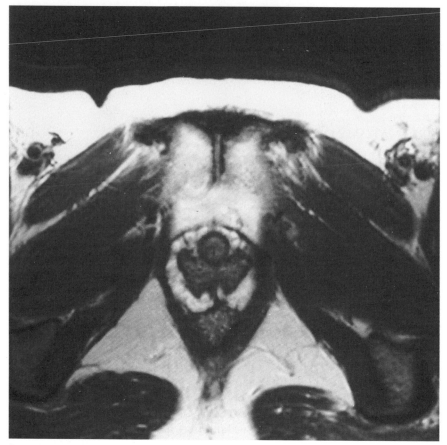

A

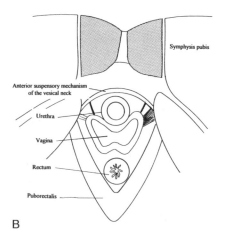

B

Fig. 13.3A. An axial section of the anterior pelvis at the level of the proximal urethra. The urethra, vagina and the rectum are enclosed within the sling of pubococcygeus and the obturator internus occupies the lateral pelvic side wall. The anterior suspensory mechanism occupies the retropubic space and inserts between the pubococcygei anterior to the urethra. The prominent feature is the butterfly-shape of the nulliparous vagina that is formed by the attachment of the anterior sulci to the arcus tendineus by the pubocervical fasciae and the posterior sulci to the rectum. The level of the section is defined by the maximum ratio of longitudinal smooth muscle to circular striated muscle in the proximal urethra. **B**. Diagram to clarify the component parts.

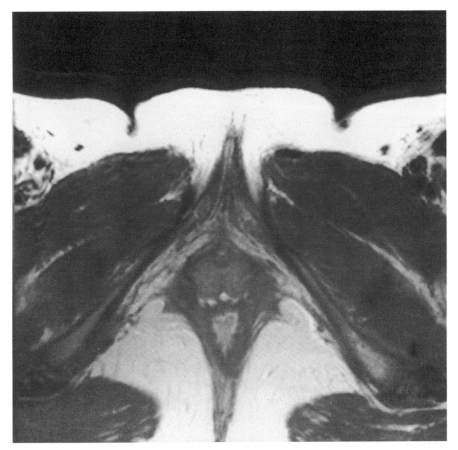

A

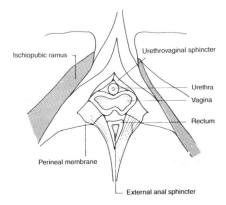

B

Fig. 13.4A. An axial section of the anterior pelvis at the level of the perineal membrane that is the prominent anatomical feature associated with the distal urethra and separates the pelvic cavity from the perineum. The urethra, vagina and the rectum penetrate the triangular shape of the perineal membrane whose posterior free edge is observed on each side of the rectum. The transverse perineal muscles arise from the external anal sphincter and insert into the posterior edge of the perineal membrane. **B**. Diagram to clarify the component parts.

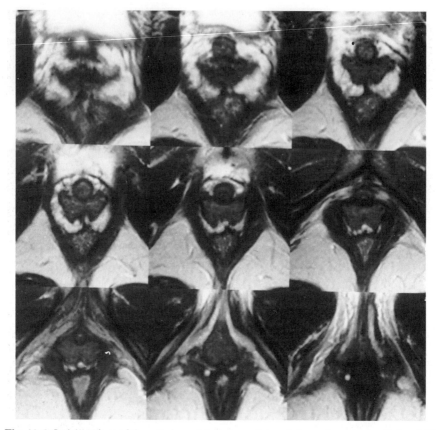

Fig. 13.5 Serial sections of the anterior pelvis at 4 mm intervals from the vesical neck (top left) to the perineal membrane (bottom left) in a nulliparous subject. The hammock of the anterior vaginal wall provides inferior support for the proximal urethra by virtue of its lateral attachments to the arcus tendineus fasciae pelvis (middle left) and the pubococcygeus (middle centre and right). Components of the anterior suspensory mechanism are demonstrated in the plates at top right and middle left and centre. The perineal membrane is the prominent axial landmark associated with the distal urethra and divides the pelvis from the perineum.

between the anterior vaginal wall and the proximal urethra. Contraction of the detrusor muscle and the longitudinal smooth muscle of the urethra causes bladder emptying through an open urethra. Pudendal neuropathy resulting from vaginal delivery may have an impact on the function of the pubococcygeus and presents with disturbances of urinary or bowel function. Previously, invasive techniques have been required to demonstrate these effects and the literature remains controversial on the precise impact of such lesions.

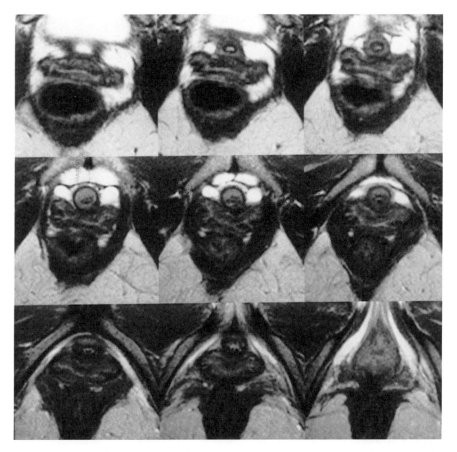

Fig. 13.6 Serial sections of the anterior pelvis at 4 mm intervals from the vesical neck (top left) to the perineal membrane (bottom centre) in a nulliparous subject. Components of the anterior suspensory mechanism are shown top right and middle left, the compressor urethrae passes anterior to the urethra in plate 6 and the urethrovaginal sphincter is shown in bottom left. The perineal body occupies the area between the fourchette and the rectum (bottom centre and right).

The perineal membrane separates the pelvic viscera, contained posteriorly by pubococcygeus, from the external genitalia, and extends between the medial borders of the ischiopubic rami to occupy a horizontal plane with the patient in an erect position (Fig. 13.5). Direct support is provided for the distal vagina and urethra, and the posterior fibres insert into the perineal body. Both the compressor urethrae and the urethrovaginal sphincter are paraurethral structures, composed of striated muscle that occupy a position immediately proximal to the perineal membrane (Fig. 13.8). They may act as secondary components in the female continence mechanism in

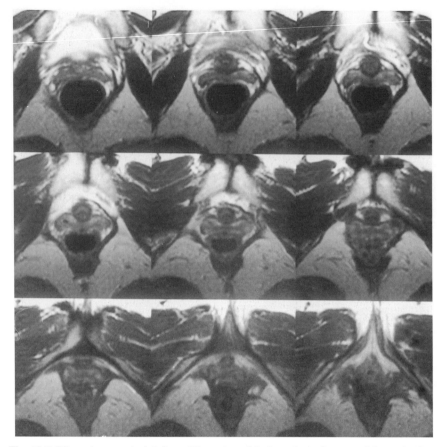

Fig. 13.7 Bilateral paravaginal defects. Disruption of the lateral attachments of the vagina in a patient with genuine stress incontinence. There is disorganization of the retropubic space, scarring of the anterior vaginal wall and an altered vaginal configuration caused by loss of the insertions into the arcus tendineus fasciae pelvis and the pubococcygeus. Continence was restored by laparoscopic colposuspension. Top right plate = proximal urethra. Bottom left plate = perineal membrane.

some circumstances. Important anatomical features in the posterior compartment of the pelvis include the external anal sphincter (EAS) together with some fibres that insert in the perineal membrane. The perineal body is not a substantive feature of perineal anatomy and has a limited role in the prevention of genital prolapse.[62]

Previous descriptions of the MRI anatomy of urinary stress incontinence have described alterations of the pubococcygeus[60] and disruption of the vaginolevator attachments.[61] In a series of consecutive patients with genuine stress incontinence, similar anatomical abnormalities have been noted (Figs 13.7 & 13.9). Disruption of the anterior suspensory mechanism and vaginol-

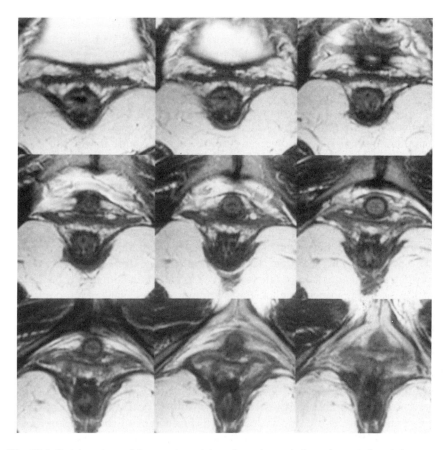

Fig. 13.8 Serial sections of the anterior pelvis at 4 mm intervals from the vesical neck (top centre) to the perineum in a patient with urinary stress incontinence and faecal urgency. The vagina is reduced in both shape and dimension (compare with Fig. 13.4) and the pubococcygeus has lost its usual sling conformation and is markedly atrophied. These observations were noted at all levels of the urethra. Middle row left = proximal urethra. Bottom row centre = perineal membrane.

evator attachments at all levels of the lower pelvis are demonstrated in a patient with genuine stress incontinence (Figs 13.7 & 13.9). The vagina has taken on an n-shape as compared to the nulliparous H-shape, and the stabilizing layer of the anterior vaginal wall and pubocervical fascia has been disrupted. The sling of pubococcygeus remains intact (Fig. 13.7). In a second patient with genuine stress incontinence and faecal urgency following the spontaneous delivery of a baby weighing 5080 g, anatomical features associated with denervation of the lower pelvis are demonstrated (Fig. 13.9). The abnormal anatomical features include:

1. disruption of the anterior suspensory mechanism of the vesical neck
2. absence of a normal vaginal configuration (H-shape) with attenuation of the vagina at all levels of the pelvis
3. attenuation of pubococcygeus in both shape and dimensions with a maximum thickness of 2 mm.

Further studies in both sagittal, axial and coronal planes are required to delineate the anatomical consequences of vaginal delivery, hysterectomy and the pathoanatomy of urinary stress incontinence and genital prolapse.

US IMAGING OF LOWER URINARY TRACT

Abdominal, vaginal, perineal and rectal ultrasound imaging have been used to image the lower urinary tract.[6,49,63-74] At present vaginal and perineal techniques provide adequate resolution of the anatomical features in a non-invasive, patient-acceptable fashion.[75] Perineal ultrasound may be limited by the acoustic impedance of the symphysis pubis, lack of a consistent relationship of the transducer to the anatomical features and the inability of the technique to be used for dynamic studies with the patient in the sitting position, although it is a simple technique for observing the effects of retrograde filling cystometry on the bladder neck and proximal urethra. Vaginal ultrasound (VUS) may be used with the patient in either supine or sitting positions to image the consequences of provocative manoeuvres and suprapubic surgery on the continence mechanism. A potential disadvantage of the vaginal route is the opportunity for displacement of the anterior vaginal wall in patients with significant genital prolapse (Type B)[4] though enhanced resolution and patient acceptance are significant advantages of the technique.[76-78] VUS is the optimal technique for the evaluation of patients following suprapubic surgery where anatomical objectives are achieved by successful operations,[79] and abnormal anatomy is associated with unsuccessful suprapubic procedures.[74]

In patients without urinary symptoms ultrasound examination demonstrates minor downwards and posterior rotation of the urethrovesical junction; there is no demonstrable urinary leakage in either supine or sitting positions. In patients with genuine stress incontinence ultrasound examination demonstrates passive opening of the bladder neck and proximal urethra concurrent with a cough (Fig. 13.9). Few patients demonstrate these findings in the supine position although they may be conveniently demonstrated with the patient in the sitting position. Almost invariably there is significant posteroinferior rotation of the urethrovesical junction that is characteristic of anatomic stress incontinence and has been demonstrated using indirect radiological techniques including bead-chain cystourethrography. Patients with a fixed urethra are rare and have invariably had multiple unsuccessful surgical procedures. Patients with neurological symptoms require formal evaluation

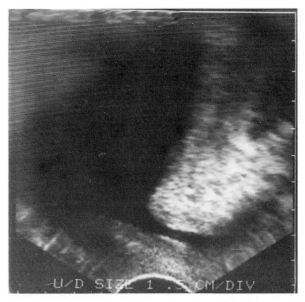

Fig. 13.9 Genuine stress incontinence. Concurrent opening of the bladder neck and proximal urethra with urinary leakage concurrent with a cough. Urinary incontinence is almost invariably associated with posteroinferior rotation of the urethrovesical junction in patients with primary stress incontinence.

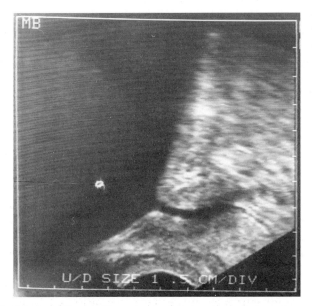

Fig. 13.10 Detrusor incontinence. The nature and timing of urinary incontinence associated with detrusor instability is different from that associated with genuine stress incontinence. Urinary incontinence is delayed relative to the cough, and the mechanism of urethral opening is an active process resulting from the effects of the cough on the detrusor muscle.

with cystometry and concurrent measurement of intravesical and intra-abdominal pressures.

Urinary incontinence associated with detrusor instability may be differentiated from genuine stress incontinence by the nature and timing of urinary leakage relative to the cough (Fig. 13.10). Urinary leakage is delayed relative to the cough and is associated with active contraction of the detrusor muscle that accounts for the phasic increase in intravesical pressure. In a prospective comparison of traditional urodynamic techniques and vaginal ultrasound the ultrasound technique was both sensitive and specific for the diagnosis of genuine stress incontinence without the necessity for urethral and rectal catheterization.[6] Imaging studies to detect the effects of detrusor instability on the continence mechanism have not been performed because additional provocative manoeuvres including retrograde bladder filling may be required to provoke detrusor activity whose clinical significance remains uncertain.[26]

Surgical treatment of genuine stress incontinence has included many different surgical procedures which can be segregated into three approaches: colposuspension, needle suspension operations and sling procedures. Laparoscopic techniques for colposuspension are becoming increasingly popular because they combine surgical accuracy with reduced morbidity.[37] The often-stated, central principle of suprapubic surgery for genuine stress incontinence – elevation of the bladder neck – has been based on theories of pressure transmission so that a displaced urethrovesical junction is restored to an intra-abdominal pressure zone. This approach has been associated with effective treatment of primary stress incontinence, but has been accompanied by significant rates of postoperative detrusor instability, voiding difficulties and genital prolapse.[28,30,42,80] Vaginal ultrasound of the postoperative results of suprapubic surgery is a simple, non-invasive, clinical technique that confirms that the anatomical objectives of the operation have been achieved.[6,51] In addition it demonstrates to the patient early in the postoperative period that she has an accurate surgical result that has converted a mobile, incontinent mechanism into a stable, continent configuration. Reproducible anatomical observations in the midline sagittal plane are independent of bladder volume because the vaginal fornices have been secured in a fixed, permanent configuration that prevents downward displacement of the urethrovesical junction. Accurate postoperative configurations following colposuspension demonstrate absence of downward displacement of the urethrovesical junction with an increase in intra-abdominal pressure and absence of fixed indentations of the trigone or bladder base.

Abnormal anatomical configurations following colposuspension may be identified by mobility of the urethrovesical junction, or fixed indentations of the trigone and bladder. Abnormal mobility of the urethrovesical junction may be observed in association with recurrent stress incontinence whereas fixed indentations are associated with frequency-urgency syndrome, postoperative detrusor instability or persistent stress incontinence (PSI). Fixed indentations of the bladder base are associated with inaccurate placement of the supporting sutures (and possibly excessive elevation of the vaginal fornices towards the iliopectineal ligaments). If the sutures are placed adjacent to the vaginal vault then no support is afforded to the urethrovesical junction and the patient has persistent stress incontinence; suture placement beneath the trigone is associated with persistent urge syndrome and postoperative detrusor instability. These observations regarding surgical technique may explain the variable incidence of postoperative detrusor instability in several series describing the long term results of colposuspension (Table 13.2) and also an explanation for the persistent and intractable symptoms that have been described in the medium term.[48]

CONCLUSIONS

Contemporary urodynamic investigations based on retrograde filling cystometry have assumed widespread application for the investigation of incontinent women; they have been extensively standardized though none have been convincingly validated. The definition of genuine stress incontinence as involuntary urinary loss in the absence of increases in intravesical pressure, does not include reference to the pathoanatomy of the condition. The significance of phasic increases in intravesical pressure that define detrusor instability, remain unclear. Much of their justification is substantiated by the misplaced analogy with bladder outflow obstruction in the high-pressure male system and anecdotal observations that have little evidence to support their implied significance e.g. 'systolic' or 'high pressure' DI. Traditional concepts of continence based on theories of pressure transmission to an intra-abdominal urethra have provided the template for many urogynaecological aphorisms; though, detailed anatomical and radiological studies have refuted the basic premise of this theory of female continence.[8]

The aetiology, diagnosis and surgical treatment of urinary stress incontinence may be coherently explained in anatomical terms.[8] Impaired support of the anterior vaginal wall is associated with urinary stress incontinence and prolapse of the anterior vaginal wall. Improved imaging techniques describe some of the anatomical alterations of the lower urinary tract caused by vaginal delivery and may result in urinary stress incontinence. In most patients suprapubic surgery has anatomical objectives that include prevention of downward displacement of the urethrovesical junction and may be evaluated with simple ultrasound techniques. New hypotheses regarding the structure and function of the lower urinary tract may be evaluated against the hammock hypothesis of female continence in the expectation of further improvements in the care of patients with urinary incontinence.

REFERENCES

1 Hodgkinson C P. Relationships of the female urethra in urinary incontinence. Am J Obstet Gynecol 1953; 65: 560–573
2 Hodgkinson C P. Urethrocystogram: metallic bead-chain technique. Clin Obstet Gynecol 1958; 1: 668–677
3 Hodgkinson C P. Urinary stress incontinence in the female. Clin Obstet Gynecol 1963; 6: 164–177
4 Green T H Development of a plan for the diagnosis and treatment of urinary stress incontinence. Am J Obstet Gynecol 1962; 83: 632–648.
5 Bates C P, Whiteside C G, Turner-Warwick R. Synchronous cine/pressure/flow cystourethrography with special reference to stress and urge incontinence. Br J Urol 1970; 42: 714–723
6 Quinn M J. MD Thesis. Vaginal Ultrasound of the Lower Urinary Tract. University of Bristol, 1994
7 Enhorning G. Simultaneous recording of intravesical and intraurethral pressure. Acta Chirurg Scand (Suppl) 1961; 276: 1–6
8 Delancey J O L. Structural support of the urethra as it relates to stress urinary incontinence: the hammock hypothesis. Am J Obstet Gynecol 1994; 170: 1713–1723
9 Richardson A C, Lyon J B, Williams N L. A new look at pelvic relaxation. Am J Obstet Gynecol 1976; 126: 568–572
10 Richardson A C, Edmonds P B, Williams N I. Treatment of stress urinary incontinence due to paravaginal fascial defect. Obstet Gynecol 1981; 57: 357–362
11 Shull R L Capen C V, Riggs M W, Kuehl T J. Preoperative and postoperative analysis of site-specific pelvic support defects in 81 women treated with sacrospinous ligaments suspension and pelvic reconstruction. Am J Obstet Gynecol 1992; 166: 1764–1771
12 Shull R L, Benn S J, Kuehl T J. Surgical management of prolapse of the anterior vaginal segment: An analysis of support defects, operative morbidity and anatomic outcome. Am J Obstet Gynecol 1994; 171: 1429–1439
13 Milley P S, Nicholls D H. The relationship between the pubourethral ligaments and the urogenital diaphragm in the human female. Anat Rec 1971; 170: 281–283
14 Nicholls D, Milley P S. Identification of the pubourethral ligaments and their role in the transvaginal surgical correction of stress incontinence. Am J Obstet Gynecol 1973; 115: 123
15 Zacharin R F. The suspensory mechanism of the female urethra. J Anat 1963; 97: 423–427
16 Zacharin R F. The anatomic supports of the female urethra. Obstet Gynecol 1968; 32: 754–759
17 Farrar D J, Whiteside C G, Osborne J L. A urodynamic analysis of micturition symptoms in the female. Surg Gynecol Obstet 1975; 141: 875–881
18 Jarvis G J, Hall S, Stamp S, Millar D R, Johnson A. An assessment of urodynamic examination in incontinent women. Br J Obstet Gynaecol 1980; 87: 893–896
19 Mundy A R. Urethral pressure profilometry. In: Drife J O, Hilton P, Stanton S L, eds. Micturition. London: Springer-Verlag, 1990: pp 104–109
20 Bates C P, Bradley W E, Glen E et al. First report on the standardisation of terminology of lower urinary tract function. Urinary incontinence. Procedures related to the evaluation of urinary storage: cystometry, urethral closure pressure profile, units of measurement. Br J Urol 1976; 48: 39–42
21 Bates C P, Glen E, Griffiths D et al. Second report on the standardisation of terminology of lower urinary tract function. Procedures related to the evaluation of micturition; flow rate, pressure measurement, symbols. Br J Urol 1977; 49: 207–210
22 Bates C P, Bradley W E, Glen E et al. Third Report on the standardisation of terminology of lower urinary tract function. Procedures related to the evaluation of micturition: pressure-flow relationships, residual urine. Br J Urol 1980; 52: 348–350
23 Bates C P, Bradley W E, Glen E et al. Fourth report on the standardisation of terminology of lower urinary tract function. Terminology related to neuromuscular dysfunction of the lower urinary tract. Br J Urol 1981; 52: 333–335
24 Abrams P, Blaivas J, Stanton S L, Andersen J T, Fowler C J, Gerstenberg T, Murray K. Sixth report on the standardisation of terminology of lower urinary tract function. Procedures related to neurophysiological investigations: Electromyography, nerve

conduction studies, reflex latencies, evoked potentials and sensory testing. Scand J Urol Nephrol 1986; 20: 161–164

25 Aagard J, Bruskewitz R. Are urodynamic studies useful in the evaluation of female incontinence? A critical review of the literature. Prob Urol 1991; 5: 12–22

26 Robertson A S, Criffiths C J, Ramsden P D, Neal D E. Bladder function in healthy volunteers: ambulatory monitoring and conventional urodynamic studies. Br J Urol 1994; 73: 242–249

26a McGuire E. Classic pages in urogynaecology. Neurourol Urodynam 1988; 7: 565

27 Delancey J O L, Wall L, Norton P. Urogynaecology. Boston: Little Brown, 1993

28 Stanton S L, Cardozo L D. A comparison of vaginal and suprapubic surgery and the correction of incontinence due to urethral shincter incompetence. Br J Obstet Gynaecol 1979; 51: 497–499

29 Cardozo L D, Stanton S L, Williams J E. Detrusor instability following surgery for genuine stress incontinence. Br J Urol 1979; 51: 204–207

30 Galloway N T M, Davies N, Stephenson T P. The complications of colposuspension. Br J Urol 1987; 60: 122–124

31 Lose G, Jorgensen L, Mortensen S O, Molsted-Pedersen L, Kristensen J K. Voiding difficulties after colposuspension. Obstet Gynecol 1987; 69: 33–38

32 Wiskind A K, Creighton S M, Stanton S L. The incidence of genital prolapse after the Burch colposuspension. Am J Obstet Gynecol 1992; 167: 406–411

33 Hilton P, Stanton S L. A clinical and urodynamic evaluation of the Burch colposuspension for genuine stress incontinence. Br J Obstet Gynaecol 1983; 90: 934–939

34 Burch J C. Urethrovaginal fixation to Cooper's ligament for correction of stress incontinence, cystocoele and prolapse. Am J Obstet Gynecol 1961; 117: 805–813

35 Stamey T. Endoscopic suspension of the vesical neck for urinary stress incontinence. Surg Gynecol Obstet 1973; 136: 547–554

36 Pereyra A J. A simplified surgical procedure for the correction of stress incontinence in women. West J Surg Obstet Gynecol 1959; 67: 223–227

37 Lyons T. Laparoscopic retropubic colposuspension. In: Garry R, Reich H, eds. Laparoscopic hysterectomy. Oxford: Blackwell Science, 1993: pp 142–147

38 Cardozo L D, Stanton S L. Genuine stress incontinence and detrusor instability: a review of 200 patients. Br J Obstet Gynaecol 1980; 87: 184–190.

39 Eriksen B C, Hagen B, Eik-Nes S, Molne K, Mjolnerod O K, Romslo I. Long term effectiveness of colposuspension. Acta Obstet Gynaecol Scand 1990; 69: 45–50

40 Langer R, Ron-El R, Newman M, Herman A, Casp I. Detrusor instability following colposuspension for urinary stress incontinence. Br J Obstet Gynaecol 1988; 95: 607–610

41 Iosif C S. Colpo-urethropexy – a simple method for the treatment of primary stress incontinence. Acta Obstet Gynecol Scand 1985; 6: 525–527

42 Alcalay M, Monga A, Stanton S L. Burch colposuspension: a 10–20 year follow-up. Br J Obstet Gynaecol 1995; 102: 740–745

43 Vierhout M E, Mulder A F P. De novo detrusor instability after Burch colposuspension. Acta Obstet Gynecol Scand 1992; 71: 414–416

44 Sand P K, Bowen L W, Ostergard D R, Brubaker L, Panganiban R. The effect of retropubic urethropexy on detrusor instability. Obstet Gynecol 1988; 71: 818–822

45 Milani R, Scalambrino S, Quadri G, Algeri M, Marchesin R. Marshall-Marchetti-Krantz procedure and Burch colposuspension in the surgical treatment of female urinary incontinence. Br J Obstet Gynaecol 1985; 92: 1050–1053

46 Jorgensen L, Lose G, Mortensen S O, Molsted L, Kristensen J K. The Burch colposuspension for urinary incontinence in patients with stable and unstable detrusor function. Neurourol Urodynam 1988; 7: 435–441

47 Webster G D, Kreder K J. Voiding dysfunction following cysoturethropexy: its evaluation and management. J Urol 1990; 144: 670–673

48 Steel S A, Cox C, Stanton S L. Long term follow up of detrusor instability following colposuspension. Br J Urol 1985; 58: 138–142

49 Quinn M J, Beynon J, Mortensen N J, Smith P J B. Vaginal endosonography in the postoperative assessment of colposuspension. Br J Urol 1989; 63: 295–300

50 Hilton P. Urinary incontinence in women. Br Med J 1987; 299: 455–460

51 Bates C P, Corney C E. Synchronous cine-pressure-flow cystography: a method of routine urodynamic investigation. Br J Radiol 1971; 44: 44–50

52 Quinn M J, Beynon J, Mortensen N J, Smith P J B. Transvaginal endosonography in the assessment of urinary stress incontinence. Br J Urol 1988; 62: 414–418

53 Delancey J O L. Correlative study of paraurethral anatomy. Obstet Gynecol 1986; 68: 91–97

54 Delancey J O L. Structural aspects of the extrinsic continence mechanisms. Obstet Gynecol 1988; 72: 296–301

55 Delancey J O L. Pubovesical ligament: a separate structure from the urethral supports (pubourethral ligaments). Neurourol Urodynam 1989; 8: 53–61

56 Delancey J O L. Anatomy of the urethral sphincters and supports. In: Drife J O, Hilton P, Stanton S L, eds. Micturition. London: Springer-Verlag, 1990: pp 3–16

57 Klutke C, Golomb J, Barbaric Z, Raz S. The anatomy of stress incontinence: Magnetic resonance imaging of the female bladder neck and urethra. J Urol 1990; 143: 563–566

58 Hricak H, Secaf E, Buckley D W, Brown J J, Tanagho E A, Mcaninch J W. Female urethra: MR Imaging. Radiology 1991; 178: 527–535

59 Plattner V, Leborgne J, Heloury Y et al. MRI evaluation of the levator ani muscle: anatomic correlations and practical applications. Surg Radiol Anat 1991; 13: 129–131

60 Kirschner-Hermanns R, Wein B, Niehaus S, Schafer W. The contribution of magnetic resonance imaging of the pelvic floor to the understanding of urinary incontinence. Br J Urol 1993; 72: 715–718

61 Huddlestone H T, Dunnihoo D R, Huddleston P M, Meyers P C. Magnetic resonance imaging of defects in DeLancey's vaginal support levels I, II & II. Am J Obstet Gynecol 1995; 172: 1778–1784

62 Snell R. Clinical Anatomy for Medical Students. Boston: Little Brown & Co., 1981

63 White R D, McQuown D, McCarthy T A, Ostergard D R. Real-time ultrasonography in the evaluation of urinary symptoms. Am J Obstet Gynecol 1980; 138: 235–237

64 Kohorn E I, Scioscia A L, Jeanty P, Hobbins J C. Ultrasound cystourethrography by perineal scanning for the assessment of female stress urinary incontinence. Obstet Gynecol 1986; 68: 269–272

65 Richmond D H, Sutherst J R, Brown M C. Screening of the bladder base and urethra using linear array transrectal ultrasound scanning. J Clin Ultrasound 1986; 14: 647–651

66 Richmond D H, Sutherst J R. Clinical application of transrectal ultrasound for the investigation of the incontinent patient. Br J Urol 1989; 63: 605–609

67 Richmond D H, Sutherst J R. Burch colposuspension or sling for stress incontinence? A prospective study using transrectal ultrasound. Br J Urol 1989; 64: 600–603

68 Richmond D H, Sutherst J. Transrectal ultrasound scanning in urinary incontinence: the effects of the probe on urodynamic parameters. Br J Urol 1989; 64: 582–585

69 Gordon D, Pearce M, Norton P, Stanton S L. Comparison of ultrasound and lateral chain urethrocystography in the determination of bladder neck descent. Am J Obstet Gynecol 1989; 160: 182–186

70 Koelbl H, Bernaschek G. A new method for sonographic urethrocystography and simultaneous pressure-flow studies. Obstet Gynecol 1989; 74: 417–422

71 Koelbl H, Bernaschek G, Deutinger J. Assessment of female urinary incontinence by introital sonography. J Clin Ultrasound 1990; 18: 370–376

72 Clark A L, Creighton S M, Pearce J M, Stanton S L. Localisation of the bladder neck by perineal ultrasound; methodology and applications. Neurourol Urodynam 1990; 9: 394–395

73 Creighton S M, Pearce J M, Stanton S L. Perineal video-ultrasonography in the assessment of vaginal prolapse: early observations. Br J Obstet Gynaecol 1992; 99: 310–313

74 Quinn M J, Farnsworth B A, Pollard W J, Smith P J B, Stott M A. Vaginal ultrasound in the diagnosis of stress incontinence: a prospective comparison to urodynamic investigations. Neurourol Urodynam 1989; 8: 291

75 Sanders R, Genadry R, Yang A, Mostwin J. Transabdominal, transvaginal, translabial and transrectal sonographic techniques in the evaluation of stress incontinence. Neurourol Urodynam 1993; 12: 304–305

76 Wise B G, Burton A, Cutner A, Cardozo L D. Effect of vaginal ultrasound probe on lower urinary tract function. Br J Urol 1990; 70: 12–16

77 Haylen B T, Golovsky D. The effect of the vaginal endoprobe on lower urinary tract function. Br J Urol 1993; 71: 240

78 Mouritsen L, Rasmussen A. Bladder neck mobility evaluated by vaginal ultrasonography. Br J Urol 1993; 71: 166–171

79 Kil P J M, Hoekstra J W, van der Neijden H P M, Smans A J, Theeuwes A G M, Schreinemachers L M H. Transvaginal ultrasonography and urodynamic evaluation after

suspension operations: Comparison among Gittes, Stamey and Burch suspensions. J Urol 1991; 146: 132–136

80 Korda A, Ferry J, Hunter P. Colposuspension for the treatment of female urinary incontinence. Aust NZ J Obstet Gynaecol 1989; 29: 146–149

14 The management of the urge syndrome

J. W. Barrington

The combination of urinary frequency, nocturia, urgency and urge incontinence is commonly referred to as 'The Urge Syndrome' since urgency is usually the cardinal symptom.[1]

Frequency is defined as voiding more than once every 2 hours, or as voiding more than 7 times per day. Nocturia is characterized only if the desire to void causes the patient to wake. It is less common under the age of 60 years, but as a general rule, one episode of nocturia can be added for each decade past that age without it being regarded as abnormal.[2] Urgency is a sudden strong almost irresistible desire to micturate because of discomfort or fear of urine leakage or both. Urgency usually occurs in conjunction with frequency in about 80% of patients[3] and a surgical cure of one usually leads to the resolution of the other symptom,[4] but urgency may also occur in isolation affecting as much as 18% of adult females aged between 30 and 60 years.[5] It is probably an underestimated condition since 33% of patients will wait between 1 and 5 years before seeking help and 25% will delay for more than 5 years.[6] Urgency only occurs alone if bladder sensation is deficient or when near-normal bladder capacity is reached.[2] If nocturia is also absent, it suggests that the patient is a heavy sleeper or that the urgency is triggered by changes in posture or by activity. Urge incontinence is usually preceded by urgency, and is estimated by the number of wet episodes and volumes of leakage per day. However, it is impossible to differentiate between urge and stress incontinence in some patients who are unaware of any sensation associated with their involuntary detrusor contractions. The patient with normal intrinsic sphincter function will not usually suffer significant urine leakage, so that if incontinence occurs, there is probably a degree of sphincter weakness.[2]

Patients complaining of frequency and urgency may be divided into three main groups, which is clinically useful since they have different aetiologies (Table 14.1):

1. Extravesical causes,
2. Sensory urgency,
3. Motor urgency.

259

Table 14.1 Aetiology of 'The Urge Syndrome'

Extravesical causes
Diabetes mellitus
Diabetes insipidus
Hypothyroidism
Chronic renal failure
Habit
Large fluid intake
Diuretic therapy
Pregnancy
Pelvic mass
Post pelvic surgery

Sensory urgency
  Bladder causes
  Urinary tract infection
  Urethrotrigonitis
  Bladder calculi
  Carcinoma in situ
  Bladder neoplasm
  Tuberculosis
  Chronic cystitis
  Interstitial cystitis
  Radiation cystitis
  Genuine stress incontinence

  Urethral causes
  Urethral syndrome
  Urethral diverticulum

  Both
  Atrophic changes
  Idiopathic sensory urgency

Motor urgency
Idiopathic detrusor instability
Detrusor hyperreflexia
Outflow obstruction

EXTRAVESICAL CAUSES

Many conditions outside the urinary tract exert their effects indirectly upon the bladder. The polyuria of diabetes mellitus, diabetes insipidus, hypothyroidism, chronic renal failure or simply from a habitually large fluid intake may manifest itself by frequency. Similarly diuretic therapy may have the same effect and is best taken in the morning to avoid nocturia. Urinary frequency may be the first sign of pregnancy. Other pelvic masses will reduce the bladder capacity and result in frequency. Pelvic surgery, particularly radical hysterectomy, can disrupt the autonomic nerves innervating the bladder and urethra. This usually presents with chronic retention and the voiding of frequent small volumes, but must be differentiated from detrusor and urethral instability.[7]

SENSORY URGENCY

Sensory urgency is caused by hypersensitivity of the bladder or urethral mucosa, or both, which causes either a constant desire to void which is unrelieved by voiding, or a desire to void at low bladder volume because of pain or discomfort, which is relieved by voiding. The commonest bladder causes of sensory urgency are urinary tract infections, urethrotrigonitis, bladder calculi and tumours. Chronic inflammatory conditions such as tuberculosis, chronic cystitis or interstitial cystitis can result in a physically reduced bladder capacity. Although the amount of radiation the bladder is exposed to during the treatment of advanced cervical and endometrial carcinoma is much lower nowadays, post-radiation cystitis is not uncommon and the resultant fibrosis also results in a physically small bladder. Sensory urgency is more common in postmenopausal women which suggests that hormonal status is important. The female lower genital and urinary tracts are embryologically similar, and the therapeutic administration of oestrogens can reduce this constant desire to void by increasing the sensory threshold of the bladder.[8]

Genuine stress incontinence (GSI) frequently occurs in conjunction with symptoms of the urge syndrome, which suggests a common mechanism. Continence in females is usually maintained at the bladder neck and not at the rhabdosphincter in mid-urethra as one would suspect.[9] This region relies on passive elastic tension since there is no sphincteric circular smooth or striated muscle. Hypermobility of the bladder neck, commonly seen in parous or postmenopausal women, allows urine to enter the proximal urethra initiating urgency, which is the basis of urethral conductance tests.[10] Many women are able to withstand reflex micturition or lose only a few drops of urine, until they reach the safety of a toilet, unless the intrinsic urethral sphincter is also weakened in which case urge incontinence will occur.

The 'Urge Syndrome' is often confused with the 'Urethral Syndrome' in which there is, in addition, dysuria in the absence of urinary infection. Treatment with antibiotics may give temporary relief but the symptoms always return and may eventually become refractory to antibiotic therapy. Several aetiologies have been proposed including infection by organisms not detected by standard microbiology techniques. Urethral swabs for chlamydia are negative. Subclinical outflow obstruction or external sphincter spasm has also been proposed which possibly explains the beneficial effects of cystourethroscopy; unfortunately this may only be temporary. A less common cause of urinary frequency and urgency is a urethral diverticulum. This is thought to result from an infection of the paraurethral glands, and is found on the posterior wall of the urethra.

Finally, there are a group of patients who do not have a bladder or urethral cause for their urgency and have stable bladders on urodynamics. Serum levels of complement factors C5–C9 are often raised[2] and therefore comparisons have been made to interstitial cystitis. However, bladder capacity and biopsy under general anaesthetic are usually normal, and this sensory urgency of unknown cause is extremely refractory to treatment.

MOTOR URGENCY

Motor urgency is caused by involuntary or unstable detrusor contractions. The International Continence Society (ICS) have defined an unstable bladder as one that is shown to objectively contract, spontaneously or on provocation, during the filling phase while the patient is attempting to inhibit micturition.[11] In the vast majority of women who suffer from detrusor instability, no cause can be found although an underlying psychological disorder is present in a significant proportion.[12] A similar urodynamic finding is seen following anti-incontinence surgery,[13-15] which is likely to be caused by an outflow obstruction similar to prostatic enlargement in men. It might, however, be also the result of extensive dissection of the bladder neck since it is more common after multiple previous operations or it was not detected preoperatively. In the presence of neuropathy, detrusor instability is termed detrusor hyperreflexia and the changes in bladder pressure seen during the filling phase of an urodynamic study are almost always because of the underlying neurological disorder.

Patients with detrusor instability without a definable cause fall into three main groups: children and young adults with nocturnal and diurnal enuresis; adult middle-aged females; and postmenopausal women. It appears in the younger group that 'congenital instability' is caused by a failure of maturation of the central nervous system resulting in a failure of development of inhibition of involuntary voiding by higher centres. In the elderly population, the aetiology is usually neuropathic or 'degenerative'. The cause of motor urgency in the large group of women in the childbearing years is idiopathic. Since recent studies using ambulatory monitoring have shown that up to 10% of the general population exhibit detrusor contractions greater than the ICS definition of 15 cm of H_2O, and are asymptomatic,[16] then it is reasonable to regard idiopathic detrusor instability as a variant of normal. The amount of caffeine drunk by some patients may increase detrusor pressure sufficient for them to become symptomatic.[17]

INVESTIGATIONS

Clinical examination is often unhelpful but is essential to exclude a local cause, particularly a pelvic mass and co-existent stress incontinence. A neurological lesion should be excluded by examining perineal sensation together with anal tone and reflexes.

A urine sample (Table 14.2) is mandatory to exclude an urinary tract infection together with microscopic haematuria, which might be caused by bladder calculi or the first manifestation of a bladder tumour. Urine cell cytology is useful in the middle-aged or elderly patients particularly if they are smokers. Blood tests and urine osmolarity may be appropriate to assess renal function.

A frequency/volume chart should be sent to all patients at least a week prior to their outpatient appointment so that the relationship between

Table 14.2 Investigations

Mid-stream urine for microscopy, culture and sensitivity
Urine cell cytology
Urinary acid-fast bacilli
Frequency/volume chart
Urinary flow rate
Urinary residual volume
Cystometry/videocystourethrography
DNEC/BNEC
Ambulatory urodynamics

urinary frequency and fluid intake and type can be assessed. It also allows the functional bladder capacity to be measured and serves as a baseline for subsequent bladder drill and biofeedback.

A flow rate and postmicturition urinary residual should be performed to determine whether the motor urgency is caused by outflow obstruction (low flow: high voiding pressure: high residual volume) or idiopathic in nature (high flow: high voiding pressure: low residual volume).

Cystourethroscopy is necessary, for cases of sensory urgency, to exclude intravesical pathology. It also enables a biopsy to be taken to exclude interstitial cystitis. The maximum bladder capacity under anaesthesia will help to distinguish a physically from a functionally small bladder. Cystoscopy and urethral dilatation may actually be curative, albeit only for a short time in some patients with urethral syndrome in particular.

Cystometry, with or without video studies, is essential to distinguish a stable (Fig. 14.1) from an unstable bladder (Fig. 14.2). A normal bladder will have a first sensation of bladder filling when approximately 150 ml has been infused, and a strong desire to void at about 450 ml, and has normal compliance i.e. no associated tonic rise in bladder pressure on filling. Detrusor instability can be diagnosed either by the presence of systolic contractions during filling as a result of bladder stimulation, or by suitable provocative tests including coughing, standing or withdrawal of the filling catheter. During the voiding study, a 'stop-test' should be performed. If the detrusor continues to contract against a closed bladder neck, an isometric contraction or pISO can be demonstrated (Fig. 14.3). A significant pISO is usually associated with detrusor instability whilst the patient with a hypersensitive bladder may not be able to interrupt her stream.[18] A steady rise in subtracted detrusor pressure on filling suggests a poorly compliant bladder, which is usually indicative of a detrusor abnormality. The reduced compliance of detrusor instability can be differentiated from that of a physically reduced bladder or an extravesical cause since the pressure usually subsides exponentially as the detrusor muscle relaxes after filling. Patients with sensory urgency caused by hypersensitivity of bladder and/or urethra may complain of severe discomfort during the insertion of the filling and pressure transducer lines. They have an early first

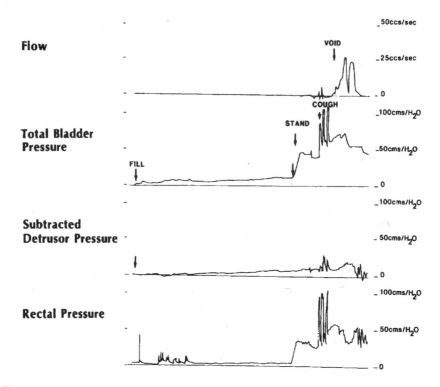

Fig. 14.1 Normal female urodynamic study. (Reproduced with permission of Mr T. Stephenson.)

sensation, which often co-exists with a first desire to void, and usually have a greatly reduced functional bladder capacity.

Videocystourethrography may reveal a wide open bladder neck especially in those patients with concomant GSI, or a failure of 'milk-back' of urine from the proximal urethra when voiding is interrupted. A stable cystometrogram is, however, found in 70% of patients with urgency[19] and 50% of patients with urge incontinence.[20,21] These findings may be explained by the distal urethral electrical conductivity (DUEC)[22] or bladder neck electrical conductivity (BNEC) tests.[10] The bladder is first filled with 250 ml of isotonic saline at room temperature and two gold plated ring electrodes mounted on a fine 7F gauge silastic catheter is placed at the bladder neck or distal urethra. A high frequency AC voltage is then applied between the electrodes. The presence of urine in the proximal urethra owing to opening of the bladder neck is seen as an increased electrical impedance across the electrodes which can occur not only with unstable contractions, but also in their absence (Fig. 14.4). Holmes has shown[23] that there is a highly significant correlation between the symptoms of urgency and urge incontinence and if the maximum amplitude of bladder neck activity exceeds 13 μA. This test has a sensitivity and specificity of 100% and 77%, respectively, for the detection of

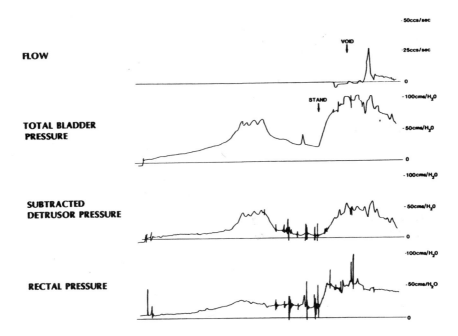

FLOW

TOTAL BLADDER
PRESSURE

SUBTRACTED
DETRUSOR PRESSURE

RECTAL PRESSURE

Fig. 14.2 Idiopathic instability. (Reproduced with permission of Mr T. Stephenson.)

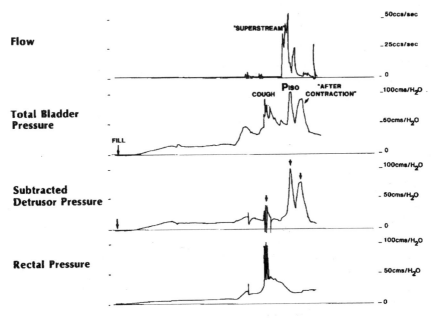

Flow

Total Bladder
Pressure

Subtracted
Detrusor Pressure

Rectal Pressure

Fig. 14.3 The high pISO 'after contraction' and superstream in the urge syndrome.
(Reproduced with permission of Mr T. Stephenson.)

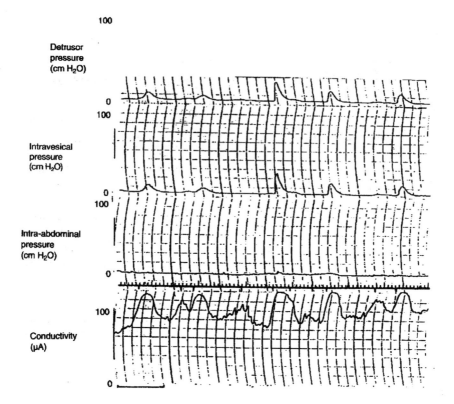

Fig. 14.4 Bladder neck conductivity variations associated with and without unstable bladder contractions in a patient with marked urinary urgency. (Reproduced with permission of Mr D. Holmes.)

an abnormality associated with urgency compared with corresponding values of 58% and 92% for conventional cystometry, which is similar to other cystometric studies.[21]

The low sensitivity of conventional urodynamics to define an underlying disorder has questioned the role of such studies. Ambulatory monitoring is a more physiological method of measuring bladder function. Although this technique was first described in 1978,[24] it was only with the introduction of solid state transducers that the sensitivity has improved. Webb[25] has shown that 31 out of 52 patients (60%) suspected on clinical grounds of having detrusor instability had this diagnosis confirmed on ambulatory monitoring (20 on filling and 11 on provocation) despite having normal conventional cystometrograms (Fig. 14.5). It has been suggested that ambulatory monitoring will replace artificial filling CMG in the assessment of urinary incontinence in women.[26]

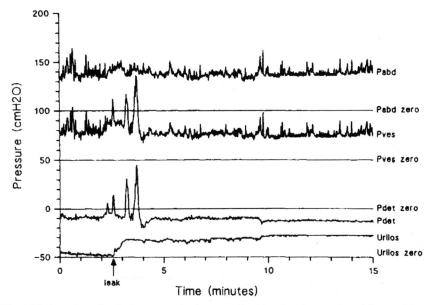

Fig. 14.5 A section of ambulatory monitoring recording showing detrusor instability resulting in loss of urine in a patient who had a stable CMG. (Reproduced with permission of Professor D. Neal.)

TREATMENT

Extravesical causes

The treatment of the underlying pathological disorder or modification of fluid intake is sufficient to cure most of the patients in this group.[27]

Sensory urgency with a known cause

Patients with an urinary tract infection or bladder calculus should have been diagnosed without the need for specialist tests. Following the diagnosis of a bladder tumour, an IVU should be requested to exclude a lesion elsewhere in the urinary tract and an urgent referral made to a urological surgeon.

The aetiology of interstitial cystitis is unclear and therefore treatment is empirical. Parsons[28] has suggested that there is a deficiency of glycosaminoglycans (GAG), which constitute a barrier on the luminal side of the transitional epithelium. This abnormal surface GAG layer leads to the leakage of toxic urinary substances deep into the transitional cells, ultimately inducing inflammation in the bladder wall. The administration of a synthetic GAG such as pentosanpolysulphate sodium (PPS) has therefore been suggested as a treatment for interstitial cystitis.[29] Other chronic inflammatory fibrotic conditions are treated by the same techniques as for refractory idiopathic detrusor instability.

Atrophic cystitis and urethritis responds well to hormone replacement therapy, which may be administered vaginally or systemically. A recent innovation is the development of a slow-release oestrogen-containing ring (Estring, Pharmacia), which only requires replacement every 3 months and thereby ensures good compliance.

The successful treatment of genuine stress incontinence may also cure symptoms of the urge syndrome.[4] Stephenson and colleagues in Cardiff[30] have shown that a fascial sling procedure using autologous rectus sheath carries a 94% subjective and 92% objective cure rate of GSI. In addition, 78% of patients were improved or cured of their urge component postoperatively, which was objectively seen by videourodynamics to be caused by closure of the previously noted dilated proximal urethra.

Sensory urgency of unknown cause

Drug treatment for this condition is ineffective[31] with poor patient compliance.[32] Bladder retraining has been suggested as an appropriate form of treatment[33] and a 60% improvement claimed.[34]

Transvesical subtrigonal infiltration of the pelvic plexuses with phenol was first described by Ewing[35] for the treatment of refractory detrusor instability. Blackford[36] demonstrated a 68% symptomatic response in women with idiopathic sensory urgency and this response was sustained for more than 12 months in 65%. The technique fell out of favour in 1990 when Rosebaum[37] failed to show a significant improvement, and a high complication rate was also described;[38] particularly the development of vesico-vaginal fistulae, periureteric fibrosis and a substantial (10%)[39,40] risk of paralysing the bladder, condemning the patient to lifelong intermittent self-catheterisation. A long-term follow-up study by McInerney[40] showed a 31% short-term and 28% long-term improvement in sensory urgency treated by this method. There were no fistulaes in this series of 97 patients in contrast to other reports,[41] which was thought to be a result of placing the phenol too medially. There would therefore still appear to be a place for subtrigonal phenolization in selected patients with severe intractable bladder hypersensitivity of unknown cause.

Motor urgency of known cause

If motor urgency still persists after a 6 month period of treatment, it is best treated as for the idiopathic variety.

Motor urgency of unknown cause

Since the pathophysiology of this condition is unknown[42] with considerable overlap with normal voluntary voiding, treatment is often empirical and therefore unsatisfactory. Treatment usually involves one or more of the following methods listed in Table 14.3.

Table 14.3 Treatment of motor urgency

Psychotherapy
Bladder retraining
Biofeedback
Hypnotherapy
Acupuncture

Electrical stimulation

Drug therapy
Anticholinergic agents
Antispasmodic agents
Tricyclic antidepressants
Vasopressin analogues

Transvesical phenol

Surgery
Bladder transection
Clam enterocystoplasty

Psychotherapy

Bladder drill was first described nearly 30 years ago[43] and improved by Frewen in the 1970s.[44] This technique assumes that detrusor instability is the result of the frequency and urgency rather than the cause. Retraining the bladder to a normal voiding pattern as suggested by Jarvis[45] corrects the urgency and urge incontinence. Although Frewen[44] suggested this treatment was equally effective whether performed as in-patient or out-patient, several authors suggest the initial treatment should take place under supervision in hospital.[2] The addition of drug treatment is not always necessary and may have an adverse effect in bladder retraining. The initial results of bladder retraining are excellent with subjective cure rates[46,47] of up to 70% and objective cure rates of 50% evaluated 3 months after treatment.[46] However, there is a high relapse rate[48] of up to 40% unless the patient maintains her regime. Although the use of bladder drill has become underused in most centres, the high success rate and minimal costs involved[49] suggest this should be the first-line treatment for motor urgency.

Biofeedback involves a similar process of re-educating the patient as in bladder retraining but by a more specific means.[50] Between four and eight 1 hour urodynamic evaluations are performed in which a rise in bladder pressure is converted into auditory and/or visual signals. The patient can then try to suppress that pressure rise by any suitable means and can recognize the effect of suppression by a reduction in the intensity of the transmitted signal. Initial reports[50] suggested an 80% subjective and 60% objective cure rate but again a high relapse rate was seen[51] and its use has now declined except in children.[52]

Freeman and Boxby[53] treated 61 women by 12 sessions of hypnosis over a

1 month period, followed by 12 sessions at home using a prerecorded cassette. They reported an 86% subjective and 50% objective cure rate but again a high relapse rate was seen.[54]

Acupuncture has also been used to treat motor urgency.[55] It is thought that endogenous opioid release may reduce or block the autonomic innervation of detrusor and urethral sphincter muscles[56] and a 76% subjective cure rate has been reported.[55]

Electrical stimulation   80 % improve

Electrical stimulation is thought to work by artificially restoring detrusor muscle inhibitory reflexes. Activation of the inhibitory pathways to the micturition centre via pudendal afferents has no effect on efferent pathways and hence very few recognized side-effects.[57] The stimulation may be either short-term or long-term: in the former the patient is stimulated for 20–30 minutes at maximum tolerable intensity for up to 10 sessions over a 2–3 week period. In long-term stimulation, a lower more comfortable frequency is used but the treatment time is increased as a consequence. These treatments are usually carried out in out-patient physiotherapy departments but may also be carried out at home, using small personal devices, with no loss of efficacy.[58] Whatever mode of stimulation is used, the results are fairly consistent with 80% of patients symptomatically improved or cured,[59] and this technique requires further development and usage.

Drug therapy

Anticholinergic drugs, such as propantheline, competitively blockade acetylcholine (M_2) receptors at postganglionic parasympathetic receptor sites. Unfortunately its action is not specific for detrusor muscle, which is reflected in its side-effects including dry mouth, constipation, blurred vision, nausea and facial flushing; these are the reasons usually cited for poor patient compliance of 10–23%.[60] Relaxation of smooth muscle, and hence detrusor pressure, usually occurs at dosages ranging between 15–60 mg qds.

The most commonly used drug for motor urgency is oxybutynin hydrochloride which acts in two ways on detrusor muscle: it possesses both anticholinergic activity and also a direct spasmolytic effect. Its side effect profile is similar to propantheline and may precipitate urinary retention. At an oral dose regimen of 5 mg bd/tds, up to 70% of patients show a subjective improvement and this improvement will be confirmed by urodynamic studies[2] in 60%. However, it is more appropriate to start at a lower dose of 2.5 mg bd and increase gradually to improve patient compliance.[61] It may also be administered intravesically with equal efficacy[62,63] and although it is absorbed from the bladder, the peak serum concentration is lower and achieved later, which may explain its reduced incidence of side effects.

Tricyclic antidepressants, e.g. imipramine, are thought to work by blocking the reuptake of presynaptic neurotransmitters such as noradrenaline and serotonin. It may also have a local anaesthetic action. It primarily has anticholinergic activity similar to the previously mentioned drugs. It is particularly useful for the treatment of nocturia and for coital incontinence.[64]

Desmopressin (DDAVP) is a synthetic analogue of vasopressin available in oral form or as an intranasal spray. It reduces urine production[65] by up to 50% and is taken at night for the effective treatment of nocturia. DDAVP should be used with caution in elderly patients to avoid fluid retention and there is a compensatory diuresis in the daytime.

Transvesical phenol

Although useful for sensory urgency, the results of transvesical phenolization for detrusor instability are disappointing with only a 40% response rate.[36] However, when grouped according to age, only 14% of patients less than 55 years showed a response compared with 69% in the over 55 years group in whom the response was not sustained.[36] There would appear to be little place for transvesical phenol injection in the management of the unstable bladder.[38]

Surgery

Overall, about 90% of patients will be symptomatically improved or cured by conservative treatments already discussed or will cease to attend for follow up.[2] For the remaining refractory patients, surgery may be indicated if the patient is suitably motivated. Bladder transection has been widely used in the past[66] but this procedure has a high complication rate and at best a short period of effectiveness.

The 'clam enterocystoplasty' procedure was first described by Bramble in 1982[67] and elaborated by Mundy and Stephenson in 1985.[68] A questionnaire sent to pelvic reconstruction units in the UK in 1994[69] revealed that 67 units were using this technique compared with only 8 in 1982, and that they were widely distributed around the country. Approximately 400 clam enterocystoplasties are presently carried out in this country annually which would equate to over 3000 enterocystoplasties having been performed in total.[69] The majority of patients are female (82%) with the major indication being refractory idiopathic detrusor instability (78%). The average age distribution at operation varied widely, but was usually performed between the ages of 31–45 years, which is the age at which idiopathic detrusor instability commonly presents in females.

The operation comprises incising the bladder coronally so that the bladder opens up like a 'clam shell' (Figs 14.6–14.9). It is important to extend the incision well in front of the ureteric orifices to within a centimetre of the trigone so that efficient bivalving of the bladder occurs, preventing the development of a pseudo-diverticulum. In the original description, sigmoid colon

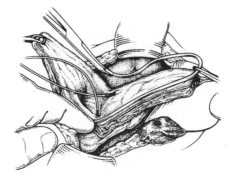

Fig. 14.6 The bladder is bisected in the coronal plane and the bladder circumference is measured. (Reproduced with permission of Professor A. Mundy.)

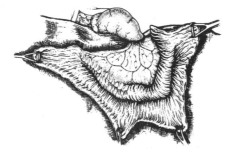

Fig. 14.7 A section of ileum equal in length to the measured bladder circumference is isolated on its vascular pedicle and opened to form a patch. (Reproduced with permission of Professor A. Mundy.)

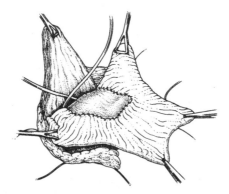

Fig. 14.8 The ileal patch has been sewn on to the posterior bladder wall. (Reproduced with permission of Professor A. Mundy.)

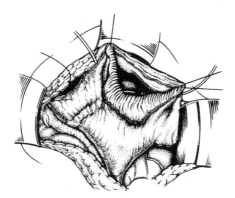

Fig. 14.9 The ileal patch has been flipped over and sutured to the anterior bladder wall. (Reproduced with permission of Professor A. Mundy.)

was used, but now a distal segment of ileum is standard in most units except in the occasional case where the mesentery is too short to reach into the pelvis. A measured segment of terminal ileum (about 25 cm) is isolated and opened along its antimesenteric border and this detubularised segment is sutured into the 'clammed' bladder. In older women the pedicle is brought anteriorly to the broad ligament whilst in the young female the pedicle is passed through the broad ligament to reduce the risk of potential damage to the blood supply should any obstetrical or gynaecological surgery be necessary.[70] The mechanism by which this procedure abolishes unwanted contractions or at least greatly reduces their amplitude is not absolutely clear, but it is probable that the contractions continue and the potential pressures are dissipated by the high compliance of the ileal segment. The continence success rate is approximately 90% but, not surprisingly, the voluntary voiding contractions are also often affected and hence 25% of patients will have to void by clean intermittent self-catheterization (SIC).[2]

However, there is a substantial morbidity following a clam enterocystoplasty. The need to self-catheterize to reduce the urinary frequency rate and also to reduce urinary stasis and the resulting urinary tract infections has already been mentioned. There is also a significant increase in urinary tract infections amongst patients who have undergone clam enterocystoplasty irrespective of stasis.[71] Approximately 12% of patients will develop profuse diarrhoea postoperatively, which is caused by disruption of the enterohepatic circulation of bile salts which responds to cholestyramine.[72] There are also concerns regarding metabolic changes, and there is a metabolic acidosis with respiratory compensation and hyperchloraemia, the long-term consequences of which are uncertain.[73]

By far the major concerns are development of a malignancy either in the bladder remnant or in the incorporated bowel segment,[74] which seems to be localized to the anastomotic site of these tissues.[75] This appears to be similar to the urocolic tumours originating at or in close proximity to the anastomotic site of ureterosigmoidostomy.[76] Tumour within an augmentation was first described in 1971 and since then a further 34 such tumours have been noted (29 malignant and 5 benign).[77] In the only global study, the interval between augmentation and diagnosis of tumour ranged from 5 to 29 years (mean 18 years) and most of these were stitch line adenocarcinomas.[75] The increased risk of tumour in ureterosigmoidostomy has been variously quoted and is increased by a factor of 100-fold,[78] 500-fold[79] and 7000-fold.[80] If there is a similar malignant transformation for the clam procedure, this would equate to a carcinoma induction rate of up to 29% and an estimated polyp adenoma rate[77] of up to 40%.

The mechanism of malignant change is unclear but it has been shown that nitrosamines are elevated in the urine of these patients.[69] It has also been shown that the incorporation of these carcinogenic compounds into the DNA of the transitional epithelium but not the bowel mucosa results in formation of the promutagenic adduct O^6-methyl guanine,[69] which is known to be expressed in other nitrosamine-dependent tumours.[81] There appears to be a deficiency of the repair enzyme O^6-alkyl transferase in the transitional epithelium but not the bowel mucosa, which predisposes this tissue to alkylation damage.[69] Following initiation, it is possible that there is promotion of tumorigenesis by the elevated amount of urinary growth factors, in particular basic fibroblast growth factor,[82] which may be reduced using pentosanpolysulphate sodium.[83] If the effect of this operation is in the short term to cure an often benign, if socially unacceptable condition, but in the long term leads to the development of a tumour which would otherwise not have developed, then the indications for this procedure may have to be revised in the future.

CONCLUSIONS AND THE FUTURE

The management of the 'Urge Syndrome' is a common and vexing challenge for both gynaecologists and urologists. With increasing patient awareness, it will be seen with increasing frequency in out-patient clinics and a logical treatment approach as outlined will be required.

Future developments will centre upon defining the true aetiology of this condition and the development of new pharmacological agents. Brading[84] has suggested that drugs which reduce detrusor excitability by hyperpolarization, e.g. pinacidil, are likely to be more effective than the current neurotransmitter blocking agents if their action could be localized to the bladder. For the refractory case, long-term follow-up of new surgical techniques such as detrusor myomectomy are indicated before they can be suggested as an appropriate form of treatment.[85]

REFERENCES

1 McGuire E J. Clinical evaluation of the lower urinary tract. Clin Obstet Gynaecol 1985; 12: 311–317
2 Stephenson T P, Mundy A R. The urge syndrome. In: Mundy A R, Stephenson T P, Wein A J, eds. Urodynamics: principles, practice and application. 2nd edn. London: Churchill Livingstone, 1994: pp 263–276
3 Cardoza L D, Stanton S L. Genuine stress incontinence and detrusor instability. Br J Obstet Gynaecol 1980; 87: 184–190
4 Stanton S L, Williams J E, Richie D. The colposuspension operation for urinary incontinence. Br J Obstet Gynaecol 1976; 83: 890–895
5 Bungay G T, Vessey M P, McPherson C K. Study of symptoms in middle life with special reference to the menopause. Br Med J 1980; 281: 181–183
6 Norton P A, McDonald L D, Sedgwick P M, Stanton S L. Distress and delay associated with urinary incontinence, frequency and urgency in women. Br Med J 1988; 297: 1187–1189
7 McGuire E J. Reflex urethral instability. Br J Urol 1978; 50: 200–204
8 Fantl J A, Wyman J F, Anderson R L, Matt D W, Bump R C. Post menopausal urinary incontinence: comparison between non-estrogen-supplemented and estrogen-supplemented women. Obst Gynaecol 1988; 71: 823–828
9 Hilton P. Anatomy and physiology of the lower urinary tract and pathophysiology of urinary incontinence and sensory disorders of the lower urinary tract. In: Smith A R B, ed. Urogynaecology. The investigation and management of urinary incontinence in women. London, RCOG press, 1995: pp 1–16
10 Holmes D M, Plevnik S, Stanton S L. Bladder neck electrical conductivity in female urinary urgency and urge incontinence. Br J Obstet Gynaecol 1989; 96: 816–820
11 Bates C P, Bradley W, Glen E et al. International continence society: Fourth report of the standardisation of terminology of lower urinary tract function. Br J Urol 1981; 53: 333–335
12 Freeman R M, McPherson F M, Baxby K. Psychological features of women with idiopathic detrusor instability. Urologia Internationalis 1985; 40: 247–259
13 Cardoza L D, Stanton S L, Williams J E. Detrusor instability following surgery for genuine stress incontinence. Br J Urol 1979; 51: 204–207
14 Steel S A, Cox L, Stanton S L. Long-term follow-up of detrusor instability following the colposuspension operation. Br J Urol 1985; 58: 138–142
15 Copcoat M J, Charag C, Pope A, Cumming J, Shah P J R, Worth P H L. Changes in bladder function after endoscopic bladder neck suspension in female stress incontinence. Neurourol Urodynam 1987; 6: 193–194
16 Robertson A S, Griffiths C J, Ramsden P D, Neal D E. Bladder function in healthy volunteers: ambulatory monitoring and conventional urodynamic studies. Br J Urol 1994; 73: 242–249
17 Creighton S M, Stanton S L. Caffeine: does it affect your bladder? Br J Urol 1990; 66: 613–614
18 McInerney P D. The practice of urodynamics. In: Mundy A R, Stephenson T P, Wein A J, eds. Urodynamics: principles, practice and application. 2nd edn. London: Churchill Livingstone, 1994: pp 101–110
19 Abrams P H. The clinical contribution of urodynamics. In: Abrams P H, Fenley R C L, Torrens M, eds. Urodynamics. London: Springer-Verlag, 1983: p 142
20 Cantor T J, Bates C P. A comparative study of symptoms and objective urodynamic findings. Br J Obstet Gynaecol 1980; 87: 889–892
21 Jarvis G J, Hall S, Stamp S, Millar D R, Johnson A. An assessment of urodynamic examination in incontinent women. Br J Obstet Gynaecol 1980; 87: 893–896
22 Peattie A B, Plevnik S, Stanton S L. Distal urethral electrical conductance (DUEC) test: a screening test for female urinary incontinence? Neurourol Urodynam 1988; 7: 173–174
23 Holmes D M. Clinical and research application of conductivity measurement in the female lower urinary tract. MD thesis. University of Wales, 1987
24 James E D. The behaviour of the bladder during physical activity. Br J Urol 1978; 50: 387–394
25 Webb R J, Ramsden P D, Neal D E. Ambulatory monitoring and electronic measurement of urinary leakage in the diagnosis of detrusor instability and incontinence. Br J Urol 1991; 68: 148–152
26 Neal D E. Ambulatory monitoring. In: Mundy A R, Stephenson T P, Wein A J, eds.

Urodynamics: principles, practice and application. 2nd edn. London: Churchill Livingstone, 1994: pp 133–144

27 Griffiths D J, McCracken P N, Harrison G M, Gormley E A. Relationship of fluid intake to voluntary micturition and urinary incontinence in geriatric patients. Neurourol Urodynam 1993; 12: 1–7

28 Parsons C L, Boychuk D, Jones S et al. Bladder surface glycosaminoglycans: an epithelial permeability barrier. J Urol 1990; 143: 139

29 Parsons C L, Mulholland S G. Successful therapy of interstitial cystitis with pentosanpolysulfate. J Urol 1987; 138: 513

30 Cartledge J, Fulford S, Lloyd-Davies E, Barrington J W, Stephenson T P. The medium-term follow-up of the rectus fascial sling. Br J Urol 1996 (in press)

31 Milroy E. Pharmacological management of common urodynamic problems. In: Turner-Warwick R T, Whiteside C G, eds. The urology clinics of North America. Volume 6. Philadelphia: Saunders, 1979: pp 265–272

32 O'Boyle P J, Parsons K F. Primary vesical sensory urgency. A clinical review of bromocriptine. Br J Urol 1979; 51: 200–203

33 Frewen W K. The management of urgency and frequency of micturition. Br J Urol 1980; 52: 367–369

34 Jarvis G J. The management of urinary incontinence due to primary vesical sensory urgency by bladder drill. Br J Urol 1982; 54: 374–376

35 Ewing R, Bultitude M I, Shuttleworth K E D. Subtrigonal phenol infiltration for urge incontinence secondary to detrusor instability in females. Br J Urol 1982; 54: 689–692

36 Blackford H N, Murray K, Stephenson T P, Mundy A R. Results of transvesical infiltration of the pelvic plexuses with phenol in 116 patients. Br J Urol 1984; 56: 647–649

37 Rosebaum T P, Shaw P J R, Worth P H L. Trans-trigonal phenol failed the test of time. Br J Urol 1990; 66: 164–169

38 Chapple C R, Hampson S J, Turner-Warwick R T, Worth P H L. Sub-trigonal phenol injection. How safe and effective is it? Br J Urol 1991; 68: 483–486

39 Cox R, Worth P H. Chronic retention after extratrigonal phenol injection for bladder instability. Br J Urol 1986; 58: 237–238

40 McInerney P D, Vanner T F, Matenhelia S, Stephenson T P. Assessment of the long-term results of subtrigonal phenolisation. Br J Urol 1991; 67: 586–587

41 Wall L L, Stanton S L. Transvesical phenol injection of pelvic nerve plexuses in females with refractory urge incontinence. Br J Urol 1989; 63: 465–468

42 Mundy A R. Detrusor instability. Br J Urol 1988; 62: 393–397

43 Jeffcoate T N A, Francis W J A. Urge incontinence in the female. Am J Obstet Gynecol 1966; 94: 604–618

44 Frewen W K. An objective assessment of the unstable bladder of psychological origin. Br J Urol 1978; 50: 246–249

45 Jarvis G J. Bladder drill. In: Freeman R, Malvern J, eds. The unstable bladder. Bristol: Wright, 1989: pp 55–60

46 Elder D D, Stephenson T P. An assessment of the Frewen regime in the treatment of detrusor dysfunction in females. Br J Urol 1980; 52: 467–471

47 Jarvis G J, Millar D R. Controlled trial of bladder drill for detrusor instability. Br Med J 1980; 281: 1322–1323

48 Holmes D M, Stone A R, Bary P R, Evans C, Stephenson T P. Bladder retraining: 3 years on. Br J Urol 1983; 55: 660–664

49 Fantl J A, Wyman J F, McClish D K et al. Efficacy of bladder training in older women with urinary incontinence. JAMA 1991; 265: 609–613

50 Cardoza L D, Stanton S L, Hafner J, Allan V. Biofeedback in the treatment of detrusor function. Br J Urol 1978; 50: 250–254

51 Cardoza L D, Stanton S L. Biofeedback: a five year review. Br J Urol 1984; 56: 220

52 Van Gool J D, De Jonge G A. Urge syndrome and urge incontinence. Arch Dis Child 1989; 64: 1629–1634

53 Freeman R M, Boxby K. Hypnotherapy for incontinence caused by detrusor instability. Br Med J 1982; 284: 1831–1832

54 Freeman R M. Hypnosis and psychomedical treatment. In: Freeman R M, Malvern J, eds. The unstable bladder. Bristol: Wright, 1989: pp 73–80

55 Philp T, Shah P J R, Worht P H L. Acupuncture in the treatment of bladder instability. Br J Urol 1988; 61: 490–493

56 Murray K H A, Feneley R C L. Endorphins – a role in lower urinary tract function? The effect of opioid blockade on the detrusor and urethral sphincter mechanisms. Br J Urol 1982; 54: 638–640

57 Fall M, Lindstrom S. Electrical stimulation, a non-surgical means of cure for stress and urge incontinence. In: Smith A R B, ed. Urogynaecology. The investigation and management of urinary incontinence in women. London, RCOG press, 1995: pp 125–129

58 Plevnik S, Janez J, Vrtacnik P. Short-term electrical stimulation: home treatment for urinary incontinence. World J Urol 1984; 4: 24–26

59 Fall M, Madersbacher H. Peripheral electrical stimulation. In: Mundy A R, Stephenson T P, Wein A J, eds. Urodynamics: principles, practice and application. 2nd edn. London: Churchill Livingstone, 1994: pp 495–523

60 Gajewski J B, Awad S A. Oxybutynin versus probantheline in patients with multiple sclerosis and detrusor hyperreflexia. J Urol 1986; 135: 966–969

61 Moore K H, Hay D M, Imrie A H et al. Oxybutynin chloride (3 mg) in the treatment of women with idiopathic detrusor instability. Br J Urol 1990; 66: 479–485

62 Madersbacher H, Knoll M, Kiss G. Intravesical application of oxybutynin: mode of in controlling detrusor hyperreflexia. Neurourol Urodynam 1991; 10: 375–376

63 Enzelsberger H, Helmer H, Kurz C. Intravesical instillation of oxybutynin in women with idiopathic detrusor instability: a randomised trial. Br J Obstet Gynaecol 1995; 102: 929–930

64 Hilton P. Urinary incontinence during sexual intercourse: a common but rarely volunteered symptom. Br J Obstet Gynaecol 1988; 95: 377–381

65 Hilton P, Stanton S L. The use of desmopressin (DDAVP) in nocturnal urine frequency in the female. Br J Urol 1982; 54: 252–255

66 Mundy A R. The long term effects of bladder transection for urge incontinence. Br J Urol 1983; 55: 642–644

67 Bramble F J. The treatment of adult enuresis and urge incontinence by enterocystoplasty. Br J Urol 1982; 54: 693–696

68 Mundy A R, Stephenson T P. Clam ileocystoplasty for the treatment of refractory urge incontinence. Br J Urol 1985; 57: 641–646

69 Barrington J W. The malignant potential of clam enterocystoplasty. MD thesis. University of Cambridge, 1996

70 George V K, Russell G L, Shutt A, Gaches C G C, Ashken M H. Clam ileocystoplasty. Br J Urol 1991; 68: 487–489

71 Fenn N, Conn I G, German K A, Stephenson T P. Complications of clam enterocystoplasty with particular reference to urinary tract infection. Br J Urol 1992; 69: 366–368

72 Barrington J W, Fern-Davies H, Adams R J, Evans W D, Woodcock J P, Stephenson T P. Bile acid dysfunction after clam enterocystoplasty. Br J Urol 1995; 76: 169–171

73 Nurse D E, McCrae P, Stephenson T P, Mundy A R. The problems of substitution cystoplasty. Br J Urol 1988; 63: 423–426

74 Stone A R, Davies N, Stephenson T P. Carcinoma associated with augmentation cystoplasty. Br J Urol 1987; 60: 236–238

75 Filmer R B, Spencer J R. Malignancies in bladder augmentation and interstinal conduits. J Urol 1990; 143: 671–678

76 Husmann D A, Spence H M. Current status of tumour of the bowel following ureterosigmoidostomy: A review, J Urol 1990; 144: 607–610

77 Kalble T. The risk of malignancy after cystoplasty. In: Chisholm G D, Paulson D F, eds. Current Opinion in Urology Volume 3. Glasgow, Current Science, 1993: pp 476–479

78 Stewart M. Urinary diversion and bowel cancer. Ann R Coll Surg Eng 1986; 68: 98–102

79 Iannoni C, Marcheggianom A, Pallone F et al. Abnormal patterns of colorectal mucin secretion after urinary diversions of different types. Hum Pathol 1986; 17: 834–840

80 Gittes R F. Carcinogenesis in ureterosigmoidostomy. Urol Clin North Am 1981; 13: 201–205

81 O'Connor P J. Towards a role for promutagenic lesions in carcinogenesis. In: Lambert M W, Laval J, eds. DNA repair mechanisms and their biological implications in mammalian cells. New York: Plenum Press, 1989: pp 61–71

82 Barrington J W, Fraylin L, Fish R, Shelley M, Stephenson T P. Elevated levels of basic fibroblast growth factor in the urine of clam enterocystoplasty patients. J Urol 1996; 155(2): 468–470

83 Barrington J W, Fulford S, Fraylin L, Fish R, Shelley M, Stephenson T P. Reduction of Urinary Basic Fibroblast Growth Factor Using Pentosan Polysulphate Sodium. Br J Urol 1996 (in press)
84 Brading A F, Turner W H. The unstable bladder: towards a common mechanism. Br J Urol 1994; 73: 3–8
85 Fulford S, Carter K, Barrington J W, Davies G, Bales G, Stephenson T P. The preliminary results of detrusor myomectomy for detrusor instability and hyper-reflexia. Br J Urol 1996 (in press)

15 Contraceptive implants

L. Mascarenhas   J. Newton

Sustained-release progestogen implants are a new approach to meeting a worldwide need for more effective and acceptable birth control. This need stems from at least four background problems: rapid population growth, environmental degradation, persistent poverty and unplanned pregnancy.[1]

Over 500 000 women die each year from causes related to pregnancy and childbirth.[1] The five major causes are: haemorrhage, infection, unsafe abortion, hypertension and obstructed labour. Of these women 500 die every day from unsafe abortion. The World Health Organization (WHO) estimates that there are about 150 000 unwanted pregnancies terminated every day (40–60 million per year) corresponding to an annual rate of 32–46 abortions per thousand women of reproductive age.[1] In the UK alone in 1992 there were 170 000 terminations of pregnancy, the majority of which were for unwanted pregnancy.[2] Finally, some 12 million children under the age of five die of poverty each year.[3]

It is therefore easy to define our goals in reproductive health: to reduce the unmet need for family planning, the scarcity of family planning services and methods, and finally maternal and infant mortality and morbidity, which can all be summarized by increasing contraceptive prevalence.[1]

OVERVIEW OF CONTRACEPTIVE METHODS

Worldwide, from the quantitative point of view, female sterilization is the most frequently used method, followed by intrauterine devices (IUDs) and oral contraceptives.[1] Whereas the worldwide use of oral contraceptives seems to show a declining trend,[1] the use of injectable and implantable long-acting contraceptives is significantly increasing; most recent estimates suggest that more than 9 million women are using such formulations.[1] Among the alternative routes of administration, the subdermal, intrauterine, intramuscular and intravaginal routes have been developed into long-acting contraceptive methods that are widely used or are in clinical trials, achieving up to 8 years of highly effective yet reversible contraception.

The general household surveys in 1986, 1989 and 1991, of women in the UK aged between 16 and 49, have shown that the proportion of women using at least one method of contraception remains stable (69–71%) as well

Table 15.1 Overview of contraceptive methods

Method	First year pregnancy rate (%)		1 year/5 year continuation rate (%)	1991 UK use
	Lowest expected	Typical		
Norplant	0.04	0.2	82–95/25–78	–
Depo-provera	0.3	0.3	70	–
Female sterilization	0.2	0.4	–	12
Male sterilization	0.1	0.15	–	13
Combined pill	0.1	3	73	23
IUD	<1	3	75–95/33–41	5
Condoms	2	12	64	16
Cap	6	18	57	1
Natural family planning	1–9	20	67	1
Withdrawal	N.A.	N.A.	N.A.	1
No method	N.A.	N.A.	N.A.	21

Reproduced with permission from J. Trussell et al[4] & The General Household Survey.[5] N.A. Not available.

as the proportion of women not using any method (20–22%).[4] They show that approximately one-quarter of couples rely on very effective methods (female and male sterilization) another third rely on effective methods (oral contraceptive pill, intrauterine device) and a further one in five rely on less effective methods (barrier methods, natural family planning). Typical pregnancy rates (in contrast to lowest expected pregnancy rates) associated with methods that do not require much or any user attention are low, ranging from 3% for the IUD to less than 1% for implants, injectables or sterilization (Table 15.1).[5] Although ineffective use of contraceptives and failure of the methods account for a large fraction of unplanned pregnancies, couples who do not use contraceptives account for a higher proportion of unplanned pregnancies than those who use them.[6] There is, however, a disappointingly high number of unplanned pregnancies even where the present methods are available. This is much to do with the perceived side effects and 'nuisance value' both of which adversely affect motivation.[7]

SCIENTIFIC BASIS OF SUSTAINED-RELEASE PROGESTOGEN SYSTEMS

In order to increase contraceptive efficacy without considerable dose increases, non-oral systems for sustained release of progestogens have been developed. These systems exploit non-oral routes for drug delivery and therefore lead to an elimination of the hepatic first pass peak 'effect' and avoidance of the highest steroid peak plasma levels associated with oral intake (Fig. 15.1).[8] The higher bioavailability may lead to lower doses of steroids being administered with a parallel reduction in the possibility of adverse effects.

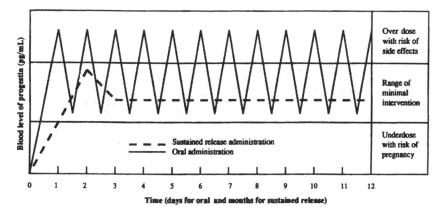

Fig. 15.1. Comparison of orally administered and sustained-release progestin blood levels. Progestin sustained-release delivery systems provide low doses that remain above the contraceptive threshold for long periods. (Reproduced with permission from P. Darney.)[8]

MODE OF ACTION, ADVANTAGES AND DISADVANTAGES OF SUSTAINED-RELEASE SUBDERMAL PROGESTOGEN IMPLANTS

The advantages of implants are that they constitute a highly effective long-acting reversible method that is easy to use and is independent of user compliance. Further advantages are that they are non-oestrogen dependent and that they are therefore suitable for women with oestrogen related side effects or contraindications. They can be used by women of all ages both pre and post family and expand the range of family planning choices available to them. The main disadvantage of the method is the disruption of the menstrual cycle but with careful counselling, continuation rates with implants can be better than with the IUD, the other multi year reversible contraceptive method.[5] However, they are expensive methods at present because both the cost of introducing the method and of providing the implants are higher than those of most other methods. However, this has to be balanced against the cost of an unwanted pregnancy and if one takes this into account, then implants are a cost-effective option.

Subdermal sustained-release progestogen implants prevent pregnancy in several ways. They make cervical mucus thicker and reduce its amount. Sperm have difficulty moving through such thick and meagre mucus, and therefore few sperm pass through the cervical canal to reach the uterus.[9–13] Ovulation occurs in approximately half the cycles.[9,13–15] If it does occur, the luteal phase is often deficient, inhibiting fertilization[15,16] and finally the endometrium is hypotrophic.[16–19] More recent research suggests that, even when ovulation occurs, endocrine dysfunction would usually prevent fertilization of the oocyte if sperm were to reach it.[20]

Table 15.2 Subdermal progestogen implants

	Efficacy
Non-biodegradable	
Norplant (6 silastic capsules with levonorgestrel)	5 years
Norplant-2 (2 silastic rods with levonorgestrel)	3 years
Implanon (1 ethylene vinyl acetate rod with 3-ketodesogestrel)	3 years
ST-1435 (1 capsule)	18 months
Uniplant (1 silastic rod with nomegestrol acetate)	1 year
Biodegradable	
Capronor (1 capsule with levonorgestrel)	1 year
Annuelle (4 pellets with 90% net & 10% cholesterol)	1 year

HISTORY AND DEVELOPMENT OF SUBDERMAL PROGESTOGEN IMPLANTS

The contraceptive implants developed until now are subdermal progestogen-only devices. Implants may be divided into two main groups: biodegradable and non-biodegradable. Non-biodegradable systems make use of a suitably inert carrier or container for the contraceptive steroid, from which it diffuses over time e.g. polydimethyl siloxane (silastic) or ethylene vinyl acetate (EVA). Biodegradable systems remain under development and have not been widely used. They are attractive in that the contraceptive steroid is incorporated into a biodegradable delivery system, which as it degrades releases the steroid for contraceptive usage over prolonged periods and does not require removal as nothing is left at the end of the effective life span.

Norplant® is a first generation implant system that consists of six silastic capsules releasing levonorgestrel, with a contraceptive efficacy of 5 years. Norplant-2®, which consists of two silastic covered rods releasing levonorgestrel, and Implanon®, which consists of one EVA rod releasing 3 ketodesogestrel, both have a contraceptive efficacy of 3 years and are classed as second generation implant systems. The ST1435 implant and Uniplant (nomegestrol acetate implant) are still in clinical trials. The main biodegradable implant, a single poly-e-caprolactone capsule with levonorgestrel (effective for 1 year) should be available by the end of the decade. Finally, biodegradable subdermal norethindrone pellets are being used in clinical trials with various ratios of norethindrone to cholesterol (Table 15.2).

This review will confine itself to implant systems that are available (Norplant®) or nearing general availability (Norplant-2® and Implanon®). Their physical properties are summarized in Fig. 15.2.

NORPLANT^R

Norplant® is currently the only commercially available contraceptive implant. By December 1990, more than 55 000 women had participated in clinical

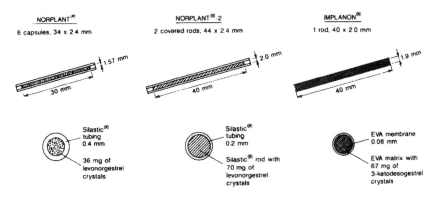

Fig. 15.2 Design and dimensions of 3 contraceptive implant systems: Norplant is of a filled capsule design, Norplant-2 and Implanon have a covered rod design. (Reproduced with permission from A.P. Sam)

trials in 46 different countries and it has now been used by around 2 million women throughout the world, including 900 000 women in the USA. To date, at least 29 countries have approved the use of Norplant®, including Finland in 1983 (the first), the USA in 1990 and the UK in 1993.

Insertion

Insertion involves a minor surgical procedure taking about 5–10 minutes by trained providers.[13] It involves subdermal insertion into the inner aspect of the upper arm, of 6 capsules in a fan shape using local anaesthetic after marking the arm using a template. Incision is not always necessary and the capsules are placed using a special trocar (Fig. 15.3)

Physical properties

Each capsule contains 36 mg crystalline levonorgestrel contained in a capsule that consists of silastic tubing sealed at either end with silastic medical adhesive type A. The release rate of levonorgestrel is determined by the total surface area of the capsule and by the thickness of the capsule walls. Since 1987, the silastic tubing and medical adhesive consists of lower density tubing, as the higher density tubing appeared to give a higher pregnancy rate in women weighing over 70 kg (see below).

Medical grade polydimethyl siloxane tubing had previously been used in over 100 000 patients as hydrocephalous drainage tubes without serious foreign body reactions or evidence of neoplasia.[13] This last experience on the use of silastic in humans without side effects was of great importance for the concept that it would be possible to develop a subdermal implant which could release steroids for contraception.

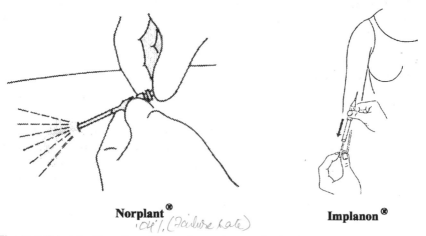

Norplant® ·04'/.(failure rate)   **Implanon**®

Fig. 15.3 Principle of insertion of first and second generation implant systems.

Pharmacokinetics

The six capsules initially release about 85 mcg/day falling to 50 mcg/day by 9 months, 35 mcg/day by 18 months and 30 mcg/day throughout the third, fourth and fifth years of use.[13] Mean plasma levels of levonorgestrel are around 0.5 ng/ml during the first year and then 0.3 ng/ml for years 2, 3, 4 and 5 owing to the sustained near zero order release rate. In comparison, oral pills reach initial plasma levels of 3 ng/ml to 5 ng/ml levonorgestrel and the area under the curve is 4 to 10 times higher than that achieved by Norplant®.[8]

Efficacy

Figures from the latest Population Council Report (1992)[13] from 2670 women in 13 countries have revealed a gross pregnancy rate ranging from 0.2 per 100 women-years after year 1, to 1.6 per 100 women-years after year 4, giving a 5 year cumulative pregnancy rate of 3.9 per 100 women-years. This gross rate includes user failure as well as method failure as the majority of pregnancies in the first year were luteal phase pregnancies, i.e. users were pregnant at the time of insertion.[21]

   With the less dense tubing, the gross cumulative 5 year pregnancy rate in women weighing more than 70 kg is only slightly higher than in lighter women. The overall average 5 year cumulative pregnancy rate is 1.6 per 100 women-years (ranging from 0 in women weighing less than 50 kg to 2.4 in women weighing more than 70 kg).[11]

   In 1990 Trussell reviewed the first year failure rates for a range of contraceptive methods.[5] It showed a first year failure rate (both lowest expected and typical) for Norplant® of 0.04. This compared favourably with the lowest expected first year failure rates for male and female sterilization of 0.1 and

0.2 respectively, and typical failure rates of 0.15 and 0.4. This rate is also 10 to 100 times lower than the rates reported for combined oral pills and copper IUDs (0.5–3%).[5]

Ectopic pregnancy

This data is reassuring; in the US Norplant® users, ectopic pregnancy occurred at an average rate of 1.3 per 1000 women-years. This should be compared to a background risk of 6.5 per 1000 women-years in women not using contraception and to 0.4 per 1000 women-years in users of the combined oral pill in the US.[13,22] This relative protection is probably a result of the fact that Norplant® interferes with ovulation but less so than the combined oral contraceptive pill.

Removal

Removal of Norplant® is slightly more difficult than insertion and takes on average less than 30 minutes, depending on how correctly the Norplant® was inserted.[13] It requires a 3 mm incision and the implants are usually removed using a mosquito forceps after infiltration of local anaesthetic under the ends of the capsules nearest the incision site. More recently the 'U' technique has been described using a modified forceps and a vertical incision, significantly reducing removal time.[23] Experience in the UK has enabled us to classify complications of Norplant® removal.[24]

Reversibility

Serum levels of levonorgestrel become undetectable within 48 hours of Norplant® removal and this normally results in a prompt return to the woman's usual level of fertility. There are no long-term effects on future fertility reported after its use. In fact, in the US International Committee for Contraceptive Research monitored study, the life table pregnancy rate after removal of Norplant® was similar to that of women not using contraception, i.e. 90% conceived within 24 months.[13]

Menstrual bleeding patterns

The most frequent side effect of Norplant® is disruption of the menstrual cycle, which affects 60–100% of users in the first year[13] and is the main reason for its discontinuation. This takes the form of irregular bleeding or spotting, prolonged bleeding or spotting, infrequent bleeding or spotting, or amenorrhoea. This disruption, however, is transient with the majority of cycles returning to a regular pattern at the end of the first year.[19] Furthermore, studies have shown that serial haemoglobin levels increase and the total amount of blood loss is reduced.[13]

Other side effects

Clinical trials comparing Norplant® and IUD users found that certain conditions are statistically associated with Norplant®. These include headaches, weight gain, acne, mood swings, breast tenderness, dizziness and functional ovarian enlargement.[13] Insertion site infection is uncommon as is expulsion of a capsule, with a frequency of 0.8% and 0.4%, respectively, in international trials. Some clinics have lower rates of infection at the insertion site than others, suggesting that some providers are more careful at maintaining aseptic conditions.[13]

Clinical pharmacology

A wide range of clinical pharmacology studies show few metabolic changes with the use of Norplant®; in particular, no clinically important changes have been noted in liver, renal, adrenal and thyroid function tests.[13] Carbohydrate metabolism studies have shown an initial increase in serum glucose levels but a maintaining of the glucose tolerance test within normal limits.[13] Later metabolism studies on serum lipoproteins have given variable results concerning HDL and LDL cholesterol. The ratio of total cholesterol to HDL cholesterol was not significantly increased in six studies and was significantly decreased in two. The clinical importance of these findings has still to be evaluated.[13] Variable effects on haemostasis have also been reported in Norplant® users regarding levels of factor VII, factor X, antithrombin III activity, fibrinogen and platelets. Changes in clotting function similar to those seen with combined oral pills are possible.[13] Finally, serum levels of oestradiol have shown non-cyclical irregular changes with base values normally between 30–70 pg/ml with occasional peaks of 200–400 pg/ml. Free testosterone concentrations were not significantly changed and there is no convincing evidence of progressive changes in endometrial histology with prolonged use of Norplant®.[13]

Acceptability

Norplant® first year continuation rates range from 76–90%.[5] First year continuation rates for oral contraceptives and IUDs average 50–74%.[5] Continuation rates during the 5th year range from 25–55%, which is greater than with the IUD (33–41%),[5] making it the most successful long-term reversible contraceptive so far marketed. The median duration of use in international trials is 3.5 years.[13]

NORPLANT-2®

To reduce the problems of insertion and removal of fixed implants, a second generation of levonorgestrel-releasing implants with a higher release rate per implant has been developed. Levonorgestrel crystals are mixed with uncured silastic type 382 without silica filler in a ratio of 1:1 and from this homogenous mixture two rods are formed by injection moulding. The two covered rods contain in total 140 mg levonorgestrel homogenously dispersed in their matrix core. Although the in vitro release rate of Norplant-2® has been published to be, in total, 70–80 mcg/day, a lower release rate can be expected towards the end of its effective lifetime of 3 years.[25]

International randomized comparisons of Norplant® and Norplant-2® have shown similar pregnancy rates and discontinuation rates (for menstrual problems, other medical problems, planning of pregnancy, and other personal reasons) with similar continuation rates at 2 and 3 years.[11,26] Norplant-2® therefore offers promising options for pregnancy spacing.

In mid-1987, the Dow Corning Corporation discontinued manufacture of the elastomeric core material. This was followed by the suspension of all preintroductory clinical trials and a reformulation of Norplant-2®. Clinical studies to support a new drug application have now been completed (H. Nash, Population Council, personal communication).

IMPLANON®

The contraceptive implant, Implanon®, developed by Organon International, consists of an EVA co-polymer device containing 67 mg of the progestogen 3-keto-desogestrel, the active metabolite of desogestrel.[25] The core of the implant consists of crystals of 3-keto-desogestrel in a matrix of EVA co-polymer. The implant is designed to release 3-keto-desogestrel, for a period of 3 years, at a level above the presumed critical level of 30 mcg/day needed for complete inhibition of ovulation. It can be administered subcutaneously from a sterile disposable inserter and the insertion procedure is very simple, minimizing the risk for insertion-related infections. Comparison of in vivo with in vitro data indicate the release rates to be quite comparable.[27] Clinical experience with implants releasing 30–40 mcg/day 3-keto-desogestrel and providing plasma levels of around 0.28 nmol/litre afford efficient contraceptive protection (Organon Laboratories, personal communication): after more than 31 000 cycles of Implanon exposure with 348 implants contributing to more than 26 cycles each, not a single pregnancy has occurred. Studies carried out in Birmingham over the last 5 years also indicate contraceptive plasma levels for more than 3 years.[28]

In the assessment of the safety of implants from EVA and releasing 3-keto-desogestrel, the following considerations were taken into account: the area under the curve for an implant releasing 60 mcg/day is considerably lower than for the oral contraceptive pill Marvelon (150 mg desogestrel/30 mg ethinyl estradiol per daily tablet). Marvelon is registered in 48 countries and has been widely available since 1981. Ethinyl vinylacetate is a polymer widely used for medical purposes such as intrauterine contraceptive devices (Progestasert, Umbrel), for occular delivery (Occusert) and for containers for

Table 15.3 Reasons for early termination of implants

	Implanon®		Norplant®	
	Europe	SE Asia *	Europe	SE Asia*
Bleeding irregularities	13	0.6	17	0.6
Amenorrhoea	1	0.1	2	–
Acne/weight/mood changes	2	0.5	3	–
Headache	0.1	0.2	–	0.2
Other medical reasons	2	0.5	1	0.4
Non-medical/personal	1	2	6	0.2

Numbers expressed as %. * China not included. Reproduced with permission from N. V. Organon, 1994.

injectable aqueous solutions (French Pharmomacopeia). There is no indication for an interaction (chemical or pharmacological) between the EVA polymer and the active substance, as implants stored for 18 months at room temperature and ambient temperature show the same 3-keto-desogestrel content as initially.[29]

Efficacy/safety studies have been started with Implanon® implants releasing initially approximately 60 mg 3-keto-desogestrel daily (Implanon®) and delivered in a disposable inserter. In these studies the following variables are being assessed: pregnancy rates, cycle control, acceptability, dropout rates, serious and minor adverse event rates, systemic and local effects of Implanon®. The general conclusion so far is that the insertion of Implanon® is very simple and in the cases where the implant had to be removed no problems were encountered; local irritation or infection, in particular, has not been encountered. In comparative studies between Norplant® and Implanon®, similar discontinuation rates and reasons for discontinuation have been observed (Organon Laboratories, personal communication) (Table 15.3). Implanon® is likely to be released at the same time as Norplant-2®

ACCEPTABILITY OF CONTRACEPTIVE IMPLANTS

The acceptability of a contraceptive method can be assessed by continuation rates, reasons for discontinuation, rates of reacceptance after discontinuation and statements made in response to interview questions about satisfaction.[5] None of these alone provides an adequate measure of acceptability. Continuation rates can be invalid indicators of satisfaction since women may continue use because they have difficulty arranging removal or because they fear the removal procedure.[5] Reasons for discontinuation may also inaccurately reflect acceptability since some women discontinue for medical problems which are unrelated to contraceptive use.[5] Statements made in open-ended interviews are probably the most sensitive indicators of user acceptance and the best reflectors of patient perceptions.[5]

Focus group discussions among users, discontinuers, potential acceptors, husbands of women in these three groups and service providers have been conducted in the Dominican Republic, Egypt, Indonesia and Thailand to expand understanding of the acceptability of Norplant[®].[30] Results suggest that factors having an impact on the acceptability of implants fall into three general categories: medical/technical, cultural/religious and informational/ educational. Users in all four countries reported satisfaction with the implants.

In the US, two studies in particular have assessed the acceptability of Norplant[®]. One study assessed socio-economic, demographic, and accepta- bility data by anonymous self-administered mail-back questionnaires to which 54 out of 75 acceptors of Norplant[®] responded[31] (2927 months of use). The group comprised caucasians (84%), blacks (12%) and hispanics (4%). Of these acceptors, all would recommend this method to others; the greatest advantages were not worrying about pregnancy, convenience and reduced risk (41% of them had become pregnant whilst using another method of birth control). The authors concluded that Norplant[®] was partic- ularly suited for women who are concerned about compliance with and/or failure of other methods.

The other US study concerned 205 acceptors of Norplant[®] and Norplant- 2[®] who were interviewed after an average of 24 months of use and after dis- continuing the method.[32] Interviews were performed by a non-Norplant[®] clinician and included contraceptive and reproductive history, sources of information, knowledge of Norplant[®], experiences using the method, and the impressions of friends and family about the method. The group comprised caucasians (37%), blacks (13%), hispanics (44%) and asian/american indi- ans (6%). The most common reasons for trying the implants were dissatis- faction with other methods and perceptions about Norplant[®]'s ease of use. A number (41%) of acceptors had anxiety prior to insertion; 49% of these feared pain, but only 5% said that they actually experienced significant pain; 74% reported little or no pain at removal. Most of the women were pleased with Norplant[®] although 95% reported side effects, with 82% reporting changes in menstruation; 95% of users said that they might like to use the implants again in the future. The authors concluded that Norplant[®] appeared to be a highly acceptable method of contraception despite the fre- quent occurrence of bothersome side effects.

More recently, negative reports about Norplant[®] have appeared in the lay and medical press.[33,34] In particular, a corporate law suit has emerged against its US manufacturers because of unrealistic expectations about removal. In the light of this, it was important to assess the acceptability of this method in the UK. Our department has currently the first and the largest clinical ex- perience with contraceptive implants in the UK. In 1993, over 250 implants have been inserted of which 110 are in prospective randomized clinical trials comparing Norplant[®] with Implanon[®]. The discontinuation rate has been 10% after 12 months of use.[35] In addition to efficacy and safety we are study- ing detailed acceptability of these two implants by means of serial interviews using a non-directive questionnaire administered by a trained interviewer. In contrast to the US studies mentioned, our study consisted of well educated caucasians who chose the method mainly because of its efficacy and who were predominately oral contraceptive pill users. All our acceptors had attended a separate counselling session prior to insertion and had received specific advice regarding the possible side effects and, in particular, the menstrual disruption. As a result, in contrast to the American experience, this was not found to be the main reason for discontinuation after 12 months. In spite of counselling, a significant number remained anxious about insertion, but this anxiety proved to be unfounded when interviewed retrospectively. In the same way, discontinuers did not experience significant pain upon removal. Our experience demonstrated in particular the advantages of a second generation implant (Implanon®) particularly with regard to ease of insertion and removal as well as the favourable acceptability of implants with careful counselling of acceptors and proper training of providers.[36] The cost of such an implant has still to be determined but there is no doubt that its duration of action (3 years) will be particularly attractive considering that the median duration of use of Norplant® is 3.5 years from the worldwide experience.[13] This successful preliminary experience awaits confirmation by long-term multicentre studies in the UK.

CONCLUSIONS

Global population is 5.3 billion today. If we take till the year 2010 to reach replacement level of fertility (around 2.1 children per couple), then global population will stabilize by the end of the 21st century at 8 billion (WHO low projection); if it is reached in 2035, population will stabilize at around 10 billion (WHO median projection); however, if it is not reached until 2065, then global population in 2100 will consist of more than 14 billion people, with major consequences on every aspect of life.[37] To restrict the final population to 10 billion, contraceptive prevalence must increase from 51% to 58% before the year 2000 and to 71% by 2020, implying an increase from the present 350 million users to 500 and 800 million users, respectively.[37] Whether or not these ambitious targets can be reached will depend not only on the availability of a wider choice of safe, acceptable and affordable contraceptives and greatly increased funding, but also on fundamental changes in behavioural, educational, socio-cultural, economic and political factors.[37] Meanwhile, in the UK where 1 in 5 conceptions results in an abortion, these methods will be a valuable addition to the armamentarium against unwanted pregnancy[38] and should increase the range of contraceptive options available to women.

REFERENCES

1 Diczfalusy E. Contraceptive prevalence, reproductive health and our common future. Obstet Gynaecol Surv 1993; 48(5): 321–332

2 Report on confidential enquiries into maternal deaths in the UK 1988–90. London: HMSO, 1994

3 Smith R, Leaning J. Medicine and global survival. Br Med J 1993; 307: 693–69

4 Goddard E. General household survey 1991. London: HMSO, 1993

5 Trussell J, Hatcher R A, Willard Cates Jr, Stewart F H, Kost K. Contraceptive failure in the United States: an update. Stud Fam Plann 1990; 21(1): 51–54

6 Harlap S, Kost K, Darroch Forrest J. Pregnancies occurring during contraceptive use. In: Preventing pregnancy, protecting health: a new look at birth control choices in the US. Chapter V. New York: Alan Guttmacher Institute, 1991: 33–39

7 Szarewski A, Guillebaud J. Contraception. Br Med J 1991; 302: 1224–1226

8 Darney P D, Klaisle C M, Tanner S, Alvarado A M. Sustained-release contraceptives. Curr Prob Obstet Gynaecol Fertil 1990; XIII (3): 90–125

9 Brache V, Faundes A, Johansson E, Alvarez F. Anovulation, inadequate luteal phase and poor sperm penetration in cervical mucus during prolonged use of Norplant implants. Contraception 1985; 31(3): 261–278

10 Croxatto H, Diaz S, Salvatierra A M, Morales P, Ebensperger C, Brandeis A. Treatment with Norplant sub-dermal implants inhibits sperm penetration through cervical mucus in vitro. Contraception 1987; 36(2): 193–201

11 Sivin I. International experience with Norplant and Norplant-2 contraceptives. Stud Fam Plann 1988; 19(2): 81–94

12 The Population Council. Norplant levonorgestrel implants – A summary of Scientific Data. New York: The Population Council, 1990

13 The Population Council. Decisions for Norplant Programs. New York: Population Report (K) Series No. 4, 1992

14 Brache V, Alvarez-Sanchez F, Faundes A, Tejada A S, Cochon L. Ovarian endocrine function through five years of continuous treatment with Norplant subdermal contraception implants. Contraception 1990; 41(2): 169–177

15 Faundes A, Brache V, Tejada A S, Cochon L, Alvarez-Sanchez F. Ovulatory dysfunction during continuous administration of low dose levonorgestrel by subdermal implants. Fertil Steril 1991; 56(1): 27–31

16 Shaaban M M, Ghaneimah S A, Sagel S, Khalifa E M, Salem H T, Ahmed A. Sonographic assessment of ovarian and endometrial changes during long term Norplant use and their correlation with hormone levels. Fertil Steril 1993; 59: 998–1002

17 Croxatto H, Diaz S, Pavez M, Croxatto H B. Histopathology of the endometrium during continuous use of levonorgestrel. In: Zatuchni GI, Goldsmith A, Shelton JD, Sciarra JJ, eds. Long-acting contraceptive delivery systems. Philadelphia: Harper & Row, 1984: pp 290–295

18 Shoupe D, Mishell D R. Norplant: sub-dermal implant system for long-term contraception. Am J Obstet Gynecol 1989; 160(5): 1286–1292

19 Shoupe D, Mishell D R, Bopp B L, Fielding M. The significance of bleeding patterns in Norplant implant users. Obstet Gynaecol 1991; 77(2): 256–260

20 Segal S J, Alvarez-Sanchez F, Brache V, Faundes A, Vilja P, Tuohimaa P. Norplant implants: the mechanism of contraceptive action. Fertil Steril 1991; 56(2): 273–277

21 Norplant Product Review. Roussel Laboratories Ltd., 1993

22 Xiao Feng Li, Newton J. Progestogen only contraceptives and ectopic pregnancy. Br J Fam Plann 1992; 8: 79–84

23 Praptohardjo U, Wibowo S. The 'U' technique: a new method for Norplant implants removal. Contraception 1993; 48: 526–536

24 Newton M P, Mascarenhas L, Xiao Feng Li, Newton J R. Classification of implant removals: Birmingham experience in insertion and removal. Br J Fam Plann 1995 (in press)

25 Sam A P. Controlled release contraceptive devices: a status report. J Controll Rel 1992; 22: 35–46

26 Wayne Bardin C. Long-acting steroidal contraception: An update. Int J Fertil 1989; Suppl 34: 88–95

27 Eenink, M J D, Maassen G C T, Sam A P, Geelen J A A, van Lieshout J B J M, Olijslager J, de Nijs H, de Jager E. Development of a new long-acting contraceptive subdermal implant releasing 3-ketodesogestrel. Proceedings of the 15th International Symposium on Controlled Release of Bioactive Materials. Lincolnshire, IL: Controlled Release Society, 1988: 402–403

28 Newton J R, Davies G, Xiao Feng Li, Mascarenhas L, Newton M P. First and second

generation subdermal contraceptive implants. In: Popkin D R, Peddle L D, eds. Women's health today: perspective on current research and clinical practice. Chapter 59, 1994: 399–404

29 Sam A P. Controlled-release contraceptive devices. In: Hincal A A, Kas S, Sumnu M, eds. Minutes of the Fifth Int Pharm Technol Symp. Paris: Editions de Sante 1990; 271–284

30 Zimmerman M, Haffey J, Crane E, Szumowski D, Alvarez F, Bhiromrut P, Brache V, Lubis F, Salah M, Shaaban M, Shawky B, Sidi I P S. Assessing the acceptability of Norplant implants in four countries: findings from focus group research. Stud Fam Plann 1990; 21(2): 92–103

31 Sinopsky F E, Pasquale S A, Gonzalez S J. Long acting contraceptive implants – Acceptance by US women. San Francisco: The American College of Obstetrics & Gynecology, 1990

32 Darney P, Atkinson E, McPherson S, Hellerstein S, Alvarado A. Acceptance and perceptions of Norplant among users in San Francisco, USA. Stud Fam Plann 1990; 21(3): 152–160

33 Rogers L. Contraceptive implants face legal challenge. Sunday Times, 3rd July 1994

34 Roberts J. Women in US sue makers of Norplant. Br Med J 1994; 309: 145

35 Mascarenhas L, Newton P, Newton J. First clinical experience with contraceptive implants in the UK. Br J Fam Plann 1994; 20(2): 60

36 Mascarenhas L, Newton P, Newton J, van Beek A, Coelingh Bennink H J T. First clinical experience with contraceptive implants in the UK. Int J Gynaecol Obstet 1994; 46(Suppl 2): 68 (Free Communication FIGO, 1994)

37 Diczfalusy E. Contraceptive prevalence, reproductive health and our common future. Contraception 1991; 43(3): 201–227

38 Mascarenhas L. Long acting methods of contraception. Br Med J 1994; 308: 991–992

16 Contraception for the over forties

A. Gebbie

Relatively little attention has been paid by scientists and clinicians over the years to the contraceptive needs of older women. On an individual level, many older women find that choice of a suitable contraceptive method poses particular difficulty and they may often have exaggerated fears or longstanding taboos concerning use of some methods at their age. Advice on fertility given to older women by health professionals may not be appropriate or particularly accurate and many women are tempted to take chances or abandon contraception altogether. A pregnancy for a woman in her later years can have devastating psychological or social consequences. Difficulty in the choice of available methods of contraception is reflected in the high uptake of surgical sterilization procedures in the UK.

HORMONAL FACTORS

The endpoint of the reproductive years is the menopause, which occurs on average at the age of 50.8 years and is a diagnosis made in retrospect. In the decade before the menopause, however, subtle changes occur in the relationship between the hypothalamo-pituitary axis and activity of the ovary. Longitudinal studies of endocrine changes in women over 40 years indicate a strong correlation between regular cycles and the occurrence of ovulation.[1] Regular menstruation implies regular ovulation irrespective of the age of the woman. Many women in their early forties note shortening of their cycle as the first menstrual change. The shortened cycles are ovulatory but associated with a relatively higher follicle stimulating hormone (FSH) concentration in the follicular phase of the cycle. Declining levels of the glycoprotein inhibin, produced by follicular cells of the ovary, are thought to be implicated in this early hormonal change.[2]

Thereafter, menstruation becomes more erratic in the phase of the menopausal transition with an increased frequency of longer, anovulatory cycles. Anovulatory cycles may be associated with a subsequent menstrual bleed which is heavier than normal. Spells of anovulation may still be followed by spells of regular periods and ovulation with a theoretical potential for conception. The menopausal transition is a time of fluctuating hormonal activity and women must not be advised to discontinue contraception purely

Table 16.1 Risks of pregnancy to women in their 40s compared to those in their 20s

Doubling of perinatal mortality rates
Fourfold increase in maternal mortality rates
Increased risk of chromosomal abnormalities
Spontaneous abortion rates doubled

on the basis of an isolated elevated FSH concentration or short period of amenorrhoea.

PREGNANCY IN OLDER WOMEN

According to the Guinness Book of Records (1994), the oldest woman in the world to give birth following a spontaneous conception was 57 years and 129 days (the oldest woman in the UK was 55 years). Successful pregnancies after the age of 52 years are extremely rare although advances in assisted conception techniques using donor oocytes have made pregnancies possible in postmenopausal women. Data from studies which monitored conception rates in women with azospermic husbands undergoing artificial insemination by donor (AID) have found that fertility begins to slowly decline in women over the age of 30 years. Declining oocyte quality is almost certainly responsible for this age-related decline in fertility, as 'younger' and 'older' groups of women undergoing egg donation from the same source have similar conception and pregnancy loss rates.[3]

There are increased risks and complications for both mother and fetus in a late pregnancy (Table 16.1). However, with good obstetric care and testing for fetal abnormality, these are of lesser concern to an older woman than the psychological and social distress that an unplanned pregnancy may cause. Women over the age of 40 years have the highest incidence of termination of pregnancy of any age group in the UK and almost half the pregnancies at this age will end in therapeutic abortion.

SEXUAL FUNCTION

Many women experience a mid-life decline in sexual interest and find that the novelty of their sexual relationship has long gone. Sexual function may also be affected by factors such as prolonged, frequent or heavy menstruation in women in their 40s. With the ageing process itself, both men and women may find a gradual reduction in the speed and intensity of their sexual responses.[4] As women approach the menopause, they are often moving on from motherhood and domesticity to consider new, alternative roles outwith the home. Unresolved conflicts or resentments within the marital relationship not infrequently occur at this time of life.

The frequency of coitus is strongly and inversely associated with age. In her large survey of sexual lifestyles in the British population, Wellings and

Table 16.2 Contraceptive use (%) of all women at different ages (adapted from Wellings et al 1994)[5]

Method	16–24 years	25–34 years	35–44 years	45–49 years
Pill	64	44	11	2
Condom	42	31	21	13
IUD	2	9	9	4
Diaphragm	1	2	2	3
Female sterilization	0.4	6	17	18
Male sterilization	1	7	24	15
None	10	12	16	45

colleagues[5] found frequency of coitus to peak in the mid-20s age group and thereafter show a gradual decline, more marked for women than for men. For example, the average frequency of heterosexual sex reported by married women aged 16–24 was six times in the last 4 weeks falling to twice in the last 4 weeks among those aged 45–49 years. She also found a strong association with length of relationship and frequency of sex, the number of occasions in the last 4 weeks being much lower in longer relationships. The excitement of a relatively new partnership presumably influences the frequency of sexual activity in the early years of a relationship.

The method of contraception used also has an impact on sexual function and frequency of intercourse and appears to be positively associated with the effectiveness of the contraceptive method used.[6] Many couples report that their sex life is enhanced by the removal of the fear of pregnancy by a permanent sterilization procedure.

METHODS OF CONTRACEPTION USED BY OLDER WOMEN

The various methods of contraception used by women in the UK at different ages are compared in Table 16.2.

Use of oral contraception declines steeply with age. In Wellings' survey, nearly two-thirds of women aged 16–24 reported its use compared to 1 in 10 women aged 35–44 years and 1 in 40 in the 45–59 age group. In contrast, surgical methods of sterilization increased in popularity with age and there was an abrupt reversal in popularity of the pill and sterilization in the middle years. Sterilization accounted for half of all contraceptive use in the 45–59 age group. The IUD is more popular among women in their middle years, although the proportions fall markedly among younger and older women. Condom use decreases with increasing age, and female barrier methods are infrequently used at all ages.

As the age of the woman increases, the efficacy of all methods of contraception increases significantly. Methods such as the progestogen-only pill or spermicide-only preparations, which would be not recommended for a

Table 16.3 Gynaecological advantages to older women of COC use

Good cycle control
Reduction in menstrual blood loss
Reduction in dysmenorrhoea
Improvement in premenstrual syndrome
Reduced incidence of fibroids
Reduced incidence of benign ovarian cysts
Suppression of endometriosis
Protective effect against endometrial cancer
Protective effect against ovarian cancer ↓ 40%. risk

teenager, may be perfectly appropriate for an older woman at various stages in her later reproductive years.

COMBINED ORAL CONTRACEPTION

Millions of women have taken combined synthetic oestrogen and progestogen preparations since they were first introduced in the early 1960s, and 'the pill' remains the most popular method of reversible contraception worldwide. Combined oral contraception (COC) is of very high efficacy in women of all ages when taken correctly, and its principal mode of action is by suppression of ovulation. It is primarily a method of contraception used by young women. A significant reduction in dosage of both oestrogen and progestogen components has occurred over the last three decades. The modern, low-dose preparations containing 20–35 µg oestrogen are undoubtedly safer for general health as a result. Nowadays, COC offers excellent contraceptive protection and benefits to health and well-being for the great majority of women who take it. The scope of COC extends beyond just contraception – as treatment for certain gynaecological conditions and, in the future, to prevent types of gynaecological cancers.[7]

Non-contraceptive health benefits to older women

Older women who use COC have a reduced incidence of many gynaecological problems (Table 16.3) and are less likely to require hospital admission for both major and minor gynaecological surgery. A strong protective effect against epithelial ovarian cancer has been demonstrated, reducing risk by around 40% and persisting for at least 15 years after discontinuing COC.[8] A protective effect against endometrial cancer, which is maintained for a similar length of time after discontinuing COCs, has also been demonstrated. There is evidence that use of COC prevents significant bone mineral density loss in perimenopausal women[9] although there does not appear to be any particular benefit to bone density in women who take COCs premenopausally. COCs are an excellent way of providing contraception, cycle control and relief of early menopausal symptoms in older, low-risk women.

Risk of arterial disease in COC users

There has been awareness since 1968 of a causal relationship between COC use and an increased risk of myocardial infarction (MI) and thrombotic stroke, which is potentiated by other risk factors, particularly cigarette smoking. This relationship was attributed to the effect of oestrogen increasing clotting factors and, to a lesser extent, the atherogenicity of progestogens.

There is good evidence for a gradient of risk associated with oestrogen dose. One UK study showed a relative risk of MI of only 1.1 with current use of low-dose COC compared to a risk of 4.2 with current use of preparations containing 50 μg oestrogen.[10] Another UK study found that current usage of COCs had no detectable effect on the risk of MI unless the woman also smoked.[11] Overall, smoking in women is a much stronger risk factor for MI than COC use. Unfortunately, many women and health professionals still believe that COCs must be discontinued at the age of 35 years, based on the increased risk of MI and stroke associated with older, stronger pills. There is now universal agreement that modern, low-dose COCs can be continued in healthy, non-smoking, low-risk women until the menopause, and this was endorsed by the US Food and Drugs Adminstration's Fertility and Maternal Health Drugs Advisory Committee in 1989.[12] Women who smoke must *always* be advised to discontinue COCs at the age of 35 years.

The introduction of COCs containing the third generation progestogens (desogestrel, norgestimate and gestodene) was thought to further enhance their safety profile and make these preparations particularly suitable for older women continuing COCs. Third generation progestogens are associated with fewer androgenic side effects than the second generation progestogens (norethisterone and levonorgestrel) contained in earlier low-dose pills and produce fewer adverse effects on lipid and carbohydrate metabolism. To date, COCs containing third generation progestogens are yet to be shown to have any *clinical* benefit over older pills in reduction of arterial disease and hypertension.

Risk of venous thromboembolism

The risk of deep-vein thrombosis, pulmonary embolism, and thrombosis in other veins such as mesenteric, hepatic or retinal is increased in COC users of all ages and is related to an oestrogen-induced alteration in clotting factor levels, tending to promote coagulation. The Oxford/FPA study found a sevenfold increase in risk associated with current use of COC but with a strong suggestion that the risk was less with preparations containing 30 μg oestrogen than high-dose preparations.[13]

In October 1995, the Committee of Safety of Medicines (CSM) in the UK notified all doctors that COCs containing third generation progestogens were associated with a doubling in risk of venous thromboembolism (VTE) compared with pills containing the older progestogens. This advice was based on three studies unpublished at the time, two of which were also unfinished. The risk overall of VTE was small – at worst, 30 per 100 000 women taking third generation preparations compared with 15 per 100 000 in women taking older equivalent preparations. This compared with a risk in healthy women not taking hormones of 5 per 100 000 and a risk in pregnancy of 60 per 100 000.[14] Doctors were required to advise women taking the third generation preparations to change to older, low-dose pills unless they had previously been intolerant of these preparations or were prepared to accept an increased risk of VTE. This increased risk of VTE associated with third generation pills was an unexpected finding and it is regrettable that these research studies will now almost certainly not be completed. They had the potential to demonstrate a clinical benefit in terms of reduced incidence of arterial disease with third generation preparations, a benefit particularly pertinent to older women continuing COC. The COC containing 20 µg oestrogen and the third generation progestogen, desogestrel, had been the pill of choice for older women. The uncertainty and anxiety raised by the 'pill scare' associated with third generation preparations is likely to significantly reduce the prescribing practice of COC in older women and lead to further uptake of sterilization procedures.

Breast cancer

Although a source of great anxiety to many women, numerous studies show no overall association between breast cancer and use of COC.[15] A weak association has been found between development of breast cancer in women under the age of 36 years and previous COC use. No increased risk of breast cancer associated with prior use of COC in women over 45 years of age has been found. The numbers of women continuing with COC into their late 40s have not been large enough to demonstrate any conclusive association with breast cancer.

PROGESTOGEN-ONLY CONTRACEPTION

Progestogen-only methods of contraception offer older women significant advantages in terms of safety and reliability. They are particularly appropriate for women who smoke or have cardiovascular risk factors which contraindicate COC. Although relatively overshadowed in popularity over the years by the combined pill, a variety of delivery systems now exist for giving very low to high-dose progestogen-only contraception and offering women a wide choice of hormonal contraceptives. Progestogen-only pills (POPs), injectables, subdermal implants and progestogen-releasing IUDs are all now available commercially. It is anticipated that in the next few years, vaginal contraceptive rings will be marketed, containing either progestogen alone or combined with oestrogen.

Progestogens act as contraceptives by primarily altering cervical mucus

Table 16.4 Gynaecological problems common to progestogen-only methods of contraception

Amenorrhoea and oligomenorrhoea
Irregular periods
Spotting
Functional ovarian cysts

and modifying the endometrium to inhibit sperm transport and implantation. There is varying suppression of ovulation with different progestogen dosages, which tends to disrupt the menstrual cycle in an unpredictable way. Many users experience erratic and scanty spotting or breakthrough bleeding.[16] This and other gynaecological problems are frequently the limiting factor to their acceptability to women of all ages (Table 16.4). Irregular bleeding in users of progestogen-only contraception may occasionally be associated with pathological causes, particularly in older women, which should not be overlooked.

Progestogen-only methods are not contraindicated in women with hypertension, gallstones, migraine or diabetes. They cause minimal effect on lipid levels and no evidence of an increased likelihood of thromboembolic events.[17] Myocardial infarction and stroke are not contraindications to progestogen-only use, but low-dose methods are preferable as they allow secretion of endogenous ovarian oestradiol which is important for vascular endothelial cell function and protects against further cardiovascular episodes.[18] Progestogen-only methods do not need to be discontinued prior to major surgery. At the present time, women with breast cancer should probably avoid progestogen-only contraception as it is simply not known whether progestogens could stimulate or, alternatively, inhibit the disease process.

Progestogen-only pills

A small range of progestogen-only pills (POPs) are marketed in the UK but in reality there is very little difference in efficacy, cycle control and side effects between the different brands. Efficacy of the POP increases substantially with age, and the failure rate (FR) in a woman in her 40s compares favourably with the FR of the combined pill in young women.[19] There is a wide spectrum of response of the ovary to the POP, ranging from anovulation to no effect at all. This is reflected in the unpredictable and erratic bleeding pattern in some POP users. The incidence of amenorrhoea in POP users increases with age but is not associated with significant hypo-oestrogenism until the onset of the menopause, in contrast to Depo-Provera. The POP represents only around 7% of the total oral contraceptive market reflecting poor publicity of its advantages rather than concerns about long-term risks or side effects.

Injectables

Depot medroxyprogesterone acetate (Depo-Provera, DMPA) is most widely used in the UK although norethisterone enanthate (NET-EN) is also available and has a shorter duration of action. Amenorrhoea becomes common with prolonged use of Depo-Provera and in some older women can lead to confusion about onset of the menopause and anxiety regarding pregnancy.

Over the years, Depo-Provera has been the subject of various campaigns relating to feminist and consumer concerns over its potential for misuse and abuse. These influences have had a major effect on its availability worldwide and it was only licensed for unrestricted use in the UK in 1995. Concerns have also been expressed about the relationship between Depo-Provera and breast cancer but there is now general consensus that there is no significant overall increase in the risk in Depo-Provera users but a possible very small risk in long-term users.[20] Depo-Provera, in common with all progestogen-only methods, is protective against endometrial cancer and possibly ovarian cancer.

There was also concern from one study that long-term Depo-Provera use was associated with loss of bone mineral density in premenopausal women although no osteoporotic fractures occurred.[21] In other situations, progestogens have actually been found to have a bone conserving effect. This issue is as yet unresolved but it is probably good practice to advise women to discontinue Depo-Provera at the age of 45 years to allow time for recovery of bone density prior to the menopause. In women with amenorrhoea of longer than 5 years duration, a serum oestradiol should be checked and if possible, a bone density scan performed. If either of these gives low results, an alternative method of contraception should be advised or 'add back' oestrogen replacement offered in conjunction with Depo-Provera. Transdermal 50 µg oestrogen patches applied twice weekly would conserve bone density, although this combined regimen rather diminishes the convenience and simplicity of Depo-Provera as a method of contraception.

Norplant

Norplant consists of six flexible capsules containing the progestogen, levonorgestrel, inserted subdermally in the upper arm under local anaesthesia. Current data sheets for Norplant in the UK recommend use in women aged 18–40 years. Despite this arbitrary recommendation, Norplant can be an extremely effective and acceptable contraceptive for older women offering convenience of use over a 5 year period. Irregular bleeding is the most frequently reported side effect with Norplant and affects around 60% of users in the first year.[22] Bleeding problems are unpredictable and underlying gynaecolgical abnormality in an older user must be excluded. Women must be counselled carefully about this and other progestogenic side effects prior to insertion as the cost of Norplant (currently £179 in the UK) precludes using it on a trial basis!

INTRAUTERINE DEVICES

Although worldwide, the intrauterine device (IUD) is second in popularity only to the pill; its uptake in developed countries is very variable, ranging from only 6% of married women of reproductive age in the UK to over 30% in Finland and Norway.[23] The modern IUD is a highly effective and convenient method of contraception for older women but is the subject of more prejudice and myth than most other methods of contraception. The large inert devices, the Lippes loop and the Saf-T coil, are no longer commercially available although some older women may still have them in situ.

All copper-bearing IUDs have an effective intrauterine lifespan in excess of the manufacturers' recommendations of 3 or 5 years. Trials on many of the currently available devices have shown a contraceptive effect for up to 10 years.[24] It is now generally accepted that if a woman has an IUD inserted after her 40th birthday this device may remain in situ until she reaches the menopause.[25] IUD insertions and removals are disliked by women and less frequent insertions may encourage greater acceptability by older women who wish a method of contraception that will take them up to the menopause. There is no upper age limit for an IUD – it may be inserted during the perimenopause or used in conjunction with hormone replacement therapy (HRT) if the woman is still thought to be at risk of pregnancy. It is recommended that an IUD be removed postmenopausally as occasionally it can provide a focus for sepsis and cause confusion if postmenopausal bleeding occurs.

Before an older woman considers using an IUD, account must be taken of her pre-existing menstrual pattern. Even small copper-bearing IUDs are associated with an increase in menstrual blood loss of around 50–60 ml[26] and dysmenorrhoea, which may prove unacceptable to a woman who already has dysfunctional menstrual bleeding, menorrhagia or pelvic pain.

IUDs cause neither pelvic infection nor ectopic pregnancy. When an IUD is used by a woman in a stable, mutually monogamous relationship, there is no increased risk of pelvic infection.[27] Copper-bearing IUDs do not, however, offer protection against infection in the way that hormonal contraception makes cervical mucus hostile to ascending infection. IUDs protect against all pregnancies, but in the event of an IUD-failure pregnancy, there is an increased risk of ectopic pregnancy.[28] Older women need to be carefully counselled on the risks and benefits of an IUD and reassured that it offers excellent contraception with less risk of pelvic infection, ectopic pregnancy, expulsion and perforation than in younger users. Health professionals may also need convincing that the modern IUD is worthy of reappraisal and should be included in any discussion of contraceptive methods suitable for older women.

The levonorgestrel releasing intrauterine system

The levonorgestrel releasing intrauterine system (LNG-IUS) (Fig. 16.1) was licensed for contraceptive use in the UK in 1995, although over 12 years'

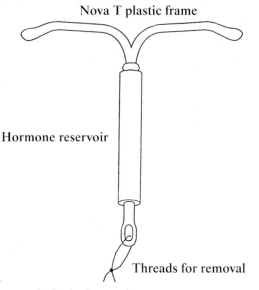

Nova T plastic frame

Hormone reservoir

Threads for removal

Fig. 16.1 Levonorgestrel-releasing intrauterine system

Table 16.5 Daily doses of levonorgestrel in contraception

Levonorgestrel-releasing IUD	20 μg
Progestogen-only pill	30 μg
Norplant	70 μg the first year
	30 μg thereafter
Combined pill (Microgynon 30)	150 μg

experience exists in Scandinavian countries. Based on the Nova-T plastic frame, it has a central reservoir which contains 52 mg levonorgestrel, released at a steady rate of 20 μg per 24 hours. This gives the lowest dose of progestogen of any progestogen-containing contraceptive (Table 16.5). The LNG-IUS combines the advantages of both hormonal and intrauterine contraception and has particular benefits for older women. In contrast to conventional IUDs, it is associated with a dramatic reduction in menstrual blood loss of as much as 90%.[29] Its efficacy approaches that of female sterilization and there is no increase in rate of ectopic pregnancy. A significantly lowered incidence of pelvic infection has been found with the LNG-IUS compared to the Nova-T.[30] Although currently licensed in the UK for only 3 years, it is effective for at least 5, possibly 8 years, and many women are likely to view it as a real alternative to sterilization procedures.

No method of contraception is perfect. Irregular bleeding and spotting are very common in the first 3–6 months of use of the LNG-IUS but improve significantly thereafter. Good counselling about this prior to insertion is essential. Hormonal side effects include acne and headache and those in common with other progestogen-only methods (Table 16.4). The LNG-IUS is broader within its insertion tube than the Nova-T (4.8 mm versus 3.7mm) but in parous women insertion should not pose any practical difficulty. Other applications for the LNG-IUS include medical treatment of menorrhagia, treatment of endometrial hyperplasia and as the progestogen component of HRT. A perimenopausal woman might therefore use a LNG-IUS for contraception, treatment of her dysfunctional bleeding and add systemic oestrogen for her early menopausal symptoms.

BARRIER METHODS

Female barriers

For centuries, women have tried to prevent pregnancy by placing various devices into the vagina. The diaphragm or Dutch cap is the most commonly used female barrier in the UK and there have been no significant improvements or variations in diaphrams for many decades. Older women use diaphragms more reliably and have significantly lower failure rates. Adjunctive spermicide is always recommended to improve efficacy and may provide additional lubrication if vaginal dryness is a problem. The presence of utero-vaginal prolapse, particularly a cystocoele, may make secure retention of a diaphragm difficult and a cervical or vault cap may overcome this problem. It is well established that diaphragms offer significant protection against ascending pelvic infection and neoplasia of the cervix, although symptomatic urinary tract infection is commoner in diaphragm users. Diaphragms offer no protection against viral infections of the vulva and vagina, including HIV.

Condoms

Individuals should be advised, irrespective of age, to consider use of condoms in new relationships for personal protection against sexually transmissible infection. Older couples are generally better at using condoms correctly but rarely find condoms sufficiently user-friendly to start using them for the first time in later life. Some older men find that condoms help them to maintain an erection although others find they may exacerbate erectile importence. Various oil-based vaginal products, including some oestrogen and antifungal creams, can drastically affect the tensile strength of latex condoms and lead to condoms splitting. Sensitivity to condoms can occasionally occur in either partner and hypoallergenic condoms are available.

Other barrier methods

Various spermicide-only preparations can be effective at times of extremely low fertility. The 'Today' contraceptive sponge has never been widely used in the UK because of a reported high failure rate but is highly acceptable and convenient for many women. The female condom (Femidom), launched in the UK in 1992, offers extremely good protection against both pregnancy and sexually transmissible infection. Many women find its appearance extremely unaesthetic although initial adverse reactions become less with familiarity.[31] It is unlikely to appeal to older couples in established relationships.

NATURAL METHODS OF FERTILITY REGULATION

Natural family planning involves a continual awareness of fertility status so that intercourse can be avoided during the fertile phase of the menstrual cycle, which can be identified by measuring basal body temperature, assessing the position of the cervix, the state of the cervical mucus (Billing's method) or using a multiple index system.[32] Effectiveness depends largely on motivation. Older couples are more likely to comply with periodic abstinence from intercourse and natural methods may sometimes be the only method of contraception acceptable for religious or ethical reasons. Difficulty with interpretation of the signs of ovulation occurs when the menstrual cycle becomes shortened or anovulatory during the menopausal transition.

Some couples value the increased self-awareness and knowledge of their own fertility which natural family planning involves. Health professionals are frequently sceptical about natural family planning and rarely offer it as an option in a discussion about contraceptive choices.

STERILIZATION

In the UK, 50% of couples aged over 40 years rely on a sterilization procedure for contraception. Vasectomy is slightly commoner in the younger age groups and therafter female sterilization is commoner.[5] Individuals seeking sterilization must be carefully counselled on the permanency of the procedure and the possible, albeit very small, failure rate. Sterilization of older individuals is less likely to lead to regret and request for reversal. The choice of which partner opts for sterilization is of course a personal decision. However, couples should be reminded that male fertility is conserved well into old age whereas female fertility naturally declines after the age of 40 years. More than 30% of marriages now end in divorce and men may wish to keep their options open in the event of remarriage to a younger partner.

Female sterilization involves the blockage of both Fallopian tubes and is generally performed laparoscopically under general anaesthesia as a day case procedure. There is no evidence that sterilization alters menstruation thereafter,[33] although women discontinuing combined oral contraception at the time of sterilization may find a substantial increase in subsequent menstrual blood loss. Pelvic examination must be performed prior to surgery to exclude pelvic pathology such as fibroids or ovarian lesion. Sterilization can be performed in women of any age up to the menopause, but common sense dictates that those approaching the menopause should probably be advised to use an alternative method for the short period before they achieve natural sterility.

Vasectomy is most often performed under local anaesthesia and involves division of the vas deferens. It is undoubtedly technically easier and associated with less risk than female sterilization although there is concern about a possible long-term association with cancer. A recent large study of Danish men concluded that the risk of testicular cancer was not increased by vasectomy.[34] Several large American studies have suggested an increased risk of prostate cancer following vasectomy.[35] At the present time, there is not enough evidence to change clinical practice.

STOPPING CONTRACEPTION

By convention, women are advised to continue contraception for 1 year following their last spontaneous menstrual period if over the age of 50 years. Women under the age of 50 years are advised to continue with contraception for 2 years following their last period to exclude the likelihood of a further ovulation.

Hormonal contraception

In women taking COC, the oestrogen component will relieve menopausal symptoms and suppress gonadotrophin levels. Diagnosis of the menopause will therefore be masked until COC is stopped at the recommended age of 50 years. A barrier method of contraception or the POP should be instituted at this stage to allow evalution of the menstrual cycle, and gondotrophin levels can be checked after approximately 6 weeks.

If a POP user is amenorrhoeic beyond the age of 45 years, then annual gonadotrophin estimation is recommended to detect the onset of the menopause and to give accurate advice on when the POP can be discontinued. The POP does not suppress gonadotrophin secretion. In the presence of elevated gonadotrophin levels, the woman should be advised to continue with POP for one further year. The presence of regular cycles in an older POP user indicates cyclical ovarian activity and the need to continue contraception.

There is considerable interest in the development of COC containing natural oestrogens which would be free from any thromboembolic risk. These regimens would be ideal for women with risk factors who wished to continue COC in their later years and to bridge the gap between COC and HRT. Although combinations have been found which will suppress ovulation reliably (see below), the poor cycle control with preparations containing the less potent natural oestrogens is a major factor limiting their clinical application.[36]

Hormone replacement therapy

Many women now start hormone replacement therapy (HRT) for relief of menopausal symptoms prior to their last menstrual period. Once established on HRT, it becomes impossible to assess accurately when the natural menopause has occurred and when contraception can safely be discontinued. Conventional HRT cannot be relied on for contraception as the dose of natural oestrogen within it does not reliably suppress ovulation.[37] Higher dose HRT regimens, particularly using the transdermal route for oestrogens, have been demonstrated to suppress ovulation.[38] Although their fertility is low, women who commence HRT prior to the menopause should be advised to continue contraception. Barrier methods can be used. An IUD can be left in situ or be inserted. The POP can be continued in conjunction with HRT. Although there is no scientific data to confirm efficacy of the POP in this context, it is now widely recommended and there have been no reports of failure.[39]

Advising women on HRT when to stop contraception is not simple. It depends on their menstrual pattern at the time of starting HRT, their age and for how long they have been taking HRT. Women can be advised to have a short break from HRT of around 6 weeks to assess their menstrual pattern and have FSH measured to give more accurate information on their risk of pregnancy. If the woman is not willing to discontinue HRT for a brief period (and many are not), contraception can be arbitrarily continued to the age of 55 years. A pregnancy beyond this age in the UK would be worthy of the Guinness Book of Records!

CONCLUSIONS

- Women should be advised to continue contraception for 1 year following their last menstrual period if aged 50 years or more, and for 2 years if aged less than 50 years.
- An unplanned pregnancy in an older woman can have devastating social and psychological consequences. Older women have the highest incidence of therapeutic abortion of any age group.
- Combined oral contraception can be continued in low-risk, non-smoking women until the menopause.
- Progestogen-only contraception is particularly suitable for older women who smoke or have cardiovascular risk factors
- The levonorgestrel releasing intrauterine system offers excellent contraception in conjunction with a dramatic reduction in menstrual blood loss
- HRT does not reliably suppress ovulation and cannot be relied on for contraception. Women who commence HRT prior to the menopause should be advised to use contraception in conjunction with HRT.

ACKNOWLEDGEMENTS

With thanks to Dr Nancy Loudon for her expert help in checking the manuscript.

REFERENCES

1 Metcalf M G. The approach of the menopause: A New Zealand study. NZ Med J 1988; 101: 103–106
2 MacNaughton J, Banah M, McCloud P, Hee J, Burger H. Age related changes in follicle stimulating hormone, luteinizing hormone, oestradiol and immunoreactive inhibin in women of reproductive age. Clin Endocrinol 1992; 36: 339–345
3 Navot D, Drews M R, Bergh P A et al. Age-related decline in female fertility is not due to diminished capacity of the uterus to sustain embryo implantation. Fertil Steril 1994; 61: 97–101
4 Bancroft J. Sexuality and family planning. In: Loudon N, Glasier A, Gebbie A, eds. Handbook of family planning and reproductive health care. 3rd edn. London: Churchill Livingstone, 1995: pp 339–362
5 Wellings K, Field J, Johnson A, Wadsworth J. Sexual behaviour in Britain. The national survey of sexual attitudes and lifestyles. London: Penguin Books Ltd., 1994
6 Trussell J, Westoff C F. Contraceptive practice and trends in coital frequency. Fam Plann Persp 1980; 12: 246–249
7 Ratnam S S, Choolani M. The health benefits of the pill. IPPF Med Bull 1995; 29: 8
8 Cancer and steroid hormone study. The reduction in the risk of ovarian cancer associated with oral contraceptive use. N Eng J Med 1987; 316: 650–655
9 Gambacciani M D, Spinetti A, Taponeco F, Cappagli B, Piaggesi L, Fioretti P. Longitudinal evaluation of perimenopausal vertebral bone loss: Effects of a low dose oral contraceptive preparation on bone mineral density and metabolism. Obstet Gynecol 1994; 83: 392–395
10 Thorogood M, Mann J I, Murphy M, Vessey M P. Is oral contraceptive use still associated with an increased risk of fatal myocardial infarction? Report of a case control study. Br J Obstet Gynaecol 1991; 98: 1245–1253
11 Croft P, Hannaford P C. Risk factors for acute myocardial infarction in women: evidence from the Royal College of General Practitioners' Oral Contraceptive Study. Br Med J 1989; 298: 165–168
12 Fortney J A. Oral contraceptives for older women. IPPF Med Bull 1990; 24(3): 3–4
13 Vessey M P, Mant D, Smith A, Yeates D. Oral contraceptives and venous thromboembolism: findings in a large prospective study. Br Med J 1986; 292: 526
14 Guillebaud J. Leader: Advising women on which pill to take. Br Med J 1995; 311: 1111–1112
15 World Health Organisation. Oral contraceptives and neoplasia. Report of a WHO scientific group. WHO Technical Report Series 1992; 817.
16 Belsey E. Task force on long-acting systemic agents for fertility regulation. Vaginal bleeding patterns among women using one natural and eight hormonal methods of contraception. Contraception 1988; 38: 181–206
17 Thorogood M, Vessey M P. An epidemiological survey of cardiovascular disease in women taking oral contraceptives. Am J Obstet Gynecol 1990; 163: 274–281
18 Fraser I. Progestogen-only contraception. In: Louden N, Glasier A, Gebbie A, eds. Handbook of family planning and reproductive health care. London: Churchill Livingstone, 1995: pp 91–118
19 Vessey M P, Lawless M, Yeats D, McPherson K. Progestogen-only oral contraception. Findings in a large prospective study with special reference to effectiveness. Br J Fam Plann 1985; 10: 117–121
20 Meirik O. Updating DMPA safety. Preface to an issue on DMPA and cancer. Contraception 1994; 49: 185–188
21 Cundy T, Evans M, Roberts H, Wattie D S, Arnes R, Reid I R. Bone density in women receiving depot medroxyprogesterone acetate for contraception. Br Med J 1991; 30: 13–16.

22 Population Council, New York. Norplant levonorgestrel implants: a summary of scientific data. 1990.
23 Population Information Program. IUDs – A new look. Population Reports Series 1988 B5.
24 Sivin I. Should collared copper T intrauterine devices be replaced before eight years? Br J Fam Plann 1992; 18: 9–11
25 Tacchi D. Long term use of copper intrauterine devices. Lancet 1991; 336: 182
26 Tatum H J, Connell E B. Intrauterine contraceptive devices. In: Filshie M, Guillebaud J, eds. Contraception – science and practice. London: Butterworths, 1989, pp. 144–171
27 Chi I. What we have learned from recent IUD studies: A researcher's perspective. Contraception 1993; 48: 81–108
28 Sivin I. Dose- and age-dependent ectopic pregnancy risks with intrauterine contraception. Obstet Gynecol 1991; 78: 291–298
29 Andersson K, Rybo G. Levonorgestrel-releasing intra-uterine device in the treatment of menorrhagia. Br J Obstet Gynaecol 1990; 97: 690–694
30 Toivonen J, Luukainen T, Allonen H. Protective effect of intrauterine release of levonorgestrel on pelvic infection: Three years comparative experience of levonorgestrel- and copper-releasing intrauterine devices. Obstet Gynaecol 1991; 77(2): 261–264
31 Editorial. The female condom. Br J Fam Plann 1992; 18: 71–72
32 Flynn A, Bonnar J. Natural Family Planning. In: Filshie M, Guillebaud J, eds. Contraception—science and practice. London: Butterworths, 1989, pp. 203–223
33 Kasonde J M, Bonnar J. Effect of sterilisation on menstrual blood loss. Br J Obstet Gynaecol 1978; 83: 572–575
34 Moller H, Knudsen L B, Lynge R. Risk of testicular cancer after vasectomy: a cohort study of over 73 000 men. Br Med J 1994; 309: 295–299
35 Editorial. Vasectomy and Prostate Cancer. Lancet 1991; 337: 1445–1446
36 Wenzl R, Bennink H C, Van Beek A, Spona J, Huber J. Ovulation inhibition with a combined oral contraceptive containing 1 mg micronized 17 – B oestradiol. Fertil Steril 1993; 60(4): 616–619
37 Gebbie A E, Glasier A, Sweeting V. Incidence of ovulation in perimenopausal women before and during hormone replacement therapy. Contraception 1995; 52: 221–222
38 Smith R N J, Studd J W W, Zamblera D, Holland E F N. A randomised comparison over 8 months of 100 μg and 200 μg twice weekly doses of transdermal oestradiol in the treatment of severe premenstrual syndrome. Br J Obstet Gynaecol 1995; 102: 475–484
39 Whitehead M, Godfree V. Hormone replacement therapy – Your questions answered. Chapter 12. 1992: 213–221

17 Abnormal uterine bleeding: diagnosis and medical management

A. D. Weeks   S. R. G. Duffy

INTRODUCTION

The social and economic cost of menorrhagia is considerable. Twenty-eight percent of the female population consider their menstruation excessive and will plan their social activities around their menstrual cycle, and nearly 10% of employed women will need to take time off work because of excessive menstrual loss.[1] Six percent of women aged 25 to 44 consult their GPs about excessive menstrual loss every year.[2] Of the 35% of these referred to hospital,[3] 60% will have a hysterectomy in the next 5 years.[4] Over 75 000 hysterectomies are now carried out every year with 30% of them carried out for menstrual disturbances alone.[5]

Over the years, menorrhagia has become an increasingly frequent complaint for two main reasons. Firstly, the woman of today experiences about 10 times more menstrual cycles than her ancestor did. This is related to a decrease in lactational amenorrhoea with the advent of effective contraception. Secondly, women are increasingly unwilling to accept menstrual difficulties. There has been a rise in expectations, and increasing intolerance of the inconvenience of menorrhagia. These factors have both led to an increased demand on the health services.

DEFINITION

The word menorrhagia is derived from the Greek and literally means 'to burst forth monthly' (*mene*, 'the moon' and *rhegnymi*, 'to burst forth'). A range of Greek derivatives stem from this (Table 17.1).

WHAT IS NORMAL?

Heavy periods can be defined in terms of menstrual blood loss. It is commonly accepted that 80 ml per cycle is the upper limit of normal. In 1964 Hallenberg reported a method of measurement of the menstrual blood loss.[6] This method uses collected sanitary pads which are soaked overnight in a sodium hydroxide solution to produce alkaline haematin. The resulting fluid

Table 17.1 Common Greek names for menstrual symptoms

Menorrhagia	Regular, heavy periods
Polymenorrhoea	Frequent periods
Polymenorrhagia	Frequent, heavy periods
Oligomenorrhoea	Infrequent periods
Oligomenorrhagia	Infrequent, heavy periods
Amenorrhoea	Absent periods

is analysed by absorption spectrophotometry and compared with a sample of the patient's venous blood. This technique led to two large population studies in Sweden and the UK. In a study of 476 Swedish women, the median menstrual blood loss was found to be 33 ml, with a 95th centile of 76 ml per cycle.[6] In a more recent study of women in the UK the mean and 95th centile were found to be 38 ml and 100 ml, respectively.[7] The incidence of iron deficiency anaemia rises steeply to nearly 70% once menstrual loss reaches more than 80 ml per cycle.[6]

Whilst menstrual blood measurements may identify the cause of anaemia in women with menorrhagia, it does not always correlate with the patient's perception of the problem. Studies have persistently shown that only 32 to 62% of women with a clear history of menorrhagia have more than 80 ml of loss per cycle.[8-11] Conversely, only 60% of women with a measured blood loss of more than 80 ml consider their periods to be heavy.[6] It may be that those with subjective menorrhagia but menstrual blood loss of less than 80 ml per cycle have a greater discharge of menstrual fluids along with blood. In the absence of underlying pathology or iron deficiency anaemia, however, the exact volume of loss is not as important as the woman's reaction to it. In everyday practice women decide themselves what level of menstrual loss is acceptable and at what stage to seek treatment.

HISTORY OF TREATMENT

The earliest reference to the problems of menorrhagia are in ancient Hindu works dating around 1400 BC. Hippocrates (c. 460–377 BC) also wrote on the subject and suggested cupping, applied to the breast, as a cure. Jesus Christ is recorded as healing a woman with bleeding when she touched his cloak, whilst Soranus of Ephesus (AD 98–138) suggests that ligatures be applied to the armpits and groins to reduce bloodflow to the uterus. The first of the present-day medical treatments was progesterone, first described by Albright in 1938.

AETIOLOGY

Menorrhagia has multiple causes (see Table 17.2). The menorrhagia resulting from those listed in Table 17.2 is sometimes referred to as secondary

Table 17.2 Causes of secondary menorrhagia (secondary DUB)

Systemic disorders
Hypothyroidism
Systemic lupus erythematosis
Chronic liver failure

Clotting dysfunction
Congenital deficiencies
Thrombocytopenia
Leukaemia

Uterine causes
Fibroids
Endometriosis
Adenomyosis
Endometrial or cervical polyps
Endometrial hyperplasia/carcinoma
Pelvic inflammatory disease

Iatrogenic causes
Intrauterine contraceptive device
Progesterones – oral or depot injection
Warfarin

---

menorrhagia. Primary menorrhagia (also known as dysfunctional uterine bleeding or DUB) is a term given to the group of disorders which are left following exclusion of these abnormalities. Up to 40% of women with primary menorrhagia will eventually end up with some other diagnosis if intensively investigated.[12] It may be that as medical science advances and identifies more causes of menorrhagia, the diagnosis of primary menorrhagia will no longer be required.

Menorrhagia is a common complaint in women with clotting disorders,[13-15] but the finding of a clotting disorder in women with menorrhagia is rare. The only exception is in teenagers with menorrhagia severe enough to warrant hospital admission who were found to have clotting disorders in 29% of cases.[16]

There are very few studies on the effect of hypothyroidism on menstrual function. Scott found that 56% of women with hypothyroidism had abnormal menstrual patterns with menorrhagia being the most common.[17] Higham reported a case of hypothyroidism in which the menstrual loss was measured.[18] An initial loss of 480 ml decreased to 58 ml following a 3 month treatment with thyroxine.

There may be a high incidence of early or potential hyopthyroidism in women presenting with menorrhagia. Wilansky performed thyrotrophin-releasing hormone (TRH) tests in 67 women who complained of excessive menstrual loss.[19] All had normal levels of thyroxine and thyroid-stimulating hormone (TSH). They found that 22% had abnormal TRH tests and they treated these women with thyroxine. At follow-up between 12 and 36

Table 17.3 Patterns of dysfunctional uterine bleeding with associated endocrine and histological changes

Ovulation	Phase changes	Endometrial histology	Menstrual pattern
Normal	Shortened FP	Normal	Polymenorrhoea Menorrhagia
Normal	Long FP	Normal	Oligomennorhoea Menorrhagia
Abnormal corpus luteum	Short luteal phase	Deficient secretory endometrium	Premenstrual spotting Menorrhagia
Persistent corpus luteum	Long luteal phase	Well developed secretory endometrium	Prolonged cycles
Anovulation (insufficient follicles)	Short cycle	Deficient proliferative endometrium	Polymenorrhoea Metrorrhagia
Anovulation (polycystic ovaries)	Prolonged cycle	Proliferative or hyperplastic endometrium	Oligomenorrhoea Metropathica haemorrhagica

Reproduced with permission from Davey.[20] FP = follicular phase

months later, all considered their menstrual loss to be normal. In the 16 women with normal TRH tests, 56% still complained of menorrhagia. These findings were confirmed by Blum & Blum who studied 40 women with menorrhagia secondary to an intrauterine contraceptive device.[20] They all had normal free thyroxine and TSH levels. The 10 patients who had the highest TSH levels were given a TRH test and all proved to have early hypothyroidism. All patients reported a significant improvement with thyroxine treatment. This recent development deserves further study.

Primary DUB can have its origin in an endocrine imbalance or can occur in normal menstrual cycles (ovulatory DUB). The endocrine abnormalities associated with primary DUB are set out in Table 17.3.

Women with menorrhagia and regular cycles show no abnormalities of the hypothalamo-pituitary-ovarian axis.[22] The underlying abnormality is thought to be with the paracrine control of the endometrial spiral arteries.

The onset of menstruation is normally preceded by intense constriction of the spiral arterioles. Microscopic examination of the uterus shortly after menstruation reveals that haemostasis has been achieved predominantly by vasoconstriction.[23] It is clear that a vasoactive substance is vital for haemostasis, and that disruption of its production or function could lead to menorrhagia. Prostaglandins are the most likely candidates for this role. These unstable fatty acids are not stored but synthesized and released as required from cell membranes (see Fig. 17.1). In primary menorrhagia the levels of total prostaglandins are raised, and PGE_2 is always increased relative to PGF_{2a}. The reason for this is not clear and research is now focused on other vasoactive groups like leukotrienes, cytokines and endothelins which act both alone and via the prostaglandins. Recently, the role of nitric oxide (NO) has been under investigation. This highly unstable gas is produced as a by-product of the conversion of arginine to cysteine. NO is present throughout the

Phospholipids

(in cell membranes)

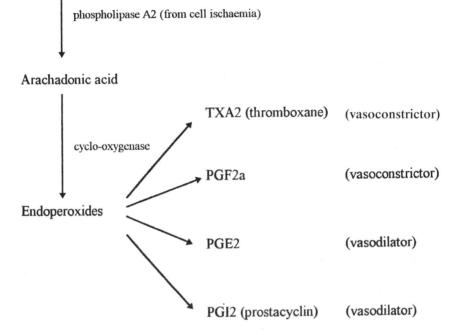

Fig. 17.1 Pathway of prostaglandin synthesis

uterus and acts as a potent vasodilator and inhibitor of platelet aggregation. It appears to mediate the vasodilatory actions of both oestrogen and PGE_2 in the uterus[24,25] and a disturbance in its function has been implicated in the cause of menorrhagia.[26]

Abnormalities of the local coagulation cascade are also implicated in the pathogenesis of primary menorrhagia. There is increased local fibrinolysis at the time of menstruation. Analysis of menstrual blood shows that it contains no fibrinogen, but high levels of fibrin degradation products are present. This is also supported by clinical experience where it takes excessively heavy menstrual loss before clots are produced vaginally – menstrual blood does not usually clot either in vivo or in vitro. Tissue plasminogen activator (TPA) is a fibrinolytic enzyme which is significantly increased in the menstrual blood and endometrium of women with primary menorrhagia. TPA can be inhibited by fibrinolytic inhibitors, e.g. tranexamic acid. The success of tranexamic acid in the treatment of menorrhagia is further evidence that excessive fibrinolysis is important.

Psychiatric morbidity is also associated with primary menorrhagia. Community studies have shown that women who score highly on psychiatric scores are more likely to complain of menstrual disturbances.[27,28] Greenberg interviewed 50 women referred to a gynaecology clinic with menorrhagia and found that 53% were suffering from mild to moderate depression.[29] These findings lead to speculation about the timing of the development of psychological symptoms. Which comes first? Does menorrhagia cause depression or does depression predispose to an inability to cope with increased menstrual loss? Furthermore, how much does a depressed state contribute to an overestimation of menstrual blood loss? The latter question was considered by Iles and Gath in a survey of 199 women awaiting hysterectomy.[30] They found that psychological factors did not affect the accuracy of women's estimation of their menstrual loss, although the accuracy of estimation by all the women in the Oxford community that made up the study population was much better than in other studies.

It has been thought for many years that previous sterilization is associated with the development of menorrhagia. The only trial to study this objectively, however, found that there was no increase in loss.[31]

It is unclear at the present time how the various abnormalities that have been discovered fit together to cause primary menorrhagia. It may be that they represent different causes of menorrhagia rather than different aspects of the same initial abnormality.

ASSESSMENT

Any woman with a complaint of excessive or changed pattern of menstrual loss should be assessed to establish risk factors and arrange investigations as appropriate. An alogrithm for investigation and treatment is shown in Fig. 17.2.

Women with irregular cycles should be investigated for abnormalities of the hypothalamic-pituitary axis and uterine cavity. Correction of the underlying abnormality will usually resolve the symptoms. Women with intermenstrual and postcoital bleeding should always have the cervix and uterine cavity investigated as the yield of underlying pathology is high.

Those with regular cycles are likely to have a normal hypothalamic-pituitary axis. The decision of whether to investigate further will depend on medical history of the patient and examination. Other symptoms accompanying menorrhagia will often give clues to the underlying disease process. Heavy painful periods with dyspareunia suggests endometriosis, while menorrhagia with vaginal discharge and abdominal pain points towards pelvic inflammatory disease. Careful questioning will usually identify those with clotting disorders and overt hypothyroidism. The woman's age is also important in determining the need for investigation. Patients under 40 years old have a very low risk of developing endometrial carcinoma[32] and so pathological examination of the endometrium is not mandatory.[33] Medical treatment can be used as a first line treatment with investigation only if symptoms persist. The risk of endometrial carcinoma in those with perimenopausal menorrhagia, however, is around 1% and so endometrial sampling is vital.

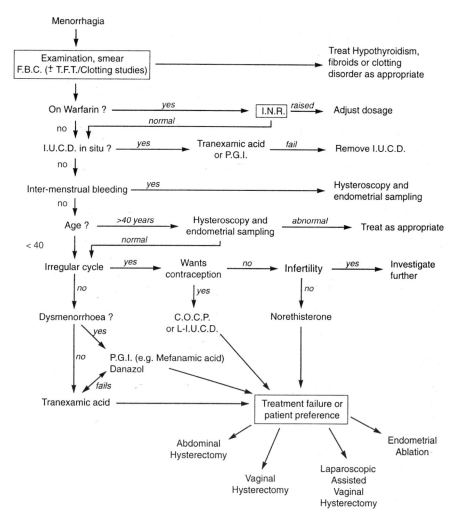

Fig. 17.2 Investigation and treatment of menorrhagia. FBC = Full blood count; TFT = Thyroid function tests; INR = International normalized ratio; IUCD = Intrauterine contraceptive device; L-IUCD = Levonorgestrel-releasing intrauterine contraceptive device; PGI = Prostaglandin inhibitors; COCP = Combined oral contraceptive pill.

A general examination may reveal signs of hypothyroidism, anaemia or clotting disorders. On pelvic examination one may find fibroids, or a tender, fixed uterus typical of pelvic inflammatory disease or endometriosis. All women must have a speculum examination of the cervix and vagina, and a cervical smear if not recently performed.

The volume of blood loss is proportional to the risk of pathology. However, volume assessment is very difficult. The alkaline haematin technique is the assessment method of choice, but is cumbersome and difficult to perform in normal clinical practice. Sanitary towel counting has been shown to be of no use in the quantifying of menstrual loss[34] as women use a varying amount of towels and tampons to collect similar amounts of menstrual blood.[10] Furthermore, the blood content of menstrual loss varies between 2% and 82%.[35] Fraser has shown that a detailed menstrual history can improve the assessment, but even then about one-third of women estimated to have menstrual loss of more than 80 ml had normal menstrual loss.[36] A pictorial blood loss assessment chart[37] was found to have a specificity and sensitivity of over 80%. It does, however, depend on use of a specific make and type of sanitary protection, which makes the method complicated in practice. Despite this, it is by far the best non-collection method for assessing menstrual loss and deserves further research and use.

In women with intermenstrual bleeding at any age or with menorrhagia at 40 years or more, the uterine cavity needs to be examined to exclude abnormalities. Dilatation and curettage (D&C) alone has been shown to miss many lesions and the optimum method for investigation is now hysteroscopy combined with endometrial biopsy. With the introduction of out-patient hysteroscopy, guided biopsy by forceps is possible, removing the need for a general anaesthetic. Pipelle sampling of the endometrium is now widely used, but will miss intrauterine polyps. Transvaginal ultrasound scanning (TVS) has also been found to be a good non-invasive method of screening. A recent study compared TVS in 279 women with hysteroscopy and D&C.[38] The study reported a sensitivity and specificity of 96% and 89%, respectively. The TVS was as useful as hysteroscopy if the cavity was normal, but not as useful if pathology was present in the cavity. It remains to be seen if these results can be repeated when the ultrasound is performed outside the research setting. The use of contrast TV scanning with fluid in the endometrial cavity may improve the reliability of TV scanning as a screening method.

TREATMENT

The range of treatment options for primary menorrhagia has multiplied in recent years, especially in the field of minimally invasive surgery. There is now a range of 7 medical and over 8 surgical options to choose from. The decision of which option to choose often reflects the physician's own preferences rather than those of the patient[3] even though in the absence of known pathology or anaemia treatment is purely symptomatic. Gynaecologists have been criticized for overdependence on surgery. A recent cohort trial, however, showed that women undergoing hysterectomy for abnormal menstrual bleeding had made significantly more improvement over a range of health indices after 12 months than those treated medically,[39] although the women treated surgically had worse symptom scores prior to treatment. A randomized trial of medical against surgical treatment is needed to assess this further. Studies are also urgently needed into the duration of medical treatment needed, and the relapse rate following cessation of therapy.

Reassurance

Many women will be satisfied just from the knowledge that their menstrual loss is not abnormal compared to others. Only one study has evaluated this approach to treatment.[40] A cohort of 17 women were investigated, found to have blood loss of less than 80 ml per cycle, and reassured. After 3 years they were contacted again. Fourteen were not taking any treatment, two were using mefanamic acid and one had had a hysterectomy.

Other women will be satisfied with the knowledge that there is no sinister underlying cause of their menorrhagia. Following investigation, non-anaemic women with primary menorrhagia should understand that the treatments offered are for symptomatic control and are not performed out of medical necessity.

Medical

Anti-fibrinolytics (e.g. tranexamic acid)

Tranexamic acid has been used for many years in Scandanavia. It acts by inhibiting tissue plasminogen activator, a fibrinolytic enzyme which has raised levels in women with DUB. It is given at the time of menstruation and has been found to be highly effective, reducing menstrual blood loss by around 50%.[11,41] Only danazol, the progesterone intrauterine device, and gonadotrophin-releasing hormone agonists are more effective (Fig. 17.3). Preson et al[11] studied 46 women with confirmed menorrhagia and randomly allocated women to tranexamic acid or norethisterone (5 mg twice daily, days 19–26). They found a reduction of mean menstrual loss of 45% with tranexamic acid against a 20% *increase* with norethisterone. Bonnar et al[42] randomized 81 women with DUB to receive tranexamic acid, mefanamic acid or ethamsylate. Over the study period of 3 months a reduction in menstrual loss of 58% was found with tranexamic acid against 25% with mefanamic acid and no change with ethamsylate.

There has been some concern over the side effects associated with tranexamic acid. The most common are nausea and diarrhoea, but it was the possibility of systemic thrombotic events that concerned many. Three cases of arterial thrombosis reported in association with its use[43] initially provoked anxiety. Analysis of adverse reports from tranexamic acid use in Sweden over 19 years, however, have shown that the incidence of thromboembolic events in users is the same as that of the general population (E Bastow, personal communication).

Recently, an ester prodrug of tranexamic acid (Kabi 2161) has been produced in order to increase the bioavailability of tranexamic acid when taken orally. This should lead to less frequent gastrointestinal side effects and a decreased frequency of administration. Edlund et al[44] found a 41% mean decrease in menstrual loss, when compared to placebo, in 68 women with

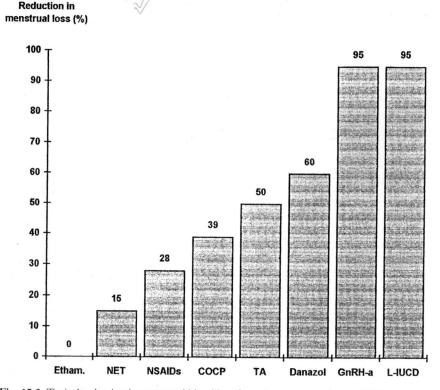

Fig. 17.3 Typical reduction in menstrual blood loss from the largest randomized trials. Etham. = ethamsylate; NET = norethisterone; NSAIDs = non-steroidal anti-inflammatory drugs; COCP = combined oral contraceptive pill; TA = tranexamic acid; GnRH-a = gonadotrophin-releasing hormone agonists; L-IUCD = levonorgestrol-releasing intrauterine contraceptive device.

menstrual loss of more than 80 ml/cycle. There was no difference in frequency of side effects between the study group and the controls.

Non-steroidal anti-inflammatory drugs

The non-steroidal anti-inflammatory groups of drugs (NSAIDs) are the most investigated of all the drugs used to reduce menstrual loss. They act by inhibiting cyclo-oxygenase, thereby reducing the production of endoperoxides. The fenamates (e.g. mefanamic acid, meclafenamate) also block myometrial PGE_2 receptors. It is for this reason that they have been the focus of most of the trials although it is now recognized that most of the NSAIDs (excluding aspirin) are effective. In addition they also have an analgesic action that is useful for concurrent dysmenorrhoea.

There are at least 13 randomized trials of mefanamic acid. Those containing over 15 women and using objective blood loss measurements are shown

Table 17.4 Mean reduction in menstrual blood loss using mefanamic acid

Number randomized to mefanamic acid	Mean reduction in blood loss (%)	Reference
69	28*	Fraser[45]
38	32*	Fraser[46]
35	46	Hall[47]
25	25	Bonnar[42]
20	20	Dockeray[9]
16	24	Cameron[8]
15	28*	Fraser[48]

*Women with initial blood loss of less than 80 ml included in trial.

in Table 17.4. They show a reduction of blood loss of around 25%. The degree of reduction is proportional to initial blood loss,[46,49] so women with severe menorrhagia get the most benefit. Analgesic action is as effective as that found with danazol,[9] and the benefits are maintained over at least 15 months.[45] Meclofenamate, which is not available in this country, has been studied in a randomized, placebo-controlled crossover trial by Vargyas et al.[50] They found a reduction in blood loss of 51% in the 29 women studied.

Naproxen, flurbiprofen and ibuprofen have not been studied in as great detail. Hall et al[47] found naproxen to be as effective as mefanamic acid in a crossover trial of 35 women. The twice daily dosage regimen and suppository option make this a useful alternative. Two smaller crossover trials found a mean reduction of blood loss of 21% and 24% using flurbiprofen.[51,52] One small randomized trial of ibuprofen found a reduction in blood loss of 25% with 1200 mg daily, but not with 600 mg daily.[53]

The NSAIDs are effective, well tested and well tolerated drugs which many use as first-line treatments, especially in the presence of dysmenorrhoea.

Progesterones

Norethisterone, used in the luteal phase, is one of the most widely used treatments for menorrhagia, but studies show that it is probably the least effective. A number of randomized trials have now shown that it has little effect on blood loss, the change in blood loss being between +20% and -16% in the only three trials that have randomized over 15 women.[8,11,54] The only role for progesterones is in women with irregular cycles where prolonged endometrial stimulation leads to heavy and irregular shedding, or in luteal phase deficiency with premenstrual spotting. Progestogen support from days 5–26 regulates irregular cycles, although this has been subjected to very few trials. The only available randomized trial is of six women with non-ovulatory cycles who were randomized to receive either norethisterone or medroxyprogesterone acetate.[55] Both treatments were equally effective, reducing blood loss by 51% over three cycles as well as reducing the number of days of blood loss.

Ethamsylate ↓B↓ 2o %↓

The mode of action of ethamsylate is not well understood although it appears to act by preventing the breakdown of capillaries. There has only been one randomized controlled trial with objective menstrual loss measurement.[42] This trial found no overall change in the 29 women allocated the drug. This is disappointing as smaller, earlier cohort trials[56] and non-randomized controlled trials[57] had suggested that it was effective. A randomized placebo-controlled trial[58] found a decrease of 20% in number of tampons used and duration of bleeding. This suggests that ethamsylate deserves further attention before being rejected on the basis of just one trial.

Danazol ↓ 6o %, B↓

Danazol is a synthetic steroid that acts in a number of ways. It inhibits sex steroid synthesis, blocks the androgen and progesterone receptors, and at higher doses it inhibits pituitary gonadotrophins. These actions combine to inhibit endometrial growth. Use of danazol, however, is limited by the androgenic side effects.

There are three large trials of danazol use. The first is that of Chimbera et al[59] who performed observational studies on 50 women using three different doses of danazol (400 mg, 200 mg and 100 mg daily). All doses were effective in reducing blood loss, the reduction being proportional to the dosage used. The 400 mg dose reduced loss from a mean of 230 ml/period to 3.6 ml/period over 3 months, with half the women becoming amenorrhoeic. The 200 mg and 100 mg doses reduced the loss by 86% and 57%, respectively. They also found that there was a 'carry-over' effect – the decrease in blood loss continued for many months after stopping the drug. The number of women reporting side effects was dependent on the dosage. Many women on the 100 mg dosage, in addition, developed metrorrhagia.

Docheray et al[9] used the 100 mg dose of danazol on 20 women in a randomized trial against mefanamic acid. They found a 60% decrease in mean blood loss compared to 20% with mefanamic acid. Interestingly, the improvement in symptoms in those women with dysmenorrhoea was the same in both arms of the trial. Seventy-five percent of the women reported side effects. Forty percent considered these unacceptable.

Subsequent trials have tended to use the 200 mg dose of danazol as a compromise between effectiveness and side effects. Higham and Shaw,[54] in a randomized trial of 57 women, compared three groups: continuous 200 mg danazol, danazol used in a decreasing dose, and norethisterone 5 mg twice daily (days 19–26). They found that the mean decrease in blood loss was greatest with the continuous 200 mg dose of danazol, although it was lower than that reported in other trials at only 39%. The mean decrease after two cycles in the decreasing danazol dose group was 30% whilst there was a mean increase of 9% in the norethisterone group.

Combined oral contraceptive pill (COCP)

It is well known that menstrual blood loss is decreased when taking the pill but there have only been two trials that objectively assess its use in DUB. Fraser & McCarron[46] performed a double-blind randomized crossover trial on 45 women, comparing the COCP with mefanamic acid. The 12 women who received the COCP (ethinyloestradiol 30 mg/levonorgestrel 15 mg) had a mean decrease in blood loss of 43% compared with 38% in the mefanamic acid group. When the women were asked whether they preferred the combined pill to the mefanamic acid, 7 of the 10 expressing a preference chose the combined pill. Nilsson & Rybo[41] used various 50 mg contraceptive pills in a series of 164 women and found a mean decrease in blood loss of 53% when compared with initial control cycles. Apart from a decrease in blood loss, the pill also has the advantages of regulating the cycle and providing contraception. The only disadvantages of the COCP are the restrictions on its use in older women who smoke, and those with risk factors for either thrombosis or heart disease.

Gonadotrophin-releasing hormone analogues (GnRH analogues)

The GnRH analogues are synthetic analogues of the 10 amino acid gonadotrophin-releasing hormone. Single amino acids are replaced to form a range of drugs. When used in a single dose they stimulate the production of leutinizing hormone and follicle stimulating hormone, but with continued administration they downregulate the pituitary and inhibit their production. Most of the preparations come as depot injections in order to facilitate this. They are highly effective in producing amenorrhoea in the presence of fibroids or endometriosis and have been used in severe dysfunctional bleeding.[60-62] The treatment, however, is limited to 6 months use because of the risk of osteoporosis. Bone loss after 6 months is only between 2% and 6% but there are conflicting studies as to whether this is completely reversible.[63-65] Early studies using oestrogen 'add-back' supplementation in combination with a GnRH-a to prevent osteoporosis are encouraging, but there is still uncertainty as to which add-back regimen is optimal, and further studies are awaited.

Levonorgestrol-releasing intrauterine device

The progesterone-releasing intrauterine devices (IUD) were initially developed in the 1970s to counteract the menstrual side effects experienced by IUD users. Now widely available, they have been found to have a very low intrauterine and ectopic pregnancy rate, and to decrease menstrual blood loss.[66,67] Although not yet licenced for the treatment of menorrhagia, the levonorgestrol-releasing IUD (Mirena) has been studied in three cohort trials.[52,67,68] Andersson & Rybo[68] followed 19 women with monthly loss of more than 80 ml prior to insertion. The loss was decreased by 86%, 91% and 97% at 3, 6 and 12 months, respectively. Milsom et al[52] followed-up 20 women with menorrhagia and reported similar results, although 4 women were excluded from the trial before the end of 12 months. One woman was excluded because of IUD expulsion, two because of intermenstrual bleeding and one because of systemic progesterone side effects. This drop-out rate is similar to that found in the larger trials of all women using the device for contraception which show continuation rates of 80% after the first year of use.[66] The marked reduction in blood loss combined with effective contraception makes this an exciting development in the treatment of menorrhagia. This could replace the need for surgery in many women. A randomized controlled trial is soon to commence comparing the levonorgestrel IUD (Mirena) with endometrial ablation.

IUCD-induced menorrhagia

The results of treatment regimens in IUCD-induced menorrhagia are similar to those from primary DUB. Tranexamic acid causes a fall of about 54% in blood loss,[69] and NSAIDs a fall of 20–30% depending on the dosage used.[53,69,70] Women, therefore, should be offered the chance of medical therapy prior to removal of an IUCD for menorrhagia.

Menorrhagia secondary to fibroids

Three randomized trials have looked at the efficacy of NSAIDs in the treatment of fibroid-induced menorrhagia and none has shown any effect on menstrual blood loss.[53,71,72] The gonadotrophin-releasing hormone agonists are highly effective, causing a reduction in fibroid volume and menstrual blood loss.[73] However, after cessation of therapy the fibroid soon returns to its pretreatment size. The benefits are therefore transient and limited to a maximum of 6 months because of the problem of associated osteoporosis. GnRH agonists may be useful, however, as a pretreatment prior to endoscopic surgery for the treatment of fibroids.

Minimally invasive surgical options

Around 15% of women want a surgical solution to menorrhagia.[3] With the introduction of minimally invasive techniques, surgery is set to become a more attractive alternative for many. Recovery from endometrial resection is only 2–4 weeks compared with 2–3 months for abdominal hysterectomy and gives satisfaction in 78% of women with menorrhagia.[74] Attempts are being made to improve these figures by refining the techniques, and endometrial ablation by microwave, heat and freezing techniques are all being evaluated.

Table 17.5 Monthly cost of medical treatment for menorrhagia.*

Tranexamic acid (1 g four times daily for 5 days)	£9.07
Mefanamic acid (500 mg twice daily for 5 days)	£2.36
Norethisterone (5 mg twice daily days 19–26)	£2.25
Danazol (200 mg once daily continuously)	£17.67
Ethamsylate (500 mg four times daily for 5 days)	£4.43
Nafarelin acetate (1 spray twice daily)	£53.01
Combined oral contraceptive pill (Brevinor)	£0.56

* Based on the price of the cheapest preparation available in Mimms, Feb 1995.

Cost considerations

The various prices of the medical therapies are outlined in Table 17.5. Surgery is much more expensive but this has to be weighed up against its permanence. The cost of an abdominal hysterectomy is estimated at £1060 and an endometrial resection at £560.[75]

SUMMARY

The treatment of menorrhagia has advanced greatly in recent years. It should now be possible to meet the needs of most women suffering from menorrhagia. Increasingly, randomized controlled trials are providing the clinician with comparative success rates thus allowing informed patient choice. There is an increasing range of therapeutic options which allow us to tailor the treatment to individual needs and preferences. The lack of effective reversible long-term therapies has been a problem for many years, but with the introduction of the progesterone-releasing IUCD, even this problem may have been solved.

REFERENCES

1 Edlund M, Magnusson C, Von Schoultz B. Quality of life – a Swedish survey of 2200 women. In: Smith S K, ed. Dysfunctional uterine bleeding. London: Royal Society of Medicine Press, 1994: pp 36–37
2 Royal College of General Practitioners and the Office of Population Surveys. Morbidity Statistics from General Practice, 1981–2. London: HMSO, 1986
3 Coulter A, Peto V, Doll H. Patients' preferences and general practitioners' decisions in the treatment of menstrual disorders. Fam Prac 1994; 11: 67–74
4 Coulter A, Bradlow J, Agass M, Martin-Bates C, Tulloch A. Outcomes of referrals to gynaecology outpatient clinics for menstrual problems: an audit of general practice records. Br J Obstet Gynaecol 1991; 98: 789–796
5 Coulter A, McPherson K, Vessey M. Do British women undergo too many or too few hysterectomies? Soc Sci Med 1988; 27: 987–994
6 Hallenberg L, Hogdahl A, Nilsson L, Rybo G. Menstrual blood loss – a population study. Acta Obstet Gynecol Scand 1966; 45: 320–351
7 Cole S K, Billewicz W Z, Thomson A M. Sources of variation in menstrual blood loss. J Obstet Gynaecol Br Commwlth 1971; 78: 933–939
8 Cameron I T, Haining R, Lumsden M A, Thomas V R, Smith S K. The effects of mefenamic acid and norethisterone on measured menstrual blood loss. Obstet Gynecol 1990; 76: 85–88

9 Dockeray C J, Sheppard B L, Bonnar J. Comparison between mefenamic acid and danazol in the treatment of established menorrhagia. Br J Obstet Gynaecol 1989; 96: 840–844

10 Fraser I S, McCarron G, Markham R. A preliminary study of the factors influencing perception of menstrual blood loss volume. Am J Obstet Gynecol 1984; 149: 788–793

11 Preston J T, Cameron I T, Adams E J, Smith S K. Comparative study of tranexamic acid and norethisterone in the treatment of ovulatory menorrhagia. Br J Obstet Gynaecol 1995; 102: 401–406

12 Beazley J M. Dysfunctional uterine haemorrhage. Br J Hosp Med 1972; 7: 573

13 Fraser I S, McCarron G, Markham R, Resta T, Watts A. Measured menstrual blood loss in women with menorrhagia associated with pelvic disease or coagulation disorder. Obstet Gynecol 1986; 68: 630–633

14 Greer I A, Lowe G D, Walker J J, Forbes C D. Haemorrhagic problems in obstetrics and gynaecology in patients with congenital coagulopathies. Br J Obstet Gynaecol 1991; 98: 909–918

15 Van Eijkeren M A, Christiaens G C, Geuze H J, Haspels A A, Sixma J J. Effects of mefenamic acid on menstrual hemostasis in essential menorrhagia. Am J Obstet Gynecol 1992; 166: 1419–1428

16 Claessens E A, Cowell C A. Acute adolescent menorrhagia. Am J Obstet Gynecol 1981; 139: 277–280

17 Scott J C, Mussey E. Menstrual patterns of myxoedema. Am J Obstet Gynecol 1964; 90: 161–165

18 Higham J M, Shaw R W. The effect of thyroxine replacement on menstrual blood loss in a hypothyroid patient. Br J Obstet Gynaecol 1992; 99: 695–696

19 Willansky D L, Greisman B. Early hypothyroidism in patients with menorrhagia. Am J Obstet Gynecol 1989; 160: 673–677

20 Blum M, Blum G. The possible relationship between menorrhagia and occult hypothyroidism in IUD-wearing women. Advanc Contracep 1992; 8: 313–317

21 Davey D A. Dysfunctional uterine bleeding. In: Whitfield C R, ed. Dewhurst's textbook of ob-stetrics and gynaecology for postgraduates, 5th edn. London: Blackwell Scientific, 1995: p 599

22 Haynes P J, Flint A P, Hodgson H et al. Studies in menorrhagia (a) mefanamic acid (b) endometrial prostaglandin concentrations. Int Obstet Gynecol 1980; 17: 567–572

23 Christiaens G C M L, Sixema J J, Haspels A A. Morphology of haemostasis in menstrual endometrium Br J Obstet Gynaecol 1980; 87: 425–439

24 Kimura T, Yoshida Y, Toda N. Mechanisms of relaxation induced by prostaglandins in isolated canine uterine arteries. Am J Obstet Gynecol 1992; 167(5): 1409–1416

25 Van Buren G A, Yang D S, Clark K E. Estrogen-induced vasodilation is antagonised by L-nitroarginine methyl ester, an inhibitor of nitric oxide synthesis. Am J Obstet Gynecol 1992; 167(3): 828–833

26 Telfer J F, Lyall F, Norman J E, Cameron I T. Identification of nitric oxide synthetase in human uterus. Hum Reprod 1995; 10(1): 19–23

27 Ballinger C B. Psychiatric morbidity and the menopause: screening of a general population sample. Br Med J 1975; iii: 344–346

28 Gath D, Osborn M, Bungay G et al. Psychiatric disorder and gynaecological symptoms in middle-aged women: a community survey. Br Med J 1987; 294: 213–218

29 Greenberg M. The meaning of menorrhagia: an investigation into the association between the complaint of menorrhagia and depression. J Psychosom Res 1983; 27: 209–214

30 Iles S, Gath D. Psychological problems and uterine bleeding. In: Drife J O, ed. Dysfunctional uterine bleeding and menorrhagia. Baillière's Clinical Obstetrics and Gynaecology. London: Baillière Tindall, 1989: pp 375–389

31 Kasonde J, Bonnar J. The effect of sterilisation on menstrual blood loss. Br J Obstet Gynaecol 1975; 83: 572

32 Mackenzie J Z, Bibby J G. Critical assessment of dilatation and curettage in 1029 women. Lancet 1978; ii: 566–569

33 Grimes D A. Diagnostic dilatation and curettage: a reappraisal. Am J Obstet Gynecol 1982; 142: 1–6

34 Chimbira T H, Anderson A B M, Turnbull A C. Relation between measured menstrual loss and the patients subjective assessment of loss, duration of bleeding, number of sanitary towels used, uterine weight and endometrial surface area. Br J Obstet Gynaecol 1980; 87: 603–609

35 Fraser I S, McCarron G, Markham R, Resta T. The blood and total fluid content of menstrual discharge. Obstet Gynecol 1985; 65: 194–198

36 Fraser I S. Treatment of menorrhagia. In: Drife J O, ed. Dysfunctional uterine bleeding and menorrhagia. Baillière's Clinical Obstetrics and Gynaecology. London: Baillière Tindall, 1989: pp 391–402

37 Higham J M, O'Brien P M S, Shaw R W. Assessment of menstrual blood loss using a pictoral chart. Br J Obstet Gynaecol 1990; 97: 734–739

38 Emanuel M H, Verdel M J, Wamsteker K, Lammes F B. A prospective comparison of transvaginal ultrasonography and diagnostic hysteroscopy in the evaluation of patients with abnormal uterine bleeding: clinical implications. Am J Obstet Gynecol 1995; 172: 547–552

39 Carlson K J, Miller B A, Fowler F J. The Maine Women's Health Study: II. Outcomes of nonsurgical management of leiomyomas, abnormal bleeding and chronic pelvic pain. Obstet Gynecol 1994; 83: 566–572

40 Rees M C P. Role of menstrual loss measurements in management of complaints of excessive menstrual bleeding. Br J Obstet Gynaecol 1991; 98: 327–328

41 Nilsson L, Rybo G. Treatment of menorrhagia. Am J Obstet Gynecol 1971; 110: 713–720

42 Bonnar J. Review of medical treatment in dysfunctional uterine bleeding. In: Smith S K, ed. Dysfunctional uterine bleeding. London: Royal Society of Medicine Press, 1994: pp 100–101

43 Agnelli G, Gresele P, De Curto M, Galli V, Nerci G G. Tranexamic acid, intrauterine contraceptive devices and fatal cerebral arterial thrombosis. Br J Obstet Gynaecol 1982; 89: 681–682

44 Edlund M, Andersson K, Rybo G, Lindoff C, Astedt B, Schoultz B. Reduction of menstrual loss in women suffering from idiopathic menorrhagia with a novel anti-fibrinolytic drug (Kabi 2161). Br J Obstet Gynaecol 1995; 102: 913–917

45 Fraser I S. McGarron G, Markham R, Robinson M, Smyth E. Long-term treatment of menorrhagia with mefanamic acid. Obstet Gynecol 1983; 61: 109–112

46 Fraser I S, McGarron G. Randomized trial of 2 hormonal and 2 prostaglandin-inhibiting agents in women with a complaint of menorrhagia. Aus NZ J Obstet Gynaecol 1991; 31: 66–70

47 Hall P, Maclachlan N, Thorn N, Nudd M W, Taylor C G, Garrioch D B. Control of menorrhagia by the cyclo-oxygenase inhibitors naproxen sodium and mefenamic acid. Br J Obstet Gynaecol 1987; 94: 554–558

48 Fraser I S, Pearse C, Sheerman R P, Elliott P M, McIlveen J, Markham R. Efficacy of mefanamic acid in patients with a complaint of menorrhagia. Obstet Gynecol 1981; 58: 543–551

49 Fraser I S. The treatment of menorrhagia with mefanamic acid. Res Clin Forums 1983; 5(3): 93–99

50 Vargyas J M, Campeau J D, Mishell D R, Jr. Treatment of menorrhagia with meclofenamate sodium. Am J Obstet Gynecol 1987; 157: 944–950

51 Andersch B, Milsom I, Rybo G. An objective evaluation of flurbiprofen and tranexamic acid in the treatment of idiopathic menorrhagia. Acta Obstet Gynecol Scand 1988; 67: 645–648

52 Milsom I, Andersson K, Andersch B, Rybo G. A comparison of flurbiprofen, tranexamic acid, and a levonorgestrel-releasing intrauterine contraceptive device in the treatment of idiopathic menorrhagia. Am J Obstet Gynecol 1991; 164: 879–883

53 Makarainen L, Ylikorkala O. Primary and myoma-associated menorrhagia: role of prostaglandins and effects of ibuprofen. Br J Obstet Gynaecol 1986; 93: 974–978

54 Higham J M, Shaw R W. A comparative study of danazol, a regimen of decreasing doses of danazol, and norethindrone in the treatment of objectively proven unexplained menorrhagia. Am J Obstet Gynecol 1993; 169: 1134–1139

55 Fraser I S. Treatment of ovulatory and anovulatory dysfunctional uterine bleeding with oral progestogens. Aus NZ J Obstet Gynaecol 1990; 30: 353–356

56 Harrison R F, Campbell S. A double-blind trial of ethamsylate in the treatment of primary and intra-uterine device menorrhagia. Lancet 1976; ii: 283–285

57 Chamberlain G, Freeman R, Price F, Kennedy A, Green D, Eve L. A comparative study of ethamsylate and mefenamic acid in dysfunctional uterine bleeding. Br J Obstet Gynaecol 1991; 98: 707–711

58 Jaffe G, Wickham A. A double-blind pilot study of Dicynene in the control of menorrhagia. J Intern Med Res 1973; 1: 127–129

59 Chimbera T H, Anderson A B, Naish C, Cope E, Turnbull A C. Reduction of menstrual blood loss by Danazol in unexplained menorrhagia: lack of placebo effect. Br J Obstet Gynaecol 1980; 87: 1152–1158

60 Friedman A J, Harrison-Atlas D, Barbieri R L, Benacerraf B, Gleason R, Schiff I. A randomised, placebo-controlled, double-blind study evaluating the efficacy of leuprolide acetate depot in the treatment of uterine leiomyomata. Fertil Steril 1989; 51: 251

61 Henzl M R, Corson S L, Moghissi K et al. Administration of nasal nafarelin as compared to oral danazol for endometriosis. N Eng J Med 1988; 318: 485–489

62 Thomas E J, Okuda K J, Thomas N M. The combination of a depot gonadotrophin releasing hormone agonist and cyclical hormone replacement therapy for dysfunctional uterine bleeding. Br J Obstet Gynaecol 1991; 98: 1155–1159

63 Fogelman I, Fentiman I, Hamed H, Studd J W W, Leather A T. Goserelin (Zoladex) and the skeleton. Br J Obstet Gynaecol 1994; 101 (Suppl 10): 19–23

64 Johansen J S, Riis B J, Hasseger C, Moen M, Jacobsen J, Christiansen C. The effect of a gonadotrophin-releasing hormone agonist (nafarelin) on bone metabolism. J Clin Endocrinol Metab 1988; 67: 701–706

65 Whitehouse R W, Adams J E, Bancroft K, Vaughan-Williams C A, Elstein M. The effects of nafarelin and danazol on vertebral trabecular bone mass in patients with endometriosis. Clin Endocrinol 1990; 33: 365–373

66 Andersson K, Odlind V, Rybo G. Levonorgestrel-releasing and copper-releasing (Nova T) IUDs during five years of use: a randomised comparative trial. Contraception 1994; 49: 56–72

67 Scholten P C, van Eykeren M A, Christiaens G C M L et al. Menstrual blood loss with levonorgestrel Nova T and Multiload CU 250 intrauterine devices. In: Scholten P C, ed. Thesis. The levonorgestrel IUD: clinical performance and impact on menstruation. University Hospital, Utrecht, 1989: pp 35–45

68 Andersson J K, Rybo G. Levonorgestrel-releasing intrauterine device in the treatment of menorrhagia. Br J Obstet Gynaecol 1990; 97: 690–694

69 Ylikorkala O, Viinikka L. Comparison between antifibrinolytic and antiprostaglandin treatment in the reduction of increased menstrual blood loss in women with intrauterine contraceptive devices. Br J Obstet Gynaecol 1983; 90: 78–83

70 Davies A J, Anderson A B M, Turnbull A C. Reduction by naproxen of excessive menstrual bleeding in women using intrauterine devices. Obstet Gynecol 1981; 57: 74–78

71 Ylikorkala O, Pekonen F. Naproxen reduces idiopathic but not fibromyoma-induced menorrhagia. Obstet Gynecol 1986; 68: 10 12

72 Ylikorkala O. Primary and myoma-associated menorrhagia: role of prostaglandins and effects of Ibuprofen. Br J Obstet Gynaecol 1986; 93: 974–978

73 Friedman A J, Hoffman D I, Comite F, Browneller R W, Miller J D. Treatment of leiomyomata uteri with leuprolide acetate depot: a double-blind, placebo-controlled, multicenter study. Obstet Gynecol 1991; 77: 720–725

74 Pinion S B, Parkin D E, Abramovich D R et al. Randomised trial of hysterectomy, endometrial laser ablation, and transcervical endometrial resection for dysfunctional uterine bleeding. Br Med J 1994; 309: 979–983

75 Sculpher M J, Bryan S, Dwyer N, Hutton J, Stirrat G M. An economic evaluation of transcervical endometrial resection versus abdominal hysterectomy for the treatment of menorrhagia. Br J Obstet Gynaecol 1993; 100: 244–252

18 Endometriosis: a review

O. A. Odukoya   I. D. Cooke

Recurrance rate 10% /year after treatment

Endometriosis is defined as the presence of tissue, histologically similar to endometrium, outside the uterine cavity and the myometrium. This definition therefore excludes adenomyosis. It is a relatively common disease, but exactly how common remains a matter for debate. Estimates of occurrence depend on the denominator and vary from 2% to 50% of all women who undergo laparoscopy.[1-3]

One of the difficulties in determining the incidence of the disease is due in part to the criteria for diagnosis. Before the advent of laparoscopy the diagnosis was based on clinical symptoms and subtle but non-specific clinical signs or findings at laparotomy. The liberal use of the laparoscope coupled with directed biopsy when necessary has reduced the error of accurate diagnosis. On balance, the prevalence of endometriosis among women aged 15–45 years is about 10%.[4] Although the cause of endometriosis has not been conclusively determined, many theories relating to its pathogenesis have been proposed. This review will focus on the various theories of pathogenesis, the clinical symptoms and the current management modalities.

PATHOGENESIS

There is a wide variety of suggestions in the literature, some of which are supported by circumstantial evidence, on the origin of endometriosis. The theories of histogenesis can be divided into four main groups (Table 18.1).

Endometrial implantation

Retrograde theory

Sampson proposed the retrograde menstruation theory in 1927.[5] This theory was ignored because reflux was thought to be a rare phenomenon and also that the menstrual effluent was made of necrotic non-viable material. However, work in experimental animals and humans has confirmed the presence of viable cells in the retrograde effluent, which has adhering and proliferating properties.[6-8] There is confirmatory evidence in humans for retrograde flow, as blood-contaminated peritoneal fluid was found at

327

Table 18.1 Theories of histiogenesis

Endometrial implantation theory
Retrograde
Vascular and lymphatic
Mechanical

In situ development
Coelomic metaplasia theory
Induction theory
Embryonic cell nest
Wolffian ducts
Mullerian ducts
Germinal epithelium of ovary

Immunological and genetic theory

Composite theory

laparoscopy performed during menstruation.[9] It is also believed that the volume of regurgitated blood, which may be a function of the uterotubal junction musculature, may influence the development of endometriosis. Indeed, uterotubal junction hypotonia had been shown in patients with endometriosis when compared with the control.[10] The retrograde implantation theory could explain the pelvic but not the extra pelvic sites of endometriosis.

Vascular and lymphatic theory

There is evidence that endometrial tissue can be transported via the haematogenous and lymphatic system. Metastasis of endometrial cells via the lymphatic system to the pleura, umbilicus, urinary tract, retroperitoneal space, diaphragm, vagina, cervix and the lower extremities explains the non-gynaecological extrapelvic sites of endometriosis. The anatomical evidence \of extensive lymphatic communication between the uterus and vagina, cervix, kidney and umbilicus and, in addition, the presence of endometrial tissues in the lymphatic channels of the pelvis, support vasculolymphatic implantation.[11,12]

Mechanical theory

Endometriosis can also occur as a result of direct mechanical transportation of the endometrial tissue to ectopic sites. This iatrogenic route explains the presence of endometriosis at episiotomy and laparotomy scars.

In situ development

Coelomic metaplasia theory

The coelomic metaplasia theory states that endometriosis develops from metaplasia of cells lining the pelvic peritoneal cavity. The fundamental principle in this theory is that the Mullerian ducts, germinal epithelium of the ovary and the pelvic epithelium are all derived from the coelomic epithelium. It also assumes that the epithelium (germinal and peritoneal) has the capacity to differentiate into any progenitor cells or contain undifferentiated cells which are able to differentiate into endometrial cells. The theory is attractive and able to explain the presence of endometriosis at any site. However, there is lack of direct evidence that peritoneal epithelium can undergo spontaneous or induced metaplasia to form endometriosis.

Induction theory

This theory presupposes that 'dying' endometrial cells liberate specific substances which may induce undifferentiated mesenchyme to form endometriosis. While this may look simple and unproven, there is accumulating data supporting the presence of various proteins such as cytokines, growth factors and cell adhesion molecules in the endometrial fluid, which may enhance the growth and development of endometrium in ectopic sites.[13] The expression of some of these proteins in ectopic endometrium has recently been demonstrated.[8] What needs to be further elucidated is the complex process by which endometrial cells attach to the peritoneal serosa.

Immunological theory

The transplantation of viable endometrial cells through the fallopian tube by retrograde menstruation can explain most peritoneal sites of endometriosis. However, as retrograde menstruation is a common phenomenon in the majority of women, why some develop endometriosis and others don't is difficult to explain. According to transplantation biology, the 'take rate' of a graft depends not only on the viability of the tissue but on the local factors of the host. In the last two decades evidence linking endometriosis with alteration in the immune system has accumulated. Changes in the cell-mediated and humoral immunity in the monkey and in humans have been observed by several research groups.

Physiologically, the refluxed menstrual debris is cleared by the cells of the immune system. These include macrophages, T-lymphocytes and Natural killer (NK) cells which are resident in the peritoneal cavity. If the amount of effluent presented to these cells is large, the resident 'garbage disposing cells' are unable to dispose of the products, thus facilitating growth and development. Indeed, factors which promote an increased volume of retrograde effluent, such as outflow obstruction, are associated with the development of endometriosis.[14] Several investigators have shown the existence of some alterations in cell-mediated immune response (T-lymphocyte subsets CD4+ and CD8+ cells) in patients with endometriosis.[15,16] Furthermore, a defect in the number and functional activity of the NK cells which are responsible for endometrial cytotoxicity has been shown to occur in the peritoneal fluid of patients with endometriosis.[17] A decreased NK cell-mediated cytotoxicity in the peritoneal fluid could facilitate the implantation of endometrial cells even in the presence of a normal amount of retrograde menstruation.

Humoral (antibody) defects have also been shown to occur in the serum and peritoneal fluid of patients with endometriosis, suggesting an immuno-logical dysregulation.[18,19] The presence of a wide variety of autoantibodies in endometriosis suggest a polyclonal B-cell activation. This is comparable to those of autoimmune disease featuring tissue damage, female preponderant, multiorgan involvement and an increased association with other autoimmune disease.[20] In addition, alteration in immunomodulatory proteins (cytokines and growth factors) also occurs in the peritoneal fluid of patients with endometriosis.[21,22]

Composite theory

Currently, there is no single theory to explain the pathogenesis of endometriosis. It is believed that a combination of endometrial transplanta-tion and immunological dysregulation may explain most cases of endometri-osis. The role played by genetic and environmental factors is currently under investigation.

RISK FACTORS ASSOCIATED WITH THE DEVELOPMENT OF ENDOMETRIOSIS

Duration of menstrual cycle   *Duration / lasting*

Patients whose menstrual cycles are less than 27 days are twice as likely to develop endometriosis than their counterparts with a longer duration (Table 18.2).[23,24] Furthermore, patients with a menstrual flow of more than 1 week have two-and-a-half times the risk of developing endometriosis when com-pared with those with flows of less than 1 week.[23]

Familial and genetic factors

In a study of 123 patients with endometriosis, not only was there a higher prevalence of disease severity with positive family history but 6.9% of all first degree and 2% of second degree relatives were affected when compared with the same pedigree of the partners.[25,26] Indeed, an apparently unaffected woman with an affected first degree relative has a 7% risk of developing

Table 18.2 Risk factors for endometriosis

Associated	Unproven (inconclusive)	Not associated
First degree relations	Obesity	Age
Second degree relations	Smoking	Race
Menstrual cycle ≤ 27 days	Exercise	Social class
Menstrual duration ≥ 7 days	Height\weight	Age and duration of marriage
Genital outflow obstruction	Age at menarche	Miscarriage
	Combined contraceptive pill	Intrauterine contraceptive device
	Uterine retroversion	

endometriosis.[27] This does not follow the Mendelian theory and it is possible that a polygenic or multifactorial inheritance may be the most likely mode of transmission.

Genital obstruction

There is evidence that patients who have an obstructed lower genital tract as a result of either congenital or acquired factors are at a higher risk of developing endometriosis.[28,29] This can be explained by the cyclical retrograde menstrual flow into the peritoneal cavity which might overwhelm the capacity of the 'peritoneal disposal system' to evacuate the menstrual debris.

Uterine retroversion

Another peritoneal factor, uterine retroversion/retroflexion, which enhances retrograde menstrual flow and occurs more commonly in patients with endometriosis, has not been shown significantly to increase the risk of endometriosis development.

Obesity

Obese women tend to have a higher concentration of serum oestrogen and should theoretically be expected to be at increased risk when compared with slim patients. Current data do not seem to support this hypothesis. However, Darrow and his colleagues[30] have shown that women with an altered waist-hip ratio have six times increased risk and suggested that a specific somatotype with a predominance of peripheral body fat distribution was a risk factor for endometriosis. Postmenopausal endometriosis, although rare, often involves the large bowel and tends to occur in women receiving hormone replacement therapy.[31] Similarly, adolescent endometriosis is rare but more common in those who complain of dysmenorrhea and chronic pelvic pain.

Infertility

The liberal use of the laparoscope has dramatically increased the diagnosis of endometriosis even in the fertile asymptomatic population. The unexpectedly high prevalence of minimal and mild lesions in this group raises doubts about the true prevalence and risk of endometriosis in the general population. Most authors express the view that the subtle or minimal lesions may be a paraphysiological or self-limiting condition which probably exist in all reproductive women as a result of the common denominator, retrograde menstruation. More detailed studies on the risk factors could help in the identification of the factors responsible for disease progression in some women thus further elucidating the natural history of endometriosis.

MORPHOLOGICAL CLASSIFICATION

Several classification methods have been used to provide standardization and prognostic significance in the last two decades. The latest method was that introduced in 1985 by the American Fertility Society[32] which primarily used the implant size (volume) and the location of endometriosis as indicators of severity of the disease. Basically, it divides endometriosis into various stages, the severity increasing with ovarian involvement and adhesion formation. The aim was to correlate the stage of severity with fertility outcome. This does not seem to incorporate pain as a major symptom, revealing the inadequacy of that classification. Some patients who are diagnosed as having severe disease lack pain symptoms, conversely, some patients with mild disease are infertile and suffer severe pain.

The relatively easy access to the peritoneal cavity in the investigation of patients with pelvic pain and infertility has resulted in the identification of distinct physical and morphological characteristics of endometriosis. These appearances are the subtle or typical (classical) lesions (Table 18.3). The subtle group can be subclassified into two broad groups: petechial or red

Table 18.3 Laparoscopic appearances of endometriosis

Classical lesions
'Powder-burn', puckered black

Subtle lesions
Vesicular
Haemorrhagic
Papular
Nodular
Discoloured
  yellow-brown
  white
  blue
Peritoneal defects
Cribriform peritoneum
Subovarian adhesions

implants, and intermediate or brown implants. The classical type is usually described as 'powder-burn' or black lesions. It has been shown that metabolic activity is related to the histological and gross appearance of ectopic endometrium. There is evidence that the subtle lesions are biochemically and morphologically more active than the powder-burn or black lesions. The subtle lesions which were not recognized until the last decade, synthesize more prostaglandin $F_{2\alpha}$ (PGF) and are known sometimes to invade the peritoneal matrix to a depth of more than 5 mm and cause pain by irritation of a nociceptive receptor.[33,34] While endometriosis may regress, there is some evidence of natural progression from the subtle to the classical lesions. In one study, women less than 25 years had a preponderance of the subtle lesions, while those over 30 years tended to have the powder-burn or puckered lesions.[31] In the clinical setting it is common to observe a variety of lesions in a patient.

ENDOMETRIOSIS AND INFERTILITY

The relationship between endometriosis and infertility is complex and poorly understood. The prevalence of endometriosis within the infertile population[35] is between 20–40%. Advanced forms of the disease based on the revised American Fertility Society[32] score (rAFS; III and IV) can understandably cause infertility by mechanical interference with ovulation, ovum pick up, tubo-ovarian adhesions, severe pelvic adhesions and distorted tubal anatomy. Where fallopian tubes are normal and there are no adhesions around the ovaries (rAFS I and II), the exact mechanism by which endometriosis impairs fertility, if at all, remains speculative. It is postulated that this could be a result of coital problems (dyspareunia/apareunia), altered peritoneal environment (biochemical and immunological), disturbance of follicular maturation (luetinized unruptured follicle, anovulation, luteolysis caused by PGF), implantation failure and early abortions. However, prospective placebo-controlled randomized studies have so far failed to show a beneficial effect on pregnancy rates in infertile patients with minimal or mild endometriosis.[36,37]

CLINICAL FEATURES

The fact that endometriosis does not always present with a classic set of symptoms often leads to a delay in diagnosis resulting in worsening sequelae. The main symptoms of endometriosis are dysmenorrhoea, pelvic pain, dyspareunia and infertility (Table 18.4). The dysmenorrhoea (congestive) usually begins some days before the onset of menstruation and continues throughout the menses. The pelvic pain described as dull and aching is poorly localized in the lower abdomen. The pain is typically bilateral but may be unilateral. It may occasionally radiate to the back or to the legs. Although the clinical presentation depends on the location and extent of the disease, the severity of the symptom does not correlate with the extent of the disease.

Table 18.4 Clinical features of endometriosis

Common symptoms
Pelvic pain
Dysmenorrhoea
Dyspareunia
Infertility
Dyschesia

Less common symptoms
Haematuria
Rectal bleeding
Urgency
Haemoptysis
Cutaneous nodules
Hyperprolactinemia

Signs
Pelvic tenderness and induration
Nodules in the cul-de-sac
Adnexal mass
Uterine fixity
Nodules along the uterosacral ligament

Severe pain may be seen in association with minimal or mild disease while severe or extensive disease may have no associated symptoms.

A recent study, however, showed a significant association between the intensity of pain and the number of both subtle and classical ectopic endometriotic implants.[38] Dyspareunia, commonly positional at deep penetration coupled with postcoital discomfort is quite common. This is often associated with endometriotic deposits in the ovaries and uterosacral ligaments, retroversion and fixity of the uterus, and deposits in the recto-vaginal septum and cul-de-sac. Dyspareunia is twice as common in patients with endometriosis when compared with controls and becomes more severe as the disease advances.[39]

Menorrhagia, premenstrual genital bleeding or spotting can also occur in endometriosis. These are more common in the older age group. Loin pain, secondary to ureteric involvement, or an acute abdominal presentation caused by rupture of endometriotic cysts are rare but require a high index of suspicion. Massive ascites sometimes occur in association with endometriosis, and usually the patients are young and nulliparous.[40] Less commonly the uterus, small bowel, ureters and bladder are involved. Adhesion formation tends to follow the same frequency. Symptoms of irritable bowel syndrome are often associated with endometriosis.

The physical findings are variable and depend on the severity and extent of the disease as well as the location of ectopic endometrium. The uterus may be fixed, retroverted and tender. There may be adnexal masses caused by endometriomas of the ovaries. Such masses may be adherent to the uterus. Tender nodules may be palpated in the utero-sacral ligaments. These nodules often become prominent and more tender before and during menstruation. Nodules in the pouch of Douglas are often discerned by simultaneous vaginal and rectal examination.

INVESTIGATIONS

The ancillary investigations can de divided into three categories: laparoscopy, serum immunoassays and imaging techniques.

Laparoscopy

The diagnosis of endometriosis is based on the visualization of the lesion. Directed biopsy of such lesions may complement the diagnosis. Since it is the main diagnostic technique, it should be performed early in the investigation of the patients whose clinical features are suggestive of endometriosis. The accuracy of diagnosis depends on the skill of the laparoscopist, the presence of co-existing pelvic inflammatory disease and adhesions and the 'special interest bias' of the operator. This is an invasive procedure, which should be performed, with meticulous attention to detail, as a double-puncture technique by a competent laparoscopist. A 2 month prelaparoscopy clinical therapeutic trial with drugs has been suggested for patients with symptoms and signs indicative of endometriosis. We believe it is inappropriate to initiate treatment for endometriosis without proper visual and histological documentation.

Serum immunoassays

The need to develop a non-invasive method of diagnosing endometriosis has resulted in the clinical evaluation of CA-125. This is a glycoprotein which is expressed by epithelial ovarian tumours as well as other tissues of Mullerian origin. This antigen has been investigated in the serum, peritoneal fluid and menstrual discharge of patients with endometriosis. The concentrations of CA-125 are elevated in women with advanced endometriosis, and this raised the possibility of developing a blood test for screening and clinical follow-up of patients with endometriosis.[41] The increase is thought to be caused by a higher level of antigen expression in ectopic than eutopic endometrium because of greater membrane concentration in the former. In addition, local inflammation associated with endometriosis increases the rate at which CA-125 is shed from the membranes into the circulation.[42] This test is not specific enough to be used as a non-invasive method of diagnosis and is better used to monitor treatment.

A variety of polyclonal humoral antibodies have been described in the serum of patients with endometriosis. One of these is endometrial antibody, but again these are neither sensitive nor specific in the diagnosis of endometriosis and have no correlation with the severity of the disease.[19,43] A combination of serum CA-125 and endometrial antibody has not been shown to improve the sensitivity of diagnosis.

Imaging techniques

The use of the transvaginal ultrasound scan has improved the diagnosis of clinically undetectable ovarian cysts. However, there are no satisfactory ultrasonographic diagnostic criteria for the differentiation of endometriotic cysts from any other benign ovarian cysts. It has a poor sensitivity and can best be used to monitor endometriotic cysts rather than as a means of diagnosis. The use of magnetic resonance imaging has been suggested to improve the diagnostic sensitivity, but this is not readily available and is expensive.[44] Immunoscintigraphy, using iodinated monoclonal antibody to OC-125 to detect implants greater than 2 cm, has been described but the sensitivity is poor and it also excludes the minimal form of the disease.[45] Other ancillary investigations which may be of importance include cystoscopy or intravenous urography if the renal system is involved or barium studies, sigmoidoscopy and colonoscopy if involvement of the gastrointestinal system is suspected.

TREATMENT

The wide range of presentation of endometriosis allows a variety of treatment options to be considered. This enables individualization based on the age, presenting symptoms, reproductive status, fertility demands, stage and previous response of the patient to treatment. The main goals of treatment are to relieve symptoms by removing or inducing resolution of implants and limiting progression of the disease as well as delaying recurrence and restoring fertility when necessary. The treatment of endometriosis may be medical, surgical or a combination (Table 18.5).

Table 18.5 Treatment classification of endometriosis

Medical	Surgical	Symptomatic
Combined oral contraceptive pill	Diathermy	Prostaglandin inhibitors
Progestogens	Laser vaporization	Assisted conception
Danazol	Excision	Psychotherapy
Gestrinone	Ovarian cystostomy	
GnRH-a	Presacral neurectomy	
GnRH-a with 'add-back' therapy	Hysterectomy and ovarian removal	

MEDICAL

Prostaglandin synthetase inhibitors

The severity of dysmenorrhoea, which is a common symptom in endometriosis, has been directly related to the number of implants.[38] The mechanism of endometriosis-associated dysmenorrhoea is poorly understood but may be related to prostaglandin production, which is elevated in the peritoneal fluid of patients with endometriosis. The increased production is more often associated with the non-pigmented form. Prostaglandin synthetase inhibitors are a group of non-steroidal anti-inflammatory agents that act by inhibiting the production of prostaglandins. In one study, tolfenamic acid relieved endometriosis symptoms more effectively than placebo, while acetylsalicylic acid and indomethacin did not show any difference when compared with placebo. If a patient's pain is unresponsive to prostaglandin synthetase inhibitor, consideration should be given to hormone suppression therapy.

Hormone suppression therapy

The rationale for the use of hormones is the understanding that endometriosis is hormone-dependent, requiring ovarian steroids for growth and development. It is rarely seen before menarche and postmenopause, and tends to regress during pregnancy. Endometriotic implants possess oestrogen, progestogen and androgen receptors, usually at a lower concentration than eutopic endometrium. This forms the basis of hormone treatment which is receptor mediated. Furthermore, the ectopic implants are often out of phase when compared with eutopic endometrium. This probably explains the variation in the clinical success of hormone therapy in these patients. The success of treatment also depends on the localization and depth of the implant, as superficial implants respond better than deep lesions or lesions within other organs such as the bladder or rectum. The aim, therefore, is to suppress cyclical hormone changes of ovarian steroid secretion, and inhibit pituitary gonadotrophin secretion creating a hypo-oestrogenic state with a hostile environment for tissue growth. The effects of such manipulation are shown in Table 18.6.

Oestrogen and androgens

In the early days of endocrine manipulation, oestrogens (stilboestrol) and androgens (methyltestosterone) were used for the treatment of endometriosis. Although both drugs were able to relieve pain symptoms, they had serious side effects such as thromboembolism, endometrial hyperplasia, nausea and vomiting, while methyltestosterone was associated with acne, deepening of voice, and hirsutism, which are unacceptable to patients. There is no place for these therapies in modern endometriosis treatment.

Oestrogen and progestogens

The pseudo-pregnancy regimen was based on the beneficial effect of pregnancy on endometriosis. Initial studies used the pill with a high oestrogen content and were efficacious in symptom control. Data on the cyclical

Table 18.6 Side effects of medical therapy

Hypo-oestrogenic
Flushes
Vaginal dryness
Insomnia
Breast atrophy
Night sweats

Progestogenic
Irregular bleeding
Mood changes
Nausea
Fluid retention

Androgenic
Weight gain
Acne
Hirsutism
Virilization
Voice changes

Metabolic
Lipid
Skeletal
Hepatic   *Drug of Choice OCP, Progestogen*

low-dose combined oral contraceptive pill (COC) is sparse but initial results suggest that it is efficacious in the relief of dysmenorrhoea and dyspareunia in patients with endometriosis.[46] This regimen is suitable for young symptomatic patients with mild endometriosis who are not desirous of starting a family.

Progestogens   *80% effective*

Progestogens have also been used either continuously or cyclically. Both progesterone (medroxyprogesterone-MPA, dydrogesterone) and the 19-nortestosterone derivatives (norethisterone oenanthate, lynoesterol) have been effectively used. They act by causing decidualization and atrophy of the tissue and by suppressing ovarian activity. The most commonly used is medroxyprogesterone acetate either in the oral (30 mg daily) or injectable (50 mg weekly) form. Treatment is effective in relieving symptoms in about 80% of cases. Side effects of therapy are irregular menstrual bleeding and breakthrough bleeding, which occur in about one-third of the patients. Others are decreased libido, weight gain, mood changes, breast tenderness, oedema and bloating. Prolonged use of progestogens causes a reduction in the serum concentration of high density lipoprotein cholesterol (HDL-cholesterol), which theoretically increases the risk of cardiovascular disease and atheroma formation. Some clinicians use progestogens as first line medication in symptom relief because they are relatively cheap, have minimal metabolic effects in low doses and acceptable side effects.

Danazol   3×1 course relieve symptoms.

Danazol is an isoxazol derivative of the synthetic steroid 17α-ethinyltestosterone. It has weak androgenic and anabolic properties. The mechanisms of action of danazol include interaction with intracellular steroid receptors (a high affinity for androgen and progestogen receptors in endometriotic tissue producing a local antioestrogenic effect and atrophy), competitively inhibiting multiple enzymes of steroidogenesis by a direct local action on the ovary causing inadequate ovarian follicular development. Danazol not only causes displacement of testosterone from circulating sex hormone binding globulin (SHBG) and cortisol from cortisol binding globulin but also reduces the production of SHBG by the liver causing an increase in the serum concentration of the steroid. The free testosterone binds to androgen receptors in endometriotic lesions causing atrophy. Furthermore, there are some data to suggest that danazol causes a clinical improvement in autoantibody associated autoimmune diseases such as systemic lupus erythematosus. Treatment of endometriosis patients with danazol has been shown to cause a reduction in endometrial immunoglobulin production either directly or indirectly.[47,48]

Danazol is the most commonly used medical therapy. Treatment is often commenced in oral doses of between 200 mg/day and 600 mg/day. Great care should be taken to ensure that patients are not pregnant, and treatment is initiated at the completion of the normal menses. Administration to mothers during the first and second trimester of pregnancy is associated with virilization of females. The side effects are weight gain, oedema, breast atrophy, acne, oily skin, hirsutism, deepening voice, headache, hot flushes, increased libido and muscle cramps. An estimated 75% of patients on danazol will complain of one or more side effects.[49] The metabolic effects of danazol (decrease in HDL-cholesterol and elevation in low density lipoprotein cholesterol (LDL-cholesterol) theoretically favour cardiovascular and thrombogenic accidents. These metabolic effects are reversible on stopping the drug and are thought to be dose and duration dependent. A 3 month treatment course of danazol has been shown to relieve symptoms adequately.[50] This short course may be of clinical importance in patients who require some symptom alleviation before infertility treatment. However, further clinical trials need to be done to assess symptom recurrence at follow-up.

Gestrinone   85' /

This is a trienic 19-norsteroid derivative which exhibits androgenic, antiprogestogenic, antioestrogenic as well as antigonadotrophic properties. It induces endometrial atrophy by a mechanism similar to that of danazol. It is administered orally in a dose of 2.5–5 mg twice weekly, inducing amenorrhoea in about 85% of patients. The efficacy is similar to danazol but the side effects are milder.

Gonadotrophin releasing hormone analogues (GnRH-a)

The continuous administration of such drugs causes 'medical castration'. This is achieved by the desensitization and downregulation of pituitary gonadotrophin-releasing hormone receptors, which results in the reduction in circulating serum gonadotrophin concentrations and inhibition of ovarian steroidogenesis. The resultant hypo-oestrogenic state provides a hostile environment for the development of endometriosis. A number of nona-peptide analogues (buserelin, leuprolide) and decapeptide analogues (nafarelin, tryptorelin, goserelin) are available either in the form of nasal spray or monthly depot injection. They are known to be effective in symptom relief as well as reducing endometriosis scores in about 90% of patients. Superficial lesions respond extremely well whereas ovarian endometriomas (greater than 3 cm), whilst showing significant suppression of symptoms, show at best a 20% reduction in size and are therefore best treated by surgery. The side effects are mainly caused by hypo-oestrogenicity synonymous with menopausal symptoms. They include hot flushes, reduced libido, vaginal dryness, emotional instability, depression, headaches and bone demineralization. A 6 month course of therapy reduces the trabecular bone density of the lumbar vertebrae by 5–6% while a 2–3% reduction is noted at the femoral neck. The effects on bone are reversible 9 months after discontinuation. The concept of a serum oestrogen threshold below which growth of ectopic endometrium is suppressed and above which bone demineralization occurs has been suggested but needs further elucidation. To protect the metabolic effects on bones various 'add-back' regimens have been developed (Table 18.7). There is evidence that the regimens, whilst preventing bone demineralization, do not adversely affect the efficacy of symptom control.[51,52]

Table 18.7 Various 'add-back' therapies for GnRH-a

Hormone replacement therapy
Combined oestrogen and progestogen
Tibone

Progestogens
Norethisterone/Norethindrone
Medroxyprogesterone acetate

Organic buphosphonates (± progestogens)
Sodium etidronate and calcium carbonate

Others
Tibolone
Calcitonin

Other forms of medical therapy include antiprogesterone (RU 486), antioestrogen (tamoxifen) and gosypol. It seems that these drugs are efficacious but require further clinical elucidation.

SURGERY

The main goals of surgery are to restore pelvic anatomy in the treatment of infertility and the interruption of sensory pathway in the symptomatic treatment of pelvic pain. Restoration of normal pelvic anatomy is performed by cytoreduction of ectopic endometrial implants either in the peritoneum or on the ovary, restoration of tubo-ovarian anatomy, and excision or photocoagulation of ovarian endometriomas. This is most often carried out by laparoscopy although laparotomy still has a place in certain cases. In a randomized study, laparoscopic laser vaporization or coagulation of implants was shown to improve the fertility rate when compared with expectant management.[53] Chronic pelvic pain associated with endometriosis responds to nerve ablation of the uterosacral ligaments in about 60% of patients.[54]

Superficial ovarian endometriosis can be treated by coagulation or vaporization. In the case of deep endometriomas, i.e. greater than 3 cm, drainage of the cyst (laparoscopic cystotomy and biopsy) followed by a 3 month course of GnRH-a has been shown to be effective.[55] Endometriosis of the recto-vaginal septum can be removed by laparoscopy if discrete and well localized.[54,56] It is the practice in our centre to administer a 3 month preoperative course of GnRH-a, to reduce the implant volume and vascularity, before removing the lesion by laparotomy in conjunction with a gastrointestinal surgeon. In patients with severe symptomatic endometriosis who have completed their family, hysterectomy may be the treatment of choice with removal of the ovaries and subsequent hormone replacement therapy. Such patients should be counselled regarding the risk (0.01%) of postcastration endometriosis, which often involves the gut.[31]

SUMMARY

Endometriosis is a benign gynaecological disease commonly affecting women in the reproductive age group. Its aetiology is unknown but retrograde menstruation and immunogenetic factors may be contributory. The commonest clinical presentation is pelvic pain and/or infertility. Management depends upon whether or not the disease is symptomatic. Accidentally discovered asymptomatic endometriosis should be left alone. Indeed, it is a very, very clever doctor who can make an asymptomatic patient feel better. Medical, surgical or a combination of both are the available management options for symptomatic patients. The selection of the drug of choice is based on its effectiveness, the individual patient, side effects and cost. Because of the chronicity of the disease, many patients will probably require and receive several courses of medical therapy during their reproductive life. Surgical

therapy is advocated for the management of endometriotic cysts greater than
3 cm. Recurrence rate of endometriosis is estimated at 10% per year of
therapy.

REFERENCES

1 Mahmood T A, Templeton A. The impact of treatment on the natural history of endometriosis. Hum Reprod 1991; 5: 965–970

2 Forman R G, Robinson J N, Mehta Z, Barlow D H. Patient history as a simple predictor of pelvic pathology in subfertile women. Hum Reprod 1993; 8: 53–55

3 Marana R, Pajelli F V, Muzili L, Dell' Acqua S, Mancuso S. The role of laparoscopy in the evaluation of chronic pelvic pain. Minerva Ginecologica 1993; 45: 281–286

4 Barbieri R L. Etiology and epidemiology of endometriosis. Am J Obstet Gynecol 1990; 162: 565–567.

5 Sampson J A. Peritoneal endometriosis due to menstrual dissemination of endometrial tissue into the peritoneal cavity. Am J Obstet Gynecol 1927; 14: 422–469

6 Keettel W C, Stein R J. The viability of the cast-off menstrual endometrium. Am J Obstet Gynecol 1951; 61: 440–442

7 Kruitwagen R F, Poels L G, Willemsen W N, de Ronde I J, Jap P H, Rolland R. Endometrial epithelial cells in peritoneal fluid during early follicular phase. Fertil Steril 1991; 55: 297–303

8 van der Linden P J, de Goeiji A F, Denselman G, van de Linden E P, Ramaeker F C, Evers J H. Expression of intergrins and E-cadherin in cells from menstrual effluent, endometrium, peritoneal fluid, peritoneum and endometriosis. Fertil Steril 1994; 61: 85–89

9 Halme J, Hammond M G, Hulka J F, Raj S G, Talbert L M. Retrograde menstruation in healthy women and in patients with endomeriosis. Obstet Gynecol 1984; 64: 151–154

10 Ayers J W, Friedenstab. Utero-tubal hypotonia associated with pelvic endometriosis. Proceedings of the 41st annual meeting of the American Fertility Society 1985: 131

11 Scott R B, Novak R J, Tindale R M. Umbilical endometriosis and Cullen's sign: Study of lymphatic transport from pelvis to umbilicus in monkeys. Obstet Gynecol 1958; 11: 556–558

12 Schenken R S. Pathogenesis. In: Schenken R S, ed. Endometriosis: contemporary concepts in clinical management. London: Lippincott, 1989: pp 3–48

13 Giudice I. C. Endometrial growth factors and proteins. Sem Reprod Endocrinol 1995; 13: 93–101

14 Sanfilipo J S, Wakin N G, Schikler K N, Yussman M A. Endometriosis in association with uterine anomaly. Am J Obstet Gynecol 1986; 154: 39–43

15 Dmowski W P, Radwanska E, Binor Z. Immunological aspects in endometriosis. Am J Obstet Gynecol 1981; 141: 377–383

16 Badawy S A, Cuenca V, Stitzel A, Ticce D. Immune rosettes of T and B-lymphocytes in infertile women with endometriosis. J Reprod Med 1987; 32: 194–197

17 Oosterlynck D J, Meuleman C, Waer M, Vandeputte M, Koninckx P R. The natural killer activity of peritoneal fluid lymphocytes is decreased in women with endometriosis. Fertil Steril 1992; 58: 290–295

18 Gleicher N, El-Roeiy A, Confino E, Friberg J. Abnormal autoantibodies in endometriosis. Is endometriosis an autoimmune disease? Obstet Gynecol 1987; 70: 115–122

19 Odukoya O A, Wheatcroft N, Weetman A P, Cooke I D. The prevalence of endometrial immunoglobulin G antibodies in patients with endometriosis. Hum Reprod 1995; 10: 1214–1219

20 Grimes D A, Lebott S C, Grimes K R. Systemic lupus erythematosus and reproductive function: A case control study. Am J Obstet Gynecol 1985; 153: 179–182

21 Oosterlynck D J, Meulema C, Waer M, Vandeputte M, Koninckx P R. Transforming growth factor-β in peritoneal fluid of women with endometriosis. Obstet Gynecol 1994; 83: 287–292

22 Ramey J Y, Archer D F. Peritoneal fluid: its relevance to the development of endometriosis. Fertil Steril 1993; 60: 1–14

23 Cramer D W, Wilson E, Stillman R J, Berger M J, Belisle S, Schiff I, Albrecht B, Gibson M, Stadel B V, Schoenbaum S C. The relation of endometriosis to menstrual characteristics, smoking and exercise. JAMA 1986; 55: 1904–1908

24 Matorras R, Rodriquez F, Pijoan J, Ramon O, Gutierrez de Teran G, Rodriguez-Escudero F. Epidemiology of endometriosis in infertile women. Fertil Steril 1995; 63: 34–38

25 Simpson J L, Elias S, Malinak L R, Buttram V C. Heritable aspects of endometriosis. I. Genetic studies. Am J Obstet Gynecol 1980; 137: 327–331

26 Lamb K, Hoffman R G, Nichols T R. Family trait analysis: a case control study of 43 women with endometriosis and their best friends. Am J Obstet Gynecol 1986; 154: 596–601

27 Malinak L R, Buttram V C, Elias S, Simpson J L. Heritable aspects of endometriosis. II. Clinical characteristics of familial endometriosis. Am J Obstet Gynecol 1980; 137: 332–337

28 Pinsonneault O, Goldstein D P. Obstructing malformation of the uterus and vagina. Fertil Steril 1985; 44: 214–218

29 Olive D L, Henderson D Y. Endometriosis and Mullerian anomalies. Obstet Gynecol 1987; 69: 412–415

30 Darrow S L, Vena J E, Batt R E, Zielezny M A, Michaleck A M, Selman S. Menstrual cycle characteristics and the risk of endometriosis. Epidemiology 1993; 4: 135–142

31 Redwine D. Endometriosis persisting after castration: Clinical characteristics and results of surgical management. Obstet Gynecol 1994; 83: 405–413

32 American Fertility Society. Revised American Fertility Society classification of endometriosis. Fertil Steril 1985; 43: 351

33 Vernon M W, Beard J S, Graves K, Wilson E A. Classification of endometriotic implants by morphologic appearance and capacity to synthesize prostaglandin F. Fertil Steril 1986; 46: 801–805

34 Cornillie F J, Oosterlynck J M, Koninckx P R. Deeply infiltrating pelvic endometriosis: histology and clinical significance. Fertil Steril 1990; 53: 978–983

35 Mahmood T A, Templeton A. Prevalence and genesis of endometriosis. Hum Reprod 1991; 6: 544–549

36 Thomas E J, Cooke I D. Impact of gestrinone on the course of asymptomatic endometriosis. Br Med J 1987; 294: 272–274

37 Inoue M, Kobayasi Y, Honda I, Fujii A. The impact of endometriosis on the reproductive outcome of infertile patients. Am J Obstet Gynecol 1992; 167: 278–282

38 Perper N M, Nezhat F, Goldstein H, Nezhat G H, Nezhat C. Dysmenorrhoea is related to the number of implants in endometriosis patients. Fertil Steril 1995; 63: 500–503

39 Fedele L, Bianchi S, Boccione L, Nola G, Parazzini F. Pain symptoms associated with endometriosis. Obstet Gynecol 1992; 79: 767–769

40 Halme J, Chafe W, Currie J L. Endometriosis with massive ascites. Obstet Gynecol 1985; 65: 591–595

41 Koninckx P R, Riittinen L, Sepalla M, Cornillie F J. Ca-125 and placental protein 14 concentrations in plasma and peritoneal fluid of women with deeply infiltrating pelvic endometriosis. Fertil Steril 1992; 57: 523–530

42 Barbieri R L. Ca-125 in patients with advanced endometriosis (editorial). Fertil Steril 1986; 53: 930–932

43 Wild R A, Shivers C A, Medders S. Detection of antiendometrial antibodies in patients with endometriosis: methodological issues. Fertil Steril 1992; 58: 518–524

44 Takahashi K, Okada S, Ozaki T, Kitao M, Sugimura K. Diagnosis of pelvic endometriosis by magnetic resonance imaging using 'fat saturation' technique. Fertil Steril 1994; 62: 973–977

45 Kennedy S H, Mojimoniyi O A, Soper N D W, Shepstone B J, Barlow D. Immunoscintigraphy of endometriosis. Br J Obstet Gynaecol 1990; 97: 667–671

45a Kaupilla A, Puolakka J, Yilorkala O. Prostaglandin biosynthesis inhibitors and endometriosis. Prostaglandins 1979; 18: 655–661

46 Vercellini P, Tresoidi L, Colombo A, Vendola N, Marchini M, Crosignani P. A gonadotrophin-releasing hormone agonist versus a low dose oral contraceptive for pelvic pain associated with endometriosis. Fertil Steril 1993; 60: 75–79

47 El-Roeiy A, Dmowski W P, Gleicher N, Harlow L, Radwanska E, Binor Z, Tummon I, Rawlings R. Danazol but not gonadotrophin-releasing hormone agonist suppresses auto-antibodies in endometriosis. Fertil Steril 1988; 50: 864–871

48 Odukoya O A, Bansal A, Wilson A P, Weetman A P, Cooke I D. Serum soluble CD23 in patients with endometriosis and the effect of treatment with danazol and leuprolide acetate depot injection. Hum Reprod 1995; 10: 9420–9460

49 Barbieri R L, Evans S, Kistner R W. Danazol in the treatment of endometriosis: analysis of 100 cases with a 4 year follow up. Fertil Steril 1982; 37: 737–746

50 Wright S, Valdes C, Dunn R, Franklin R. Short term lupron or danazol therapy for pelvic endometriosis. Fertil Steril 1995; 63: 504–507
51 Edmonds D K, Howell R. Can hormone replacement therapy be used during medical therapy of endometriosis? Br J Obstet Gynaecol 1994; 191 (suppl 10): 24–26
52 Surrey E S, Voigt B, Fournet N, Judd H. Prolonged gonadotropin-releasing hormone agonist treatment of symptomatic endometriosis: role of cyclic sodium etidronate and low-dose norethisterone 'add-back' therapy. Fertil Steril 1995; 63: 747–755
53 Tulandi T, Mouchawar M. Treatment-dependent and treatment-independent pregnancy in women with minimal and mild endometriosis. Fertil Steril 1991; 56: 790–791
54 Nezhat C, Nezhat F, Nezhat C H, Seidman D. Severe endometriosis and operative laparoscopy. Curr Opin Obstet Gynecol 1995; 7: 299–306
55 Donnez J, Nisolle M, Gillerot S, Anaf V, Clerckx-Braun B S. Ovarian endometrial cyst: the role of gonadotrophin-releasing hormone agonist and drainage. Fertil Steril 1994; 62: 63–66
56 Nezhat C, Nezhat F, Pennington E. Laparoscopic treatment of lower colorectal and infiltrative rectovaginal septum endometriosis by the technique of videolaseroscopy. Br J Obstet Gynaecol 1992; 99: 664–667

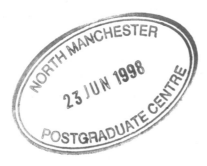

19 Laser ablation or endometrial resection?

D. E. Parkin

Whilst endometrial ablation with laser (ELA) was started in America in the late 1970s by Goldrath,[1] hysteroscopic surgery only became popular in the UK in the late 1980s and early 1990s following the introduction and popularization of transcervical resection of the endometrium (TCRE) by Magos.[2] Davis had been performing laser ablation in the UK from 1985 but this technique had failed to gain popularity at that time.[3] A third method then became available in the form of radiofrequency-induced endometrial ablation (RAFEA) in 1990.[4] The history of these techniques and the background to their use in dysfunctional uterine bleeding (DUB) is well described by Magos in Volume 9 of this series.[5]

A great expansion of both gynaecologists wishing to perform these techniques and patients asking for them occurred. This followed wide exposure in the lay press and the publication of large but uncontrolled series of both ELA and TCRE.[6,7]

They were introduced as an alternative to hysterectomy for women with dysfunctional bleeding, or menorrhagia with small fibroids which were resistant to medical treatment. One concern is that the threshold for surgery has fallen below that for hysterectomy as they were perceived as quick minor procedures. It is difficult to know who has been the most responsible for the great expansion of these techniques, gynaecologists, patients or even publicity and pressure from the equipment manufacturers.

There have, however, been anecdotal reports of deaths and major complications following these procedures,[8,9] and therefore they should not be performed for lesser indications that would not have previously merited a hysterectomy. Whether this will be the case or not still remains to be seen.

It is now 5 years since Magos described the techniques of TCRE and ELA in this series and they have now become established as part of operative gynaecology. The RAFEA is still undergoing assessment. Despite early promise, problems still remain with this technique. There were early problems with vesico-vaginal fistulae and burns from anaesthetic monitoring equipment. The manufacturer recommends that RAFEA is only suitable for a regular uterus, which excludes many patients. This technique will therefore not be discussed further.

The gynaecologist who wishes to establish an endometrial ablation service has to decide which modality should be used. More data is now available on operative hysteroscopy which this chapter will use to try and answer this question.

AIMS OF TREATMENT

Although the techniques are known as endometrial resection and endometrial ablation, this is somewhat of a misnomer as the aim is to destroy the endometrial glands efficiently and safely to prevent regeneration. A further consideration is to do this as inexpensively as possible without compromising safety and efficacy.

The endometrial glands lie up to 3 mm within the myometrium and therefore any technique that is used must be able to destroy or remove the overlying endometrium and the superficial myometrium to this depth.[10] As Duffy found that the mean thickness of the myometrium in the cornua of the uterus is 6 mm and may be as thin as 4 mm it is vital that the depth of damage can be accurately controlled and predicted to ensure adequate treatment, and to reduce the risk of perforation and full-thickness burns with possible damage to bowel or other structures.[11]

The neodynium: yttrium-aluminium-garnet (Nd:YAG) laser will cause thermal necrosis to a depth of 4–6 mm when a typical power output of 80 W is used.[12] This is of value in ensuring that an adequate depth of tissue is treated, but unsuspected full-thickness burns can occur, especially at the cornua.

Electrosurgery can be carried out in two ways. Either, tissue can be resected with a cutting loop using a blend diathermy current, or a ball-bearing electrode, the 'rollerball', can be moved across the uterine wall using either blend current or pure coagulation current. In practice many use a combination of resection and rollerball. The rollerball is used for the cornua, where the risk of perforation is greatest with the loop, and by some surgeons for the fundus which can be difficult to resect. Pure rollerball ablation is popular especially in the USA.[13] When using the resectoscope the depth of resection can be measured with the loop, but there will be thermal damage deeper than this for a distance of up to 1.8 mm.[14] With the rollerball there is often no visual guide to the depth of treatment but thermal necrosis occurs to a depth of 3.5 mm beyond any visible crater.[14]

Both ELA and TCRE require the uterine cavity to be irrigated with fluid during the procedure for uterine distension and to clear blood and debris. For ELA, electrolyte solutions such as normal saline or glycine can be used. Dextrose cannot be used as this would lead to caramelization. For TCRE an electrolyte-free solution must be used in order to prevent arcing of the current. In the UK this is almost universally glycine 1.5%.

SAFETY AND COMPLICATIONS

The risks of these procedures can be split into patient complications and staff risks. The main patient complications are trauma, fluid absorption, bleeding and infection. Following a number of anecdotal and perhaps rumoured major complications of TCRE a feeling grew that it was a more dangerous method than ELA. Although this is possible, a number of reasons for this apparent situation exist. The number of Nd:YAG lasers in the UK has always been much lower than the number of resectoscopes. In 1994 there were only 3 units in Scotland with a laser compared to 11 with resectoscopes. This meant that ELA tended to be performed by experienced and committed surgeons who might have been expected to have a relatively low complication rate. To compound this the medical equipment manufacturers widely promoted the sale of resectoscopes to gynaecologists before organized training was available, leading to a large increase in the number of inexperienced operators performing TCRE. This made TCRE appear to have a higher complication rate than ELA. However, except by comparing different personal, retrospective and uncontrolled series this could not be proven. There are theoretical reasons why TCRE may have a higher perforation rate than ELA. The resectoscope is of wider diameter, usually 9 mm or more, than the laser hysteroscope, which usually has a diameter of 7 mm, requiring greater cervical dilatation. Some surgeons used urological resectoscopes of an even larger diameter. In addition, the resectoscope needs greater manipulation than the laser hysteroscope and the uterine chips need to be removed from the cavity of the uterus, which may be damaged during this manoeuvre. TCRE also has the risk of diathermy burns to the patient if the return electrode is not correctly attached. This can be avoided by a modern diathermy machine with return electrode monitoring.

The Royal College of Obstetricians and Gynaecologists, in the report of the RCOG Working Party on Training in Gynaecological Endoscopic Surgery, however, states that: 'Laser ablation using a drag technique has a lower risk of complications than resection or electro-coagulation'.[15] Lewis, in an editorial based upon the guidelines for endometrial ablation produced by the British Society for Gynaecological Endoscopy (BSGE), also says that laser may have a lower risk of major complications, but points out that this has not been proven in controlled trials.[16]

The most accurate way to answer that question is by randomized prospective trial, or failing that, large-scale prospective audit with a high degree of reporting.

To date there is only one randomized controlled study comparing ELA with TCRE. It was performed in Aberdeen by the author's group and was part of a randomized trial of hysterectomy versus hysteroscopic surgery for patients with DUB that was resistant to medical treatment and had a uterus no larger than 10 weeks in size. Patients in the hysteroscopic arm were randomized between TCRE and ELA;[17] numbers were relatively small, 50 randomized to each method, but were well matched and operated on by the same gynaecologists to exclude bias owing to operator experience. The results showed one laparotomy for small bowel obstruction following a full-thickness cornual burn in an ELA patient, similar to that previously described by Perry et al.[18] With TCRE there was one perforation with a dilator and none with the resectoscope. A statistically significantly higher volume of fluid was absorbed in the laser group (766 ml) than in the TCRE group (414 ml), but otherwise there were no differences between the two techniques, although the numbers were too small to exclude differences in rare complications. The implication from this is that there is little, if any, difference in safety between the two techniques. We have expanded this research and completed recruitment of a large randomized study of TCRE versus ELA, of in excess of 350 patients. Although not fully analysed, early results agree with the previous study.[19] The perforation rate during TCRE is less than 1% in comparison with 3% reported in most series.[7] Possible reasons for the lack of complications in the TCRE group are that we use a small, 8 mm diameter, resectoscope, a small 3 mm deep loop and always prepare the endometrium with an LHRH analogue to ensure optimum visibility.

What other evidence is there to support the idea that ELA is safer? A Scottish National Audit of Hysteroscopic Surgery was carried out from 1991 to 1993,[20] which recruited 978 patients of whom 65% were treated with TCRE and 32% by ELA. It was estimated that reporting was 98% complete, thus providing a prospective, population-based study. There was one death from toxic shock syndrome,[9] in a patient following an uncomplicated TCRE, and significantly more cases of fluid overload with ELA than TCRE, but no other difference in any other complication rate in this series. Note that excess fluid absorption with ELA will result in fluid volume effects, rather than hyponatremia, because of the usage of normal saline. As glycine is used for TCRE both volume overload and therefore electrolyte changes leading to hyponatremia may result.[21] It is uncertain why ELA has a higher rate of fluid absorption. One factor may be that TCRE tends to be a faster procedure and reduces the time for fluid absorption to occur. For TCRE, however, the amount of fluid absorbed was not dependent upon the duration of the procedure,[21] so this may not provide the complete explanation. It may be a more fundamental difference in the degree of coagulation of blood vessels within the myometrium. Alternatively, it could be because during a TCRE the resectoscope is removed from the uterine cavity a number of times, allowing the intrauterine pressure caused by the irrigation fluid to fall. During ELA the laser hysteroscope remains within the cavity allowing the uterine pressure to remain high throughout. The use of an electronic pressure-controlled infusion system may help reduce the fluid absorption during ELA.[12]

The RCOG is running an audit of hysteroscopic surgery in England and Wales: the MISTLETOE survey. Very preliminary results on the first year's data show that only 17% of the total cases of hysteroscopic surgery were ELA. These results also showed a 7.7% complication rate for TCRE and a

5.5% complication rate for ELA, but gave no statistical analysis. Mortality rates are still awaited. To date there is no data on any difference between the two modalities on either infection rates or postoperative bleeding.

There are few staff risks regarding TCRE compared with ELA. During TCRE if the surgeon was to touch the activated loop with a punctured glove a burn may result. However, the Nd:YAG laser is potentially dangerous to anyone in the operating theatre. As the laser energy passes through the cornea, and normal glass, and becomes focused on the retina, it can cause irreversible blindness if the eye is exposed to the beam. Any part of the body can be burned if exposed to the beam. These risks can be reduced by the following precautions: ensuring that all people in the theatre wear protective goggles, not enabling the laser until it is in the uterine cavity, by covering all glass windows with a laser proof barrier and by having an interlock system that will switch off the laser if a door is opened.

RESULTS

These can be divided into menstrual symptom outcome, non-menstrual symptom outcome (including pain) and overall patient satisfaction, which may not be the same thing!

The aim of hysteroscopic surgical procedures is to reduce excessive menstrual loss and in some cases to cause amenorrhoea. Not all women presenting for surgery will have a monthly menstrual loss of more than 80 ml and these women may have a different perception on satisfaction with these techniques.

When trying to compare the results of different personal series of TCRE and ELA in the literature, to decide if one is superior, there are a number of confusing variables. The first is that the patient population may differ in the severity of symptoms, age or their perception of the likely outcome following the operation, or the experience of the surgeons may be different. The method of collecting the data may vary and if collected on a face-to-face interview with the patient may lead to under-reporting of dissatisfaction with the outcome. There may also be differences with terminology of menstrual outcome, such as whether some brown spotting counts as amenorrhoea or oligo-amenorrhoea. The other vital difference is that the duration of follow-up may vary. This would have a major effect on results as some failures appear over time. For these reasons only data that are closely comparable between ELA and TCRE will be used.

The only randomized study to date,[17] has shown identical results in all respects between ELA and TCRE. At 12 months 22% of patients were amenorrhoeic and 62% reported hypomenorrhoea. There was no dysmenorrhoea in 42% and less pain in 43%. There was no change in the dysmenorrhoea in 5% and it worsened in 10%. Interestingly, there was a large reduction in the degree of non-menstrual symptoms such as premenstrual symptoms and breast discomfort. At 12 months 78% of patients were very satisfied and 18% moderately satisfied. Long-term follow-up will continue and our expanded randomized study may reveal small differences between these methods.

The two large audit projects are worth examining. The patient selection may be different between the two treatment modalities and there may be differences in operator experience. The assessment of patient outcome and satisfaction was assessed by confidential questionnaires common to each treatment type, which were sent to a central office and therefore should be valid. They should give population-based information and have the advantage of large numbers.

The Scottish Audit,[20] has shown no difference in patient outcome, between TCRE and ELA, at 6, 12 or 24 months postoperatively. Overall, the menstrual results showed amenorrhoea in 25%, brown discharge in 18%, much lighter periods in 42%, periods a little lighter in 11% but unchanged or heavier in 5%. The duration of the bleeding was reduced and dysmenorrhoea was absent in 51%, less in 31%, unchanged in 11% and worse in 7%. Overall, at 12 months 53% of patients were very satisfied and 31% satisfied with the results of their treatment.

Relatively young age was said by the BSGE guidelines group to give a poor outcome and to be a relative contraindication.[16] In the Scottish Audit the outcome above and below the age of 40 years was compared. Although the outcome at 12 months was statistically significantly worse in the younger group there was still a satisfaction rate of 79% compared to 88% in the older group. This suggests that there are still acceptable results by both methods in the younger age group.

The preliminary results of the MISTLETOE study show a cumulative failure rate for TCRE of around 18%, but of 32% for ELA. Patients were extremely or very satisfied in 74% of TCRE cases but only 62% of ELA cases. This data is only preliminary, but if confirmed may be clinically significant.

Both techniques suffer from the same problem of menstrual results being better than patient satisfaction. This is not unexpected, as hysterectomy for menorrhagia does not give 100% satisfaction despite causing amenorrhoea.[17] In both the Aberdeen study and the Scottish Audit it appeared that some women, with what appeared to be good menstrual results, were not satisfied.[17,20] This may be because of pain, or may be that the patient's perception of her menstrual loss is inappropriate, or amenorrhoea is the patient's goal. I have performed three hysterectomies for persistent excessive menstrual loss following TCRE or ELA where the pathologist has been unable to identify any residual endometrium in the uterus.

INTRAUTERINE APPEARANCE

When Goldrath[12] introduced ELA he was aiming to reproduce Asherman's syndrome of amenorrhoea with intrauterine synechiae.[22] There has been discussion at meetings as to whether this is the case, and as to any difference between the two methods. This may be important as if one technique caused more adhesions than the other it may cause pain because of the formation of a haematometra and may, in the future, cause a focus of endometrial tissue to be hidden and not to produce the warning symptoms of postmenopausal bleeding. The women in the Aberdeen randomized study,[17] were assessed by out-patient hysteroscopy 6 months following their procedure. Hysteroscopy was possible in over 75% of patients after either treatment. The uterine cavity was reduced in length compared to the preoperative state, but intrauterine adhesions were found in only 3% of women, with no difference between ELA and TCRE.[23] The cavity was never totally occluded. This suggests that there is probably no difference between the two modalities and neither gives a 'cleaner' cavity than the other.

SPEED AND COST

Despite the current market economy in the provision of health care, the speed and cost of a procedure should not be regarded as the most important factors. When, however, as in this situation there seems little difference in safety or efficacy, then it needs to be discussed.

In our randomized study the total theatre time, including anaesthetic, for TCRE was 40 minutes compared to 50 minutes for ELA, which was statistically significant.[17] The total theatre time was relatively long in this study as we were still on the learning curve. The current study has shown a decrease in theatre time for both methods, but the differential remains.[19] The Scottish Audit showed little difference in total theatre times between the two methods; however, TCRE theatre time was 4 minutes shorter. This study may have been biased in the respect that operators may have chosen TCRE for the larger uterus, making laser seem faster.

The cost of a procedure is always difficult to assess. The basic camera and video equipment, whilst expensive, is common to both procedures. There is no evidence that recovery periods are any different, leaving theatre time, initial cost, running costs and differences in success rates as the main factors. As shown earlier TCRE is probably quicker but only marginally. The cost of a resectoscope and a laser hysteroscope are similar, as is the cost of irrigation fluid. A Nd:YAG laser will cost around £75 000, whilst the diathermy machine will be part of the usual theatre equipment. Added to this is the cost of making a theatre safe for laser use. Both methods require disposables in the form of laser fibres, and resectoscope loops and rollerballs. The cost of these probably balances out but depends partly on whether reuseable or disposable laser fibres are used. Even a large unit does no more than 300 cases per year. If all these cases were done with the laser, which probably has a life span of 10 years, the cost per case is £25. Obviously, if the laser can be used for other forms of surgery the cost is reduced.

As all the factors are in favour of TCRE it appears that it is the more economical of the two, but this does not mean that ELA is uneconomical compared to hysterectomy.

VERSATILITY

Both methods have their enthusiastic advocates and supporters. It appears that for the management of DUB in a fairly normal sized uterus similar results can be obtained with both methods. Both techniques can be used for endometrial ablation in a larger uterus, myomectomy, removal of uterine septae and the treatment of Asherman's syndrome. The use of either method for endometrial ablation in an enlarged uterus is not recommended by the BSGE guidelines,[16] but as both methods can be used for myomectomy, their use in a uterus larger than 10 weeks size is possible. I have performed more than 50 TCREs in patients with a uterine cavity length of between 10 cm and 15 cm in whom a hysterectomy was either contraindicated or was refused by the patient. In these patients the uterus was prepared with two injections of the LHRH analogue Zoladex to reduce the size of the cavity and to shrink any fibroids. The results in terms of patient satisfaction were similar to overall figures, but with a reduced amenorrhoea rate. The complication rate was no different, although 40% needed a two-stage procedure.

Myomectomy can be performed with either technique. The two main protagonists are with the resectoscope Jaques Hamou of Paris and with the laser Jaques Donnez of Brussells. Both use a LHRH analogue preoperatively and both report a high success in the ability to perform myomectomies, with good results in terms of fertility[24] and menorrhagia.[25]

Asherman's syndrome can be treated hysteroscopically. The anatomy can be very distorted with a high risk of uterine perforation and may best be performed under laparoscopic control. As the Nd:YAG laser causes deep thermal damage, hysteroscopic scissors or the straight resectoscope loop are preferable techniques.

TRAINING

Training is perhaps the most important area at present, although with talk of certification, rather contentious. Three centres have been established by the Department of Health as Minimal Access Therapy Training Units (MATTU, MATTUS in Scotland). In Scotland we have established courses in operative hysteroscopy. These are based on an initial laboratory course to teach basic motor skills and hand-eye co-ordination, which should be then followed up with supervised training on patients. Training for TCRE is relatively straightforward in the Surgical Skills laboratory as diathermy machines are already in place at every workstation, and resectoscopes are the only major additional piece of equipment needed. It is much more difficult to provide training in laser use as the cost precludes the purchase of multiple machines, but the principles can be taught. As there are fewer potential supervisors for further training on patients this may further reduce the opportunity to learn the technique of ELA.

It seems that the RCOG will introduce certification for these methods of treatment. This has its own problems of ensuring that standards are maintained, and that the holding of a certificate does not allow gynaecologists to feel that they are then completely trained.

CONCLUSION

There is probably little to choose between TCRE and ELA for the management of dysfunctional uterine bleeding in the woman with a reasonably normal-sized uterus. It seems that TCRE is faster and causes less fluid absorption than ELA but these differences are not great. The evidence that ELA is the safer technique seems to be lacking at the moment although the MISTLETOE survey may give more information.

In terms of efficacy the results seem equivalent, with TCRE perhaps having the edge if the early MISTLETOE results are maintained. The versatility of TCRE to deal with a larger uterus seems likely.

Cost seems to be an advantage of TCRE but if a laser is well used this may be only in the region of £25 per patient, which is a small proportion of the overall cost.

Any unit with a Nd:YAG laser should certainly continue to carry out ELA, but a unit contemplating starting hysteroscopic surgery would be best advised to aim for TCRE as the method of choice, but only after adequate training.

ACKNOWLEDGEMENTS

I would like to thank my research fellows Dr Sheena Pinion and Dr Siladitya Bhattacharya for their help and encouragement over the past 4 years and the Scottish Home and Health Department for funding our studies.

REFERENCES

1 Goldrath M H, Fuller T A, Segal S. Laser photovaporization of endometrium for the treatment of menorrhagia. Am J Obstet Gynecol 1981; 140: 14–19
2 Magos A L, Baumann R, Turnbull A C. Transcervical resection of the endometrium in women with menorrhagia. Br Med J 1989; 298: 1209–1212
3 Davis J A. Hysteroscopic endometrial ablation with the neodynium-YAG laser. Br J Obstet Gynaecol 1989; 96: 928–932
4 Phipps J H, Lewis B V, Roberts T, Prior M V, Hand V W, Elder M, Field S B. Treatment of functional menorrhagia by radiofrequency-induced thermal endometrial ablation. Lancet 1990; 335: 374–376
5 Magos A L. Endometrial ablation for menorrhagia. In: Studd J, ed. Progress in obstetrics and gynaecology. Vol 9. Edinburgh: Churchill Livingstone, 1991: 375–395
6 Garry R, Erian J, Grochmal S A. A multicentre collaborative study into the treatment of menorrhagia by Nd:YAG laser ablation of the endometrium. Br J Obstet Gynaecol 1991; 98: 357–362

7 Magos A L, Baumann R, Lockwood G M, Turnbull A C. Experience with the first 250 endometrial resections for menorrhagia. Lancet 1991; 337: 1074–1078

8 MacDonald R, Phipps J, Singer A. Endometrial ablation: a safe procedure. Gynaecol Endosc 1992; 1: 7–9

9 Parkin D E. Fatal Toxic Shock Syndrome following endometrial resection: Case report. Br J Obstet Gynaecol, 1995; 102: 163–164

10 Reid P C, Sharp F. Hysteroscopic Nd:YAG endometrial ablation: an in vitro and in vivo laser-tissue interaction study. Proceedings of the III European Congress on Hysteroscopy and Endoscopic Surgery. Amsterdam, 1992: 70

11 Duffy S, Reid P C, Smith J H F, Sharp F. In vitro studies of uterine electrosurgery. Obstet Gynecol 1991; 78: 213–220

12 Goldrath M H, Garry R. Nd:YAG laser ablation of the endometrium. In: Sutton C, Diamond M, eds. Endoscopic surgery for gynaecologists. London: Saunders, 1993: 317–327

13 Loffer F D. Endometrial ablation – where do we stand. Gynaecol Endosc 1992; 1: 175–179

14 Duffy S, Reid P C, Sharp F. In-vivo studies of uterine electrosurgery. Br J Obstet Gynaecol 1992; 99: 579–582

15 Royal College of Obstetricians and Gynaecologists. Report of the RCOG Working Party on Training in Gynaecological Endoscopic Surgery. London: RCOG Press, 1994

16 Lewis B V. Guidelines for endometrial ablation. Br J Obstet Gynaecol 1994; 101: 470–473

17 Pinion S B, Parkin D E, Abramovich D R, Naji A, Alexander D A, Russell I T, Kitchener H C. Randomised trial of hysterectomy, endometrial laser ablation, and transcervical endometrial resection for dysfunctional uterine bleeding. Br Med J 1994; 309: 979–983

18 Perry C P, Daniel J F, Gimpelson R J. Bowel injury from Nd:YAG endometrial ablation. J Gynecol Surg 1990; 6: 199–203

19 Bhattacharya S, Parkin D, Abramovich D, Kitchener H, Alexander D, Mollison J. A pragmatic randomised controlled trial of transcervical resection of the endometrium versus laser ablation for the treatment of menorrhagia. European Congress of Gynecologic Endoscopic Surgery, Rome. Gynaecol Endosc 1994; 3(suppl): 3–4

20 Scottish Hysteroscopy Audit Group. A Scottish Audit of hysteroscopic surgery for menorrhagia – complications and follow up. Br J Obstet Gynaecol 1995; 102: 249–254

21 Byers G F, Pinion S, Parkin D E, Chambers W A. Fluid absorption during transcervical resection of the endometrium. Gynaecol Endosc 1993; 2: 21–23

22 Asherman J G. Traumatic intrauterine adhesions. J Obstet Gynaecol Brit Emp 1950; 57: 892–896

23 Pinion S B. M D Thesis. Hysteroscopic surgery as an alternative to hysterectomy in the treatment of dysfunctional uterine bleeding. University of Edinburgh, 1994: 117–126

24 Donnez J, Gillerot S, Bourgonjon D, Clerckx F, Nisolle M. Neodynium: YAG laser hysteroscopy in large submucous fibroids. Fertil Steril 1990; 54: 99–103

25 Hamou J. Electroresection of fibroids. In: Sutton C, Diamond M, eds. Endoscopic surgery for gynaecologists. London: Saunders, 1993: 327–330

20 Laparoscopic hysterectomy

R. E. Richardson   A. L. Magos

Hysterectomy is a common operation of which approximately 20% of women living in England and Wales will have undergone before the age of 65.[1,2] Until recently, when a hysterectomy was indicated the choice was between an abdominal or vaginal operation. There is now, however, another possibility to consider. Since the first case report of laparoscopic hysterectomy (LH) by Reich in 1989[3] numerous series have been published combining laparoscopy and vaginal hysterectomy, but the role of such procedures in gynaecological practice remains poorly defined. How many LHs should be performed, how much of the procedure should be performed laparoscopically, and what methods should be used in its execution require further clarification – indeed the term 'laparoscopic hysterectomy' itself requires definition.

DEFINITION AND CLASSIFICATION

A hysterectomy may be correctly defined as 'laparoscopic' if the uterine arteries are divided laparoscopically.[4] As operative techniques have diversified, this definition has become rather restricting and various nomenclatures and classification systems have been introduced, which attempt to quantify how much of the procedure is performed laparoscopically as opposed to vaginally.[5,6] For sake of convenience, we use the term laparoscopic hysterectomy (LH) to describe all operations combining laparoscopic and vaginal surgery, and the stage of the procedure as defined by Johns and Diamond[7] to indicate how much was performed laparoscopically (Table 20.1).

TYPE OF HYSTERECTOMY AND THE ROLE OF LAPAROSCOPY

The aim of an LH is to convert an abdominal hysterectomy (TAH) into a vaginal procedure or to convert a difficult vaginal hysterectomy into an easy one. With rates for TAH rising to more than 85% in some series,[2,8] the potential for LH appears enormous.

Whilst the indications and contraindications for the vaginal hysterectomy (VH) continue to be controversial, its advantage over that of TAH, in terms of patient morbidity, has been proven.[9] The abdominal route has the

Table 20.1 Staging of laparoscopic hysterectomy

Stage	Laparoscopic procedure
0	Diagnostic laparoscopy performed before vaginal hysterectomy
1	Adhesiolysis and/or excision of endometriosis
2	Either or both adnexa freed
3	Bladder dissected from uterus
4	Uterine artery transected
5	Anterior and/or posterior colpotomy or entire uterus freed

0, neither ovary excised;
1, one ovary excised;
2, both ovaries excised.
Reproduced with permission from Johns & Diamond.[7]

advantages of better access to and visualization of the whole pelvis and abdomen. This access gives the surgeon the ability to remove large tumours, accomplish adhesiolysis, omentectomy and lymphadenectomy, and perform adnexectomy with relative ease. During most hysterectomies, however, this versatility is usually not required and laparotomy may be performed unnecessarily because the methods of predicting pelvic pathology are inadequate, or unused. By contrast the vaginal approach may be difficult because of either poor access and/or an enlarged uterus. Alternatively it may be inadequate because of the inability to assess the peritoneal cavity, obtain peritoneal washings, perform lymphadenectomy, reliably perform salpingoophorectomy or divide adhesions. Laparoscopy enables these inadequacies of VH to be overcome.

Pelvic inflammatory disease has various end-stage features and consequently it is not surprising that the extent of the end-stage disease cannot be predicted from clinical examination.[10–12] Clinical history and pelvic examination, even if the latter is performed under general anaesthetic, have also been demonstrated to be poor indicators of the extent of endometriosis,[11,13–15] the severity of adhesions and the mobility of the adnexa in patients with prior pelvic surgery.[16,17] Poor positive and negative predictive values for clinical examination were also experienced by Lundberg et al[18] in a study of women with pelvic pain. Unfortunately, contraindications to VH are still expressed in such terms[19] – the presence of such factors, however, demands further investigation rather than TAH.

Suspected adnexal pathology is also considered as a contraindication to VH but laparoscopic findings frequently prove the severity of the disease, as estimated by pelvic examination, to be in error. Although ultrasonic and Doppler evaluation of adnexal masses represents a significant step forward in defining a pelvic mass preoperatively, they cannot disclose the mobility of a mass or give an accurate assessment of its malignant potential.[20–22] Magnetic resonance imaging offers significant advantages over ultrasound and computed tomography in terms of diagnostic accuracy,[23] however, its availability and expense limit its usefulness at present. Estimation of tumour markers such as Ca125 may improve diagnostic accuracy,[24] however, laparoscopy remains the gold standard conservative investigation for adnexal masses of uncertain origin and may be performed before hysterectomy to assess whether laparotomy is really necessary.

Most of the traditional contraindications to vaginal surgery are questionable and if other investigations are inadequate laparoscopy should be performed. The surgeon can then decide on the optimum route of hysterectomy based on actual pelvic pathology and his experience and surgical skills. If the ratio of TAH to VH is to be reversed and patients to benefit, the compulsion to perform TAH must be controlled. Although laparoscopy prior to hysterectomy may lead to longer overall anaesthetic time, the reduced postoperative morbidity associated with vaginal surgery would more than compensate for this as laparotomies would be avoided.

SURGICAL TECHNIQUE

All surgery in our unit was carried out under general anaesthesia, and cephalosporin and metronidazole administered as prophylactic antibiotic cover. Laparoscopic hysterectomy was performed as previously described.[25,26] The laparoscope was inserted through a subumbilical incision, and usually two 5 mm secondary portals were used for the laparoscopic instruments. Surgery was performed by viewing the image generated by a Supercam 9050PB video chip camera (Storz) attached to a 30° forward oblique laparoscope. The principal method of haemostasis was bipolar electrosurgical desiccation (ESD) using a Force 2 electrosurgical generator (Valleylab); however, Endo-GIA 30 linear staplers (LS) (Auto Suture Ltd) were used in eight women.

The operative technique can be broken down into component parts: the laparoscopic procedure progressing as a TAH, and the vaginal procedure being commenced after varying degrees of laparoscopic surgery as described below. After inspection of the pelvis, upper abdomen, and taking pelvic washings if necessary, any distortion of the pelvic anatomy was corrected by adhesiolysis. Procedures such as ablation of endometriosis, pelvic lymphadenectomy, omental biopsy or isolation of ovarian masses using a containment technique,[27] can also be performed before hysterectomy is commenced. Careful attention is paid to the path of the ureters, but they are not routinely dissected out.

Vaginal hysterectomy can be performed after diagnostic laparoscopy (stage 0 LH), or after laparoscopic adhesiolysis has made this possible (stage 1 LH). The presence of adhesions to the body of the uterus does not necessarily exclude the possibility of vaginal hysterectomy as they may not distort the pelvic anatomy and can be divided during the hysterectomy or after the uterus has been delivered. The presence of adhesions closing the pouch of Douglas, leaving the bladder high on the uterus, or keeping the ovaries fixed in the ovarian fossae when oophorectomy is necessary, do, however, preclude a conventional vaginal approach. This is because of the risk of bowel or bladder perforation when colpotomy is performed, or ureteral injury when vaginal oophorectomy is attempted. Such adhesions, however, can be excluded and/or divided using a combined laparoscopic approach. In difficult cases when small bowel adhesions or severe endometriosis are encountered the difficulty of the adhesiolysis may exceed that of the hysterectomy itself, and if the pathology exceeds the surgeon's laparoscopic skills laparotomy must be performed.

When the ovaries were conserved, bipolar diathermy was used medially to desiccate the round and ovarian ligaments, and the fallopian tube. The approach to the ovarian pedicle when oophorectomy was performed depended on whether the uterine vessels were to be divided laparoscopically or vaginally. If the uterine pedicles were to be divided vaginally, we coagulated and divided the ovarian vessels but not the round ligaments. Dissection then proceeded along the mesosalpinx towards the uterine origin of the round ligament after which the hysterectomy was completed vaginally (stage 2 LH) or after laparoscopic mobilization of the bladder (stage 3 LH). If the bladder is mobilized it is reflected down below the level of the cervix using sharp and blunt dissection, with careful attention being paid to the vascular cervicovesical ligaments found at the lateral part of the dissection. If the uterine vessels were treated laparoscopically (stage 4 LH), the round ligaments were divided together with the ovarian vessels and fallopian tubes, and the dissection continued to the level of the uterine arteries. Time can be wasted by serial desiccation and division of the ascending branch of the uterine artery. It is not necessary to bring the dissection close to the uterus until the origin of the ascending branch of the uterine artery is identified. At this level the artery can be desiccated and cut and the dissection continued caudally, close to the uterus, until the transverse cervical ligaments laterally and uterosacral ligaments posteriorly are reached completing the laparoscopic portion of a stage 4 LH. Laparoscopic dissection only continued beyond the uterine artery in three patients (stage 5 LH), all other procedures were completed vaginally.

The vaginal components of LH procedures were performed using a modified Heaney approach.[28] Dissection commenced with a circumferential incision around the cervix below the line of the bladder. The vagina was dissected off the cervix allowing anterior and posterior colpotomies to be performed. Using retractors as necessary, the remainder of the vaginal hysterectomy was completed in a routine fashion taking each pedicle in turn. Once the uterus had been freed from its supports it was removed vaginally, using morcellation or coring techniques[29–31] if required. The vault was closed vaginally after which a pneumoperitoneum was re-established and the pelvis inspected laparoscopically to ensure haemostasis and to allow peritoneal lavage. Even after stage 5 LH the vagina was usually closed vaginally. The vagina can be closed laparoscopically; however, it is quite time consuming and care must be taken to incorporate the cervical ligaments into the closure to ensure good vaginal support, this latter point being important as the ligaments can retract from the vaginal edge leaving it relatively unsupported when the dissection has been laparoscopic.

The laparoscopic part of the operation is performed with the patient in a dorsal position with the legs abducted, and with no or minimal hip flexion. The lack of hip flexion, however, makes vaginal surgery difficult owing to poor access, and before the vaginal procedure is started the legs are moved to attain maximal hip flexion.

A linear stapler was used for eight stage 4 LH procedures involving bilateral salpingo-oophorectomy. The stapler was introduced through 12 mm cannulae and positioned to secure the major pedicles in a stepwise fashion, with care being taken to avoid inadvertent inclusion of the ureters or bladder in the jaws of the gun. As with ESD, the ureters were not routinely dissected out but the bladder was reflected caudally in all cases.

DATA COLLECTION

In addition to noting the overall operating time, 56 of the 75 laparoscopic procedures were videotaped. The tape was only stopped at the end of surgery to allow the vaginal component of the surgery to be accurately timed. Analysis of these recordings allowed the individual surgical steps of a laparoscopic hysterectomy to be timed, based on the classification scheme of Johns & Diamond.[7] (Table 20.1).

The incidence of intraoperative and postoperative complications, febrile morbidity, analgesia requirements, and postoperative in-patient stay were documented in all cases. Patients were reviewed 6–8 weeks after surgery when they completed a questionnaire regarding their recovery. Sixty patients, including all in the randomized study, also kept a prospective record of their recovery for 6 weeks using a diary. Statistical analysis was performed using the Mann–Whitney U-test, regression analysis and Student's t test.

RESULTS

Seventy five patients who underwent LH procedures performed using either electrosurgical or stapling techniques have now been followed up for at least 6 weeks.[26] The patient characteristics and primary indications for surgery are summarized in Table 20.2. Seventy (93.3%) of the 75 laparoscopic hysterectomies were completed by the intended route; five had to be converted to TAH. All stages of LH were performed although in the majority of cases the uterine artery was divided laparoscopically: stage 0, 1.3%; stage 1, 2.7%; stage 2, 20%; stage 3, 5.3%; stage 4, 60%; and stage 5, 4%; the remaining 5 (6.7%) required laparotomy and underwent TAH. The mean uterine size was 8 weeks (range 4–16) and 56 patients underwent oophorectomy. Adhesiolysis was necessary in 35 patients and other prehysterectomy procedures such as ablation of endometriosis, lymphadenectomy, omental biopsy,

Table 20.2 Patient characteristics and primary indications for LH and VH

	Observational series	Randomized study	
		LH	VH
Patient characteristics			
Number of patients	75	22	23
Mean age (years)	45 (22–71)	41 (27–51)	45 (33–68)
Mean uterine size (weeks)	8 (4–16)	9 (4–15)	8 (4–16)
Previous LSCS	9 (16%)	4 (18%)	2 (9%)
Previous pelvic surgery	44 (65%)	14 (64%)	16 (70%)
Nulliparous	23 (26%)	6 (27%)	4 (17%)
Oophorectomy performed	56 (81%)	9 (41%)	8 (35%)
Primary indications for surgery			
Fibroids/menorrhagia	38	16	16
Pelvic pain/endometriosis	10	4	3
Dysmenorrhoea	9	2	4
Early endometrial carcinoma	5	–	–
Adnexal mass	9	–	–
Other (e.g. PMS, incontinence)	4	–	–

Reproduced with permission from Richardson[26]

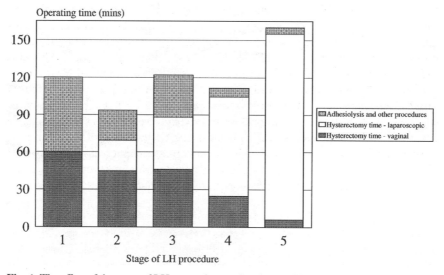

Fig. 1 The effect of the stage of LH on total operating time and hysterectomy time. Reproduced with permission from Richardson[26]

appendicectomy and 'in-a-bag' techniques[27] were performed in some patients. The mean operating time for all patients was 121 minutes (range 56–285). Video analysis showed that adhesiolysis and other pre-hysterectomy procedures considerably lengthened overall operating times (Fig. 20.1). After excluding such preparatory manoeuvres, there was a direct relationship between the stage of the procedure and time taken to complete the hysterectomy (Fig. 20.1). For instance, a stage 4 LH took significantly longer than a stage 2 procedure (105 versus 66 minutes, $P<0.001$). In contrast, neither increasing uterine size (Fig. 20.2a) nor oophorectomy (Fig. 20.2c) influenced LH procedure times.

Complications of the operation

In our series of 75 cases of LH,[26] laparotomy was necessary in five patients and occurred twice in the first 10 cases. Dense adhesions were responsible for laparotomy in two women, and large uterine size and haemorrhage were factors in two other patients. The laparoscopic approach was abandoned in a fifth patient with Turner's syndrome who had a body mass index (BMI) of 43, and her stature led to difficulties in maintaining a pneumoperitoneum. Cystotomy occurred twice in this series, once during the vaginal part of an LH and once during TAH. Other major complications included subacute bowel obstruction following extensive adhesiolysis prior to LH, vault haematoma, and intraoperative haemorrhage. Minor complications included equipment failure, persistent pyrexia, urinary tract infections, asymptomatic bacturia and prolonged nausea. The overall complication rate was 33%, but 18% after excluding complications not contributing to patient morbidity, such as equipment failure and asymptomatic pyrexia but including laparotomy, cystotomy, subacute obstruction, pelvic and vault haematomas, symptomatic urinary infection and blood transfusion.

In published series the incidence of complications varies widely and ranges between 2.4[32] and 33%[26] (Table 20.3). This is not entirely unexpected as case selection between series differs markedly, as does the consistency of reporting both major and minor complications. In addition, most series consist of less than 50 patients and will include the lower end of the surgeons' learning curve, which inflates the complication rate, and it is notable that two of our five laparotomies occurred in our first 10 cases. Therefore, further, larger, and preferably comparative, series are required before the value of LH in terms of morbidity can be judged.

In-patient stay and recovery after laparoscopic hysterectomy

Many reports of LH rely upon in-patient stay as a marker for recovery and the 'invasiveness' of the technique. In-patient stay is, however, very dependent on local policies and therefore comparison of in-patient stay between series is not useful. In our own series we have noticed that as we have become more experienced patients have gradually been discharged earlier without any special community care arrangements.[26] The average postoperative stay was 4.2 days (range 1–16), although this has shortened during the course of the series with the last 10 patients staying for only 2.5 days (range 1–4), which is in general agreement with other European groups.[47,48] American series tend to have shorter in-patient stay but this is linked with more intensive community care arrangements.[46]

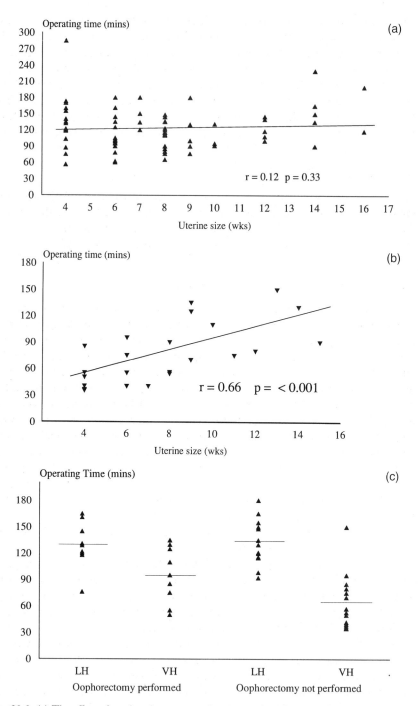

Fig. 20.2 (a) The effect of uterine size on operating time at LH; (b) the effect of uterine size on operating time at VH; (c) the effect of oophorectomy on operating times at LH and VH. Adapted with permission from Richardson[26]

Patients returned to normal activities after a mean of 26 days (range 7–56), and those employed went back to work after 6.8 weeks (range 2–13). A significant finding in our series is that the rate of postoperative recovery appears to be independent of the stage of LH performed – recovery after all stages was similar (Table 20.4). Therefore, as operative times increase substantially as more of the hysterectomy is performed laparoscopically (Fig. 20.1), without advantage in terms of recovery, the vaginal procedure should be commenced as soon as laparoscopic surgery has made this possible.

COMPARATIVE STUDIES

Although there have been numerous studies, including one of 215 cases by a single author,[43] there have been relatively few comparing LH with TAH or VH. Including our own data the number of patients enrolled into such studies is low; however, a number of important points have emerged.

Laparoscopic versus abdominal hysterectomy

In a small prospective study involving 20 patients, Nezhat et al[37] compared LH with TAH. Patients in whom pelvic pathology precluded vaginal hysterectomy were assigned to the different treatment groups alternately rather than randomly – the groups were thus poorly matched. The mean uterine weight in the TAH group was heavier as more patients had fibroids (165 versus 213 g) and grade III and IV endometriosis was more common in the LH group (7 versus 3). Mean operative time in the LH group was longer (160 versus 102 minutes) but the greater prevalence of severe endometriosis in the LH group may have accounted for some of this difference. Hospital stay and time taken to resume normal activities were, however, both shorter after laparoscopic surgery (4.2 versus 2.4 days and 5 versus 3 weeks). In addition, there were fewer minor complications in the LH group. Analgesic requirements were not compared. In this study all patients in the LH group underwent stage 5 procedures using electrosurgical desiccation (ESD) and patient characteristics suggested significant adhesiolysis, and excision of endometriotic deposits would have been necessary in most cases.

In a similar study, Phipps and Nayak[38] showed that analgesic requirements, in-patient stay and time off work were all significantly less after LH. In this study the treatment groups were better matched, the main indication for TAH being a wish to perform oophorectomy, but again the mean operating time in the LH group was significantly longer (65 versus 30 minutes). It was difficult to perform a direct comparison of the two studies owing to entirely different case selection; this was emphasized by the difference in operative times for abdominal hysterectomy between the two studies (30 versus 102 minutes). Factors contributing to a shorter operative time in the LH group in this latter study include: the use of a stapling device, the lack of ureteric dissection and significant adhesiolysis, and the fact that stage 4

Table 20.3 Morbidity after laparoscopic hysterectomy

Authors	Number of cases	Average stage of procedures	Haemostatic technique used	Mean operative time (mins) (range)	Mean in-patient stay (days) (range)	Mean estimated blood loss (ml) (range)	Laparotomies	Complication rate*	Types of major complications
Kovac et al (1990)[33]	46	0–1	–	56 (35–90)	3.8 (3–7)	–	4	15.2%	Cystotomy
Pruitt & Stafford (1992)[34]	60	3	ESD, staples, sutures	–	1–2	–	0	23%	Postoperative haemorrhage
Saye et al (1993)[32]	167	3	Staples	59 (28–142)	23h (median)	200 (25–1200)	4	2.4%	None
Howard & Sanchez (1993)[35]	15	3	ESD	169 (+/- 36)	3.7 (+/- 1.7)	532 (+/- 279)	0	13%	Laceration of inferior epigastric artery, pelvic infection
Richardson et al (1995)[26]	75	3.4	ESD, staples	121 (56–285)	4.2 (1–16)	–	5	33%	Cystotomy, subacute obstruction, haemorrhage
Minelli et al (1991)[36]	7	3.6	ESD	144 (90–180)	4	<150	0	–	–
Nezhat et al (1992)[37]	10	4	ESD	160 (130–230)	2.4 (2–3)	210 (100–350)	0	10%	None
Phipps et al (1994)[38]	114	Less than stage 4 = 52 Stage 4 or greater = 62	Staples	LAVH = 65 (50–100) LH = 82 (60–120)	48 h (36 h–8 days)	–	5	–	Haemorrhage, ureteric injury, pelvic abscess, colostomy
Reich et al (1993)[39]	123	Less than stage 4 = 30 Stage 4 or greater = 93	ESD, staples, sutures	180 (45–370)	2 (1–5)	250	2	13.8%	Fistula, ureteral injury, pulmonary embolus, cystotomy, enterotomy
Shearer (1993)[40]	35	4–5	Staples	120#	2.25#	–	3	8.6%	–
Bishop (1993)[41]	10	5	ESD	170 (105–270)	2.7	–	0	16%	Cystotomy, cuff cellulitis, postoperative haemorrhage
	15†	5	Staples	90 (60–150)	0.9	–	0		

Langebrekke et al (1992)[42]	10	5	ESD, staples	120 (85–210)	2.3 (1–5)	<150 (20–150)	0	20%	Haemorrhage, ureteric injury
Liu (1992)[43]	395	5	ESD, staples	102 (45–340)	1.2 (1–5)	85 (25–1000)	5	4.5%	Cystotomy, fistula, bowel burn, Richter's hernia, death
Maher et al (1992)[44]	17	5	ESD	152 (90–220)	3.1 (2–5)	44 (20–200)	0	5.9%	None
Padial et al (1992)[45]	75	5	ESD, staples	121	2.37 (1–5)	295 (25–1300)	0	19.6%	Haemorrhage > 500 ml
Summitt et al (1992)[46]	29	5	Staples	120.1 (50–245)	< 12 h (median)	203.8 (25–500)	1	13.8%	Cystotomy, laceration of inferior epigastric artery, hernia

* Major and minor complications, including laparotomy, described by the authors.

Excluding cases when other procedures were performed ($n = 25$).

† All cases from a single series – ESD used on the first 10 cases.

Adapted with permission from Richardson RE, Magos AL. Laparoscopic hysterectomy. In: Asch R, Studd J, eds. Progress in Reproductive Medicine Vol II, chapter 21, pp 251–266. 1995 Parthenon Publishing Group

Table 20.4 Effect of the stage of LH on recovery

Stage	n	Opiate injections	Analgesia required (days)	In-patient stay (days)	Discomfort (days)	Normal activities (days)
0	1	3	1	1	7	14
1	2	3	2	2	4	27
2	15	3.3 (3)	3 (2)	5 (2)	8 (5)	25 (14)
3	4	2	3	4	7	25
4	45	2.4 (2)	3 (3)	4 (2)	10 (6)	27 (12)
5	3	3	2	3	13	27

Numbers in parentheses are standard deviations.
Reproduced with permission from Richardson RE, Magos AL. Laparascopic hysterectomy: five years on. Contemporary Reviews in Obstetrics and Gynaecology 1995; 7: 36–43

rather than stage 5 LH procedures were carried out in all cases. This latter study also included a cost comparison revealing a 10-fold increase in intraoperative costs in the LH group. This was accounted for by the use of disposable products, with the bulk of the cost being the disposable stapling gun and staples. The advantages of LH over TAH in terms of less postoperative pain, reduced in-patient stay and sickness benefit were clearly demonstrated, but the value of the linear stapler is unclear as its use adds substantially to the cost of the operation.

Howard and Sanchez[35] performing stage 3 LH procedures, predominantly using ESD, have also compared LH with TAH. Although the patients were not randomly allocated there were no significant differences between the groups in terms of patient characteristics and pelvic pathology. The results of this study were similar in that although mean surgical time was longer (169 versus 119 minutes), in-patient stay was shorter (3.7 versus 5.2 days), and postoperative pain less in the LH group. This study failed to show any significant economic advantage of performing LH, despite the infrequent use of linear staplers, and patients were discharged earlier because of higher operating costs associated with LH. These higher costs arose because of longer operating times and the use of disposable surgical items other than linear staplers.

Laparoscopic versus vaginal hysterectomy

In our unit we have compared LH with VH in a prospective randomized trial.[26] Patients who would have normally undergone TAH were randomly assigned to undergo LH or VH. The laparoscopic cases were performed using ESD, and the VHs using a modified Heaney technique. When oophorectomy was combined with VH the technique of transvaginal endoscopic oophorectomy[49] was used in some cases. With this technique, after packing back the bowel, endoscopic instruments were used through the vagina to perform the oophorectomy. The laparoscope allowed the path of the ureter to be visualized right up to the pelvic brim and proved valuable in enabling vaginal oophorectomy to be performed safely in difficult cases.

In addition to the usual postoperative and follow-up observations all the patients in the study were requested to prospectively complete a diary of their recovery.

The two groups were well matched in terms of age, parity, previous pelvic surgery and indications for surgery (Table 20.2). The average stage of the laparoscopic procedures was 3.6 (3 stage 2, 2 stage 3, 15 stage 4 and 2 stage 5 LH). Oophorectomy was performed in nine patients in both groups, the technique of transvaginal endoscopic oophorectomy being used in three of the vaginal cases.[49]

Uterine size ranged from 4–16 weeks and although the average uterine size in the LH group was slightly larger this difference was not statistically significant. The mean operative time was significantly longer with laparoscopic surgery (LH 131 min, VH 77 min, $P<0.001$). In the VH group, increasing uterine size substantially lengthened the duration of surgery, and the time difference between LH and VH narrowed with increasing uterine size as there was a significant positive correlation between size and procedure time for VH ($P<0.001$) (Fig. 20.2b) but not for LH (Fig. 20.2a). Similarly, oophorectomy lengthened the time taken to perform VH but not LH, but it was still significantly quicker to perform oophorectomy at vaginal than laparoscopic surgery (oophorectomy performed: LH 129.7 min, VH 95.3 min, $P<0.05$; oophorectomy not performed: LH 132.7 min, VH 64.7 min, $P<0.001$) (Fig. 20.2c).

Laparotomy occurred once in each group. This was caused by haemorrhage in association with a fibroid uterus in the LH group and cystotomy in the VH group. Cystotomy also occurred during the vaginal part of an LH procedure but this was closed without the need for laparotomy. Laparoscopy was performed once in the VH group because of minor but persistent bleeding from an ovarian pedicle after vaginal oophorectomy, with haemostasis being achieved using ESD without the need for a laparotomy. Estimated operative blood loss and perioperative haemoglobin (Hb) changes were similar in the two groups (blood loss: LH 272 ml, VH 181 ml, $P>0.5$; fall in Hb: LH 1.24 g/dl, VH 1.05 g/dl, $P>0.5$). According to the definitions already given, the overall complication rate was 36% in the LH group and 30% in the VH group, but 18% and 13%, respectively, after excluding those complications not contributing to patient morbidity.

Postoperative hospital stay was similar in both groups (LH 3.2 days, VH 3.3 days) and there were no readmissions. Recovery in terms of analgesia requirements, resumption of normal activities and work was similar in each group (Table 20.5, Figs 20.3a & 20.3b).

It would be advantageous to perform dissection laparoscopically if this procedure led to a less painful or quicker recovery; unfortunately, this is not the case. Although in-patient stay after LH in many descriptive series tends to be shorter than historical data of in-patient stay after VH, in our comparative study there were no significant differences in either in-patient stay, return to normal activities or work (Table 20.5). LH takes longer than vaginal

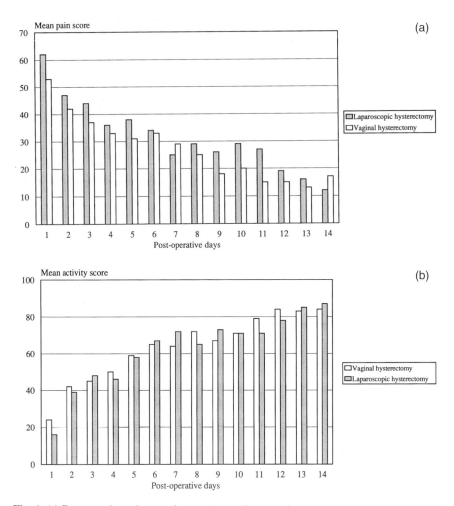

Fig. 3 (a) Postoperative pain scored on a 100 mm linear analogue scale; (b) ability to perform normal activities scored using a 100 mm linear analogue scale. Reproduced with permission from Richardson[26]

hysterectomy (VH), and as operative times increase substantially as more of the hysterectomy is performed laparoscopically, without advantage in terms of recovery, the vaginal procedure should be commenced as soon as laparoscopic surgery has made this possible or else time and effort are unnecessarily wasted. Indications to continue laparoscopic dissection include the completion of a subtotal LH, the need to secure the uterine artery laparoscopically such as when pelvic lymph node dissection is performed, or when it is preferable to perform a colpotomy under direct vision. A narrow vagina justifies a total laparoscopic hysterectomy but in our experience this is an infrequent indication. The major indication for proceeding with

Table 20.5 Operating time and recovery data from the randomized controlled study of laparoscopic hysterectomy (LH) versus vaginal hysterectomy (VH)

	VH (n = 23)		LH (n = 22)	
	Mean	Range	Mean	Range
Operating time (min)	76.7*	35–150	131.4*	76–180
Opiate injections	2.6	0–15	2.3	0–8
Analgesia required (days)	2.6	1–17	2.9	0–20
In-patient stay (days)	3.3	1–18	3.2	2–7
Discomfort (days)	9.5	2–19	10.2	1–21
Normal activities (days)	22.2	7–56	23.1	7–56
Work (weeks)	5.7	1.5–11	6.4	2–11

* P<0.001
Adapted with permission from Richardson[26]

Table 20.6 Effect of the stage of LH on mean operative times when linear staplers are used for the vascular pedicles

Authors	Number of cases	Stage of procedures	Haemostatic technique used	Mean operative time (min) (range)
Kovac et al (1990)[33]	46	0–1	–	56 (35–90)
Saye et al (1993)[32]	167	3	Staples	59 (28–142)
Phipps et al (1994)[38]	52	Less than stage 4	Staples	65 (50–100)
Phipps et al (1994)[38]	62	Stage 4 or greater	Staples	82 (60–120)
Summitt et al (1992)[46]	29	Stage 5	Staples	120 (50–245)

Reproduced with permission from Richardson RE, Magos AL. Laparascopic hysterectomy: five years on. Contemporary Reviews in Obstetrics and Gynaecology 1995; 7: 36–43

laparoscopic dissection beyond adhesiolysis necessary to allow vaginal hysterectomy is oophorectomy.

The increase in operative times as more of the hysterectomy is performed laparoscopically can also be seen in Table 20.6, where selected series using LS for haemostasis are compared.

LINEAR STAPLERS (LS) VERSUS ELECTROSURGICAL DESICCATION (ESD)

We have used both linear staplers (LS) and electrosurgical desiccation (ESD) to perform LH. ESD has the disadvantages of a moderate capital outlay, being a slower and perhaps a less haemostatic technique of securing large vascular pedicles, but the technique is more versatile and lacks the recurrent costs associated with stapling techniques. Linear stapling devices have been used in a number of series to attain haemostasis of the vascular pedicles at

Table 20.7 A comparison of bipolar and stapling techniques: operative time and postoperative recovery

Procedure step (minutes)	n	Bipolar diathermy	n	Stapling technique	
Ovarian pedicle*	45	27	8	21	P<0.05
Uterine pedicle*	32	34	8	22	P<0.001
Total operating time for stage 4 LAVH# mins	29	105	8	100	NS
Recovery					
Opiate injections		3		2	NS
In-patient stay (days)		4		4	NS
Analgesia required (days)		6		10	NS
Discomfort (days)		9		13	NS
Normal activities (days)		26		36	NS
Work (weeks)		7		6	NS

NS, not significant.
* Mean surgical time required to complete the procedure step (derived using video analysis).
# Excluding adhesiolysis and other procedures.
Reproduced with permission from Richardson RE, Magos AL. Laparoscopic hysterectomy: five years on. Contemporary Reviews in Obstetrics and Gynaecology 1995; 7: 36–43

LH.[32,38,41–43,46,50] Titanium staples are arranged in two triple-staggered rows and when the instrument is fired a blade simultaneously cuts the tissue between the two rows of staples as they are closed. Haemostasis and straight line dissection is achieved in a single action, which has potential advantages in terms of operating time, but disadvantages in terms of cost and versatility.

An attempt at comparing ESD and LS has been reported[41] and showed that when stage 5 LH procedures were performed on similar patient groups, the mean operative time with the ESD technique was much longer (170 versus 90 minutes) as was the mean length of in-patient stay (2.7 versus 0.9 days). The comparison in this study was, however, flawed as the techniques were used sequentially, with the stapling technique being used in the later cases. Therefore, the differences observed may have, in part or wholly, arisen from progress up the learning curve of operative technique and postoperative management. In our series we have certainly noticed that the length of in-patient stay has gradually decreased and postoperative stay is now significantly shorter.

In a study by Padial et al,[45] of 75 consecutive stage 5 LH procedures, both ESD and LS were used. Although the techniques were not directly compared, the average length of hospitalization in the stapling group was 2.17 days whereas it was 2.37 days for all patients. This suggests little or no benefit in terms of in-patient stay from sole use of the linear stapler.

Neither of these studies included comparative data for convalescence but in our own series we have not found any significant differences between the two operative techniques in terms of in-patient stay, analgesia requirements or time taken to resume normal activities (Table 20.7).[51]

The impact of LS devices on overall operative times depends on case selection and operator experience. From our own observations, use of the linear stapler for the ovarian or uterine pedicles reduces the time taken to perform these steps of the operation (Table 20.3). However, such devices are of little value when performing adhesiolysis, excision of endometriosis, bladder dissection or lymphadenectomy, and their impact on overall operative times in complex cases may be slight. In addition, the value of using LS to secure the uterine artery needs further clarification. Although the technique is faster, the width of the instrument and the proximity of the ureter to the artery makes its application in this area hazardous without exact clarification of ureteric position.[52,53] A transilluminating ureteric stent can be used to map the path of the ureter[54] or they can be dissected out. Both techniques, however, add to the overall operative time and contribute morbidity, which detracts from their value. Problems with bleeding between the end of the staple line and vaginal stitches have also been reported when stage 4 procedures are performed.[38] We have not encountered this problem using bipolar diathermy, although it occurred in two cases when the linear stapler was used. This complication created a need for additional haemostasis after completion of the vaginal procedure, which, together with longer bladder dissection times, accounted for similar overall operative times with both methods of haemostasis.

Current evidence suggests that the value of linear staplers is limited to their speed of application. Advantages over ESD in terms of reduced inpatient stay and speedier convalescence have not been proven. Our particular concern regarding the use of these instruments routinely is the size and location of the cannulae they require. Instrument design necessitates the use of at least 12 mm cannulae and requires them to be placed higher on the abdominal wall. This not only leads to a poorer cosmetic result but more than doubles the cannula size we currently use for ancillary ports, necessitating suture closure to prevent herniation[55,56] and probably increases postoperative pain.

With improving instrument technology and an expanding market the main disadvantages of linear staplers, namely size and expense, will almost certainly be addressed, and as ESD is not without limitations research into this area is also warranted.

NOVEL OPERATIVE TECHNIQUES INCLUDING SUBTOTAL LAPAROSCOPIC HYSTERECTOMY

Laparoscopic Doderlein hysterectomy

In this technique, described by Saye et al,[32] a stage 3 LH is performed using linear stapling and laser techniques – laparoscopic dissection stops short of the main branch of the uterine arteries. The uterus is then delivered through an anterior colpotomy and the uterine pedicles clamped before the cervical ligaments. This technique overcomes the problem of the uterine artery being avulsed if it is left intact but unsupported after vaginal division of the cervical ligaments because the artery is secured vaginally before the cervical ligaments are transected. It also keeps the linear stapler well above the ureter making routine ureteric dissection unnecessary.

In the above study the mean uterine size was 141 g, indicating that the technique is applicable only for the smaller uterus. The mean operative time was 59 minutes (Table 20.6). This demonstrates the potential of linear stapling techniques in reducing operating times when the uterine artery is not secured laparoscopically as the mean operative time, excluding prehysterectomy procedures, to perform stage 3 procedures using ESD in our study was 88 minutes (Fig. 20.1). This technique has recently been favourably reviewed as a simple, economic and secure method of performing LH.[57]

Laparoscopically assisted subtotal vaginal hysterectomy

We have modified this Doderlein technique to perform laparoscopically assisted subtotal vaginal hysterectomy. After completing a stage 3 LH the uterus is delivered through an anterior colpotomy and transected at the level of the internal os after securing the uterine artery. After haemostasis has been achieved the cervical stump is returned to the abdominal cavity. The risk of cervical stump neoplasia is low and this could be further reduced by removal of the endocervical mucosa using a reverse conisation procedure before returning the cervical stump to the abdominal cavity. This operation combines the safety of the Doderlein approach and allows the cervix to be retained without performing laparotomy in women requesting subtotal hysterectomy. The benefits of the latter operation include cervical conservation, which leaves the cervical ligaments and upper vagina anatomically undisturbed, and possibly less sexual dysfunction when compared with total hysterectomy.[58]

Donnez and Nisolle[59] have published an account of laparoscopic supracervical (subtotal) hysterectomy. They performed stage 4 procedures on 32 patients using ESD before cutting the corpus from the cervix using a monopolar knife. The detached body of the uterus was delivered through a posterior colpotomy. The average duration of surgery did not exceed 90 minutes, and all patients left hospital the day following surgery although the report did not include convalescence data. Lyons has also described laparoscopic supracervical hysterectomy (LSH).[60] His technique included various refinements such as transection of the uterus below the internal os, and removal of the endocervical mucosa. He also included data regarding convalescence and showed that, when compared with laparoscopically assisted vaginal hysterectomy, recovery after LSH was quicker, and is a finding worth further investigation. The disadvantage of both of these techniques is that as a stage 4 procedure is performed the risk of ureteral injury remains when the uterine artery is transected laparoscopically.

A totally laparoscopic subtotal hysterectomy has been described by Semm.[61] In this operation, known as CASH (Classical Abdominal Semm

Hysterectomy), laparoscopic dissection stops short of the uterine artery. The cervical transformation zone and endometrial cavity are then reamed out using a sharp edged cylinder introduced vaginally over a straight uterine probe – CURT (Calibrated Uterine Resection Tool). The resection tool is rotated and cuts through the cervix, isthmus, and then body of the uterus until the fundus is perforated. The resection tool is then withdrawn, together with the cylinder of tissue it contains, and the uterus ligated and transected in the isthmic region. The uterus is morcellated and is removed transabdominally using a SEMM set (Serrated Edged Macro-Morcellator). This operation has the advantage of not disturbing the cervical ligaments, uterine artery or ureter, and removing the transformation of the cervix, but specialized instruments are necessary which detracts from its value as a technique.

Ewen and Sutton[62] have reported the first British experience of laparoscopic supracervical hysterectomy using a modification of this technique. Operating times, hospital stay and return to full activities are comparable to our patients following LH; they were unable to confirm that recovery following supracervical hysterectomy was quicker than after LH.

THE FUTURE

Refined indications for laparoscopic hysterectomy

It is generally agreed that the main indications for LH are to convert a TAH into a vaginal operation, or a difficult VH into an easy one. The problem with these loosely described indications is that the rate of TAH is extremely high,[2] and many more hysterectomies could be performed vaginally as most contraindications to VH are only relative. This concept was explored by Kovac et al[29] who performed laparoscopy prior to hysterectomy on 46 patients in whom VH was considered inappropriate. The study confirmed the poor positive predictive powers of relative contraindications to VH as, after minimal operative laparoscopy, VH was completed in 91% of patients under the same anaesthetic. Therefore, although LH has been shown to be superior to TAH in terms of less postoperative pain, reduced in-patient stay, faster recovery and sickness benefit[35,37,63] the real comparison for the majority of cases is LH versus VH.

There are few advantages of LH over VH when the contraindications to the latter are only relative. Patients experience longer anaesthetics, require more analgesia, and do not recover more quickly. In addition, the speed of convalescence is not dependent on the amount of dissection performed laparoscopically. The only clear advantage of the laparoscopic approach to hysterectomy is in allowing pelvic surgery that cannot be completed vaginally to be performed without laparotomy, and the indications for the procedure should reflect this. Therefore, the further investigation and laparoscopic treatment of suspicious adnexal masses, the division of adhesions preventing vaginal colpotomy, ablation of symptomatic endometriosis and the need for lymphadenectomy are all good indications for a combined approach. Once these procedures have been completed we consider it unnecessary to continue with laparoscopic dissection if the procedure can be completed vaginally. This is especially true if the indication for a combined approach is oophorectomy and the only exception would be an extremely poor vaginal access.

The training necessary to acquire the skills essential to performing a stage 5 LH safely is not rewarded by quicker patient recovery when compared with VH. It is, however, easy to perform a diagnostic laparoscopy and if this then extends a surgeon's indications for vaginal surgery we would strongly recommend it. This is because LH, whatever stage, is definitely less invasive than TAH. It should always be remembered, however, that VH is the least invasive technique, and laparoscopic dissection should be discontinued as soon as the operation can be completed vaginally.

The use of laparoscopic hysterectomy in the management of gynaecological malignancies

Progress in laparoscopic surgery has made laparoscopic pelvic lymphadenectomy possible and surgically satisfactory in experienced hands. At present, experience of laparoscopic para-aortic lymphadenectomy is limited.

In cases of apparently early ovarian cancer, pelvic nodes may remain negative despite the presence of positive aortic nodes. Therefore, without adequate infra-renal para-aortic sampling, laparoscopic treatment of early ovarian carcinoma, even with containment techniques which isolate the ovarian mass from the peritoneal cavity, may be considered as surgically inadequate. The laparoscopic approach using containment techniques, however, remains a valid extension of diagnostic techniques in the management of a suspicious adnexal mass when hysterectomy is planned, as the vast majority of such cysts are benign.

In a case report on laparoscopic para-aortic node sampling, Querleu combined a stage 2 laparoscopic hysterectomy with laparoscopic pelvic and infra-renal para-aortic lymph node sampling and infra-colic omentectomy on a patient presenting with borderline serous ovarian carcinoma.[64] Twelve pelvic nodes and nine para-aortic nodes were obtained in a procedure lasting 270 minutes. All lymph tissue was negative and the patient was discharged the day following surgery.

Total lymphadenectomy with excision of the parametrial tissue is of therapeutic value in some patients with cervical carcinoma. The disease is staged surgically and provides an excellent indication for laparoscopic lymphadenectomy (LLA) allowing those who are not suitable for radical surgery to avoid laparotomy and commence radiotherapy earlier. Querleu et al have performed pelvic LLA in 39 patients to stage early (IB–IIB) carcinoma of the cervix. The procedure typically lasted 90 minutes, and between three and 22 lymph nodes were removed without significant morbidity. Five patients had metastatic nodes and were treated with radiation treatment alone, whilst the remainder underwent radical surgery; either Schauta-Amreich radical vaginal hysterectomy or Wertheims abdominal radical hysterectomy. No unexpected metastatic node was observed at laparotomy, giving a sensitivity of 100% and proving the accuracy of LLA in their hands. To go one step further in the laparoscopic management of cervical cancer, both laparoscopic radical hysterectomy and laparoscopically assisted radical hysterectomy have been described.[65–68] It remains to be proven that these radical laparoscopic hysterectomies are any better than the classic Schauta's operation preceded by laparoscopic lymphadenectomy.[69]

The value of pretherapeutic laparoscopic staging of stage I endometrial carcinoma by LLA is limited as surgery is required whatever the nodal status. Pelvic LLA can, however, be combined with LH for surgical treatment of patients with low risk stage I disease. Although such patients could be considered as inadequately staged without para-aortic sampling, the level of understaging in node negative patients would be minimal in this low risk group.

Case reports have been written proving that almost any surgical procedure can be achieved laparoscopically by experienced surgeons. The expansion of laparoscopy into the field of gynaecological oncology from second look procedures to staging and treatment must not, however, be at the expense of standards and these reports must be followed by prospective trials to assess their value and safety in the treatment of patients with early malignancy.

CONCLUSIONS

The rate of abdominal hysterectomy is undoubtably too high. The presence of contraindications to vaginal surgery demands further investigation, rather than abdominal hysterectomy, and if these are inadequate laparoscopy should be performed. Once an LH procedure has been commenced the surgeon can decide on the optimum route of hysterectomy based on actual pelvic pathology and his own particular experience and surgical skills.

The benefits and potential savings of LH over TAH in terms of less postoperative pain, reduced in-patient stay and sickness benefit have been demonstrated. When compared with vaginal hysterectomy, however, LH appears to be the inferior operation. Patients experience longer anaesthetics, require more analgesia, and do not recover more quickly – to perform an LH when simple vaginal hysterectomy is possible confers no advantage to the patient. The aim of an LH is to convert an abdominal hysterectomy into a vaginal procedure or convert a difficult vaginal hysterectomy into an easy one. However, as patients do not recover more quickly from a hysterectomy performed laparoscopically, when compared with vaginal surgery, laparoscopic dissection should be halted as soon as it is possible to complete the operation vaginally.

The stage has been set for LH to play a major role in reversing the ratio of abdominal to vaginal hysterectomy, which is currently about 4:1 in most units. Diagnostic laparoscopy (stage 0 LH) should correct the compulsion to perform abdominal hysterectomy for poor indications, and operative laparoscopy (stages 1–5 LH) convert abdominal and difficult vaginal hysterectomies into routine vaginal procedures.

REFERENCES

1 Coulter A, McPherson K, Vessey M. Do British women undergo too many or too few hysterectomies? (Review). Soc Sci Med 1988; 27: 987–994

2 Vessey M P, Villard-Mackintosh L, McPherson K, Coulter A, Yeates D. The epidemiology of hysterectomy: findings in a large cohort study. Br J Obstet Gynaecol 1992; 99: 402–407

3 Reich H, DeCaprio J, McGlynn F. Laparoscopic hysterectomy. J Gynecol Surg 1989; 5: 213–216

4 Reich H. Laparoscopic hysterectomy. Surg Laparos Endosc 1992; 2(1): 85–88

5 Garry R, Reich H, Liu C Y. Editorial. Laparoscopic hysterectomy – definitions and indications. Gynaecol Endosc 1994; 3: 1–3

6 Munro M G, Parker W H. A classification system for laparoscopic hysterectomy. Obstet Gynecol 1993; 82: 624–629

7 Johns D A. Laparoscopic assisted vaginal hysterectomy (LAVH). In: Sutton C, Diamond M, eds. Endoscopic surgery for gynaecologists. London: W B Saunders Co. Ltd, 1993: 179–186

8 El Torkey M M. Hysterectomy in patients aged 35 years and under: Indications and complications. Obstet Gynaecol Today 1990; 1: 44–49

9 Dicker R C, Greenspan J R, Strauss L T et al. Complications of abdominal and vaginal hysterectomy among women of reproductive age in the United States. The collaborative review of sterilization. Am J Obstet Gynecol 1982; 144: 841–848

10 Ledger W J. Laparoscopy in the diagnosis and management of patients with suspected salpingo-oophoritis. (Review). Am J Obstet Gynecol 1980; 138: 1012–1016

11 Lee N C, Dicker R C, Rubin G L, Ory H W. Confirmation of the preoperative diagnoses for hysterectomy. Am J Obstet Gynecol 1984; 150: 283–287

12 Morcos R, Frost N, Hnat M, Petrunak A, Caldito G. Laparoscopic versus clinical diagnosis of acute pelvic inflammatory disease. J Reproduct Med 1993; 38: 53–56

13 Friedman H, Vogelzang R L, Mendelson E B, Neiman H L, Cohen M. Endometriosis detection by US with laparoscopic correlation. Radiology 1985; 157: 217–220

14 Chatman D L. Endometriosis in the black woman. Am J Obstet Gynecol 1976; 125: 987–989

15 Williams T J, Pratt J H. Endometriosis in 1,000 consecutive celiotomies: incidence and management. Am J Obstet Gynecol 1977; 129: 245–250

16 Coulam C B, Pratt J H. Vaginal hysterectomy: is previous pelvic operation a contraindication? Am J Obstet Gynecol 1973; 116: 252–260

17 Kjer J J. Laparoscopy after previous abdominal surgery. Acta Obstet Gynecol Scand 1987; 66: 159–161

18 Lundberg W I, Wall J E, Mathers J E. Laparoscopy in evaluation of pelvic pain. Obstet Gynecol 1973; 42: 872–876

19 Thompson J D, Birch H W. Indications of hysterectomy. Clin Obstet Gynecol 1981; 24: 1245–1258

20 Meire H B, Farrant P, Guha T. Distinction of benign from malignant ovarian cysts by ultrasound. Br J Obstet Gynaecol 1978; 85: 893–899

21 DePriest P D, van Nagell J R, Jr. Transvaginal ultrasound screening for ovarian cancer. (Review). Clin Obstet Gynecol 1992; 35: 40–44

22 Bourne T, Campbell S, Steer C, Whitehead M I, Collins W P. Transvaginal colour flow imaging: a possible new screening technique for ovarian cancer. Br Med J 1989; 299: 1367–1370

23 Scoutt L M, McCarthy S M. Imaging of ovarian masses: magnetic resonance imaging. (Review). Clin Obstet Gynecol 1991; 34: 443–451

24 Schwartz P E. Ovarian masses: serologic markers. (Review). Clin Obstet Gynecol 1991; 34: 423–432

25 Broadbent J A M, Magos A L. Laparoscopically assisted vaginal hysterectomy. Contemp Rev Obstet Gynaecol 1992; 4: 154–157

26 Richardson R E, Bournas N, Magos A L M. Is laparoscopic hysterectomy a waste of time? Lancet 1995; 345: 36–41

27 Amso N N, Broadbent J A M, Hill N C W, Magos A L. Laparoscopic 'oophorectomy-in-a-bag' for removal of ovarian tumours of uncertain origin. Gynaecol Endosc 1993; 1: 85–89

28 Heaney N S. A report of 565 vaginal hysterectomies performed for benign pelvic disease. Am J Obstet Gynecol 1934; 28: 751–755

29 Kovac S R. Intramyometrial coring as an adjunct to vaginal hysterectomy. Obstet Gynecol 1986; 67: 131–136

30 Grody M H T. Vaginal hysterectomy: The large uterus. J Gynecol Surg 1989; 5: 301–312

31 Magos A, Bournas N, Sinha R, Richardson R E, O'Connor H. Vaginal hysterectomy for the large uterus. Br J Obstet Gynaecol 1996; 103(3): 246–251

32 Saye W B, Espy III G B, Bishop M R, Slinkard P, Miller W, Hertzmann P. Laparoscopic Doderlein hysterectomy: A rational alternative to traditional abdominal hysterectomy. Surg Laparosc Endosc 1993; 3(2): 88–94

33 Kovac S R, Cruikshank S H, Retto H F. Laparoscopy-assisted vaginal hysterectomy. J Gynecol Surg 1990; 6: 185–193

34 Pruitt A B, Stafford R H. Laparoscopic-assisted vaginal hysterectomy: A continuing evolution of surgical technique. J S Carolina Med Assoc 1992; September: 433–436

35 Howard F M, Sanchez R. A comparison of laparoscopically assisted vaginal hysterectomy and abdominal hysterectomy. J Gynecol Surg 1993; 9: 83–90

36 Minelli L, Angiolillo M, Caione C, Palmara V. Laparoscopically-assisted vaginal hysterectomy. Endoscopy 1991; 23: 64–66

37 Nezhat F, Nezhat C, Gordon S, Wilkins E. Laparoscopic versus abdominal hysterectomy. J Reproduct Med 1992; 37: 247–250

38 Phipps J H, John M, Hassanaien M, Saeed M. Laparoscopic- and laparoscopically assisted vaginal hysterectomy: a series of 114 cases. Gynaecol Endosc 1994; 2: 7–12

39 Reich H, McGlynn F, Sekel L. Total laparoscopic hysterectomy. Gynaecol Endosc 1993; 2: 59–63

40 Shearer R A. Laparoscopic-assisted vaginal hysterectomy: Report on 32 initial cases. Surg Laparosc Endosc 1993; 3(3): 191–193

41 Bishop M. Laparoscopic hysterectomy: How should it be done? Surg Laparosc Endosc 1993; 3(2): 127–131

42 Langebrekke A, Skar O J, Urnes A. Laparoscopic hysterectomy. Initial experience. Acta Obstet Gynecol Scand 1992; 71: 226–229

43 Liu C Y. Laparoscopic hysterectomy. Report of 215 cases. Gynaecol Endosc 1992; 1: 73–77

44 Maher P J, Wood E C, Hill D J, Lolatgis N A. Laparoscopically assisted hysterectomy. Med J Aust 1992; 156: 316–318

45 Padial J G, Sotolongo J, Casey M J, Johnson C, Osborne N G. Laparoscopy-assisted vaginal hysterectomy: Report of seventy-five consecutive cases. J Gynecol Surg 1992; 8(2): 81–85

46 Summitt R L Jr, Stovall T G, Lipscomb G H, Ling F W. Randomized comparison of laparoscopy-assisted vaginal hysterectomy with standard vaginal hysterectomy in an outpatient setting. Obstet Gynecol 1992; 80: 895–901

47 Querleu D, Cosson M, Parmentier D, Debodinance P. The impact of laparoscopic surgery on vaginal hysterectomy. Gynaecol Endosc 1993; 2: 89–91

48 Hourcabie J A, Bruhat M A. One hundred and three cases of laparoscopic hysterectomy using endo-GIA staples and a device for presenting the vaginal fornices. Gynaecol Endosc 1993; 2: 65–72

49 Magos A L, Bournas N, Sinha R, Lo L, Richardson R E. Transvaginal endoscopic oophorectomy 1995; 172(1 Pt 1): 123–124

50 Nezhat C, Nezhat F, Silfen S L. Laparoscopic hysterectomy and bilateral salpingo-oophorectomy using multifire GIA surgical stapler. J Gynecol Surg 1990; 6: 287–288

51 Richardson R E, Broadbent J A M, Bournas N G, Magos A L. Post-operative recovery following laparoscopically assisted vaginal hysterectomy. Gynaecol Endosc 1994; 3 (Suppl 1): 49 (Abstract)

52 Woodland M B. Ureter injury during laparoscopy-assisted vaginal hysterectomy with the endoscopic linear stapler. Am J Obstet Gynecol 1992; 167: 756–757

53 Kadar N, Lemmerling L. Urinary tract injuries during laparoscopically assisted hysterectomy: Causes and prevention. Am J Obstet Gynecol 1994; 170: 47–48

54 Phipps J H, Tyrrell N J. Transilluminating ureteric stents for preventing operative ureteric damage. Br J Obstet Gynaecol 1992; 99: 81

55 Kadar N, Reich H, Liu C Y, Manko G F, Gimpelson R. Incisional hernias after major laparoscopic gynecologic procedures. Am J Obstet Gynecol 1993; 168: 1493–1495

56 Milkins R C, Wedgwood K R. Incisional hernia following laparoscopic surgery: two unusual cases and literature review. Min Invas Ther 1994; 3: 35–38

57 Garry R. The evolution of a technique for laparoscopic hysterectomy: laparoscopic-assisted Doderlein's hysterectomy. Gynaecol Endosc 1994; 3: 123–128

58 Kilkku P, Gronroos M, Hirvonen T, Rauramo L. Supravaginal uterine amputation vs. hysterectomy. Effects on libido and orgasm. Acta Obstet Gynecol Scand 1983; 62: 147–152

59 Donnez J, Nisolle M. Laparoscopic supracervical (subtotal) hysterectomy (LASH). J Gynecol Surg 1993; 9: 91–94

60 Lyons T L. Laparoscopic supracervical hysterectomy using the contact Nd: YAG laser. Gynaecol Endosc 1993; 2: 79–81

61 Semm K. Hysterectomy via laparotomy or pelviscopy. A new CASH method without colpotomy. (German). Geburtshilfe und Frauenheilkunde 1991; 51: 996–1003

62 Ewen S, Sutton C J G. Initial experience with supracervical laparoscopic hysterectomy and removal of the cervical transformation zone. Br J Obstet Gynaecol 1994; 101: 225–228

63 Phipps J H, John M, Nayak S. Comparison of laparoscopically assisted vaginal hysterectomy and bilateral salpingo-oophorectomy with conventional abdominal hysterectomy and bilateral salpingo-oophorectomy. Br J Obstet Gynaecol 1993; 100: 698–700

64 Querleu D. Laparoscopic para-aortic node sampling in gynecologic oncology: a preliminary experience. Gynecol Oncol 1993; 49: 24–29

65 Nezhat C, Burrell M, Nezhat F, Benigno B, Welander C E. Laparoscopic radical hysterectomy with para-aortic and pelvic node dissection. Am J Obstet Gynecol 1992; 166: 864–865

66 Canis M, Mage G, Wattiez A, Pouly J L, Chapron C, Bruhat M A. Vaginally assisted laparoscopic radical hysterectomy. J Gynecol Surg 1992; 8: 103–105

67 Querleu D. Hysterectomies elargies de Schauta-Amreich et Schauta-Stoeckel assistees par coelioscopie. J Gynecol Obstet Biol Reproduc 1991; 20: 747–748

68 Kadar N, Reich H. Laparoscopically assisted radical schauta hysterectomy and bilateral laparoscopic pelvic lymphadenectomy for the treatment of bulky stage Ib carcinoma of the cervix. Gynaecol Endosc 1993; 2: 135–142

69 Trope C, Iverson T. Laparoscopic radical hysterectomy: technical gimmick or surgical advance? Gynaecol Endosc 1993; 2: 83–84

21 What the gynaecologist should know about breast cancer risk, management and follow-up

P. Neven

Breast cancer is one of the most common cancers among women. It is estimated that 1 in 12 women will develop breast cancer at some time in their life. Overall mortality is second only to lung cancer but breast cancer is the commonest single cause of all deaths in women aged 35–54.

This chapter on breast cancer reviews information for the obstetrician/gynaecologist treating women at risk for breast cancer development and those surviving it. Risk factors together with information on screening, diagnosis, management and follow-up are considered.

BREAST CANCER RISK

Multiple risk factors which increase a woman's breast cancer risk have been identified. These range from high-risk conditions such as lobular carcinoma of the breast in situ, to reproductive factors, such as nulliparity, with only a small increase in risk.

Reproductive factors/endogenous hormones

The breast shows dramatic changes in size, shape and function during life: growth, puberty, pregnancy, lactation, postlactational involution and involution by ageing. Female hormones play, in an interactive way with exogenous factors and lifestyle, a crucial role in the development of breast cancer.[1] Whether hormonal events, during reproductive years or after the menopause, are related to development of breast cancer or to the speed at which breast tumour grows is unknown.

A vast amount of literature on reproductive variables and breast cancer risk has been reviewed.[2,3] The age-incidence curves for breast cancer are similar with those for endometrial and ovarian cancer. Frequent cyclical hormone exposure during the years of active ovulation increases breast cancer risk. A greater number of menstrual cycles before the first full-term pregnancy[4] and a shorter menstrual cycle[5] (a women spends more time in the luteal phase) have been associated with increased breast cancer risk.

Moderate physical activity with its impact on ovarian function reduces breast cancer risk.

Oestrogens, progestins and prolactine have, together with insulin and other growth factors, a synergistic relationship in promoting breast epithelial proliferation. The degree of breast cell division during the menstrual cycle differs between the proliferative and the luteal phase; oestrogens induce some cell division, but oestradiol and progesterone together induce more.[6]

The oestrogen-augmented-by-progestogen hypothesis explains why there is a protective effect of late menarche, early menopause, early oophorectomy and premenopausal obesity (anovulation) on breast cancer risk. All are associated with a decreased breast exposure to both oestrogens and progestins. Postmenopausal obesity is a breast cancer risk factor because of elevated levels of bioavailable oestrogens (and decreased binding protein).

It should be emphasized, however, that no clear and consistent abnormality was found in urine and blood oestrogens, progesterone, prolactin, androgens, luteinizing hormone (LH), follicle-stimulating hormone (FSH), and thyroid-stimulating hormone (TSH) in women with benign or malignant breast diseases.[7,8]

Pregnancy and lactation

The effect of pregnancy on breast cancer risk is complex. An early age at first delivery reduces the risk of breast cancer. Before the age of 30 and with an increasing number of full-term pregnancies there are changes in the breast that render the tissue less susceptible to carcinogenic agents together with a protective effect caused by long-lasting changes in the hormonal milieu.[9] This decreases breast cancer risk later in life (45–54 and older) but the question as to whether there is a transiently increased risk shortly after a full-term pregnancy[10] compared to nulliparous women is unsettled and has recently been questioned.[11] The view that age at first full-term pregnancy is the principal reproductive variable related to breast cancer risk has also been challenged. Kalache et al[12] found that late age at any or last birth is a breast cancer risk factor independent of age at first birth and parity, probably by accelerating the growth of occult breast cancers. Long-term lactation slightly reduces the risk of breast cancer in young women irrespective of the duration of lactational amenorrhea.[13,14] Lactation does not reduce breast cancer risk in postmenopausal women; hormones to inhibit the flow of milk may be associated with a small increase in the risk of breast cancer.[15] Abortion prior to first full-term pregnancy, whether spontaneous or induced, has no protective effect. Uncertainty remains about premenstrual tenderness and infertility on breast cancer risk.

Family history and other gynaecological cancers

Family history is probably the most widely recognized breast cancer risk factor. Women with several affected relatives may face a lifetime risk level of

50%. The occurrence of breast cancer early in life, bilaterally or with tumours of other organs (particulary the ovary) suggests an underlying genetic susceptibility. In women with hereditary breast cancer both the mutated P53 and the BRCA1 gene have been identified. The BRCA1 gene, located on the chromosomal region 17q12–q23, has previously been associated with early-onset breast cancer. This gene is estimated to account for about 45% of families with several cases of breast cancer and up to 67% of such families where the age at onset of the cancers is less than 45.[16] Almost all families with epithelial ovarian cancer in addition to several cases of breast cancer carry the BRCA1 gene.[17] However, it has to be said that only a small proportion of breast cancers (5%) are caused by highly penetrant dominant genes.[16] In the absence of a pedigree consistent with genetic breast cancer, a woman whose mother or sister has the disease has a relative risk of 1.5 to 3.0, with a ninefold increase in risk with bilateral premenopausal breast cancer in a first degree relative.

Epidemiological studies suggest that breast and ovarian cancer share other common etiological factors because women with breast cancer have twice the expected incidence of ovarian cancer, and women with ovarian cancer have a three- to fourfold increased risk of developing carcinoma of the breast. Breast and ovarian cancer may have similar oncogenes.[18]

Endometrial cancer has also been reported in association with breast cancer both as an antecedent in individuals, and with family pedigrees. Such an association might occur because of common genetic and environmental determinants (such as diet), because of carcinogenic modalities used to treat the first neoplasm (see below) or as a statistical coincidence when two diseases share descriptive predictors, such as, in the case of breast/endometrium and endometrium/breast, parity, obesity and age at menopause.

Breast cancer can metastasize to the female genital tract and to the peritoneal surface. Uterine polyps, leiomyomata and ovaries containing breast cancer tissue have been reported.

The oral contraceptive pill

Numerous epidemiological analyses have focused on whether oral contraceptive (OC) use may increase the risk of breast cancer because most of the known risk factors for breast cancer are related to steroid hormones. Results from the Cancer and Steroid Hormone (CASH) Study, the Swedish Study, the UK National Case-Control Study, the Australian Case-Control Study and the World Health Organization (WHO) Study have been reviewed.[19] Overall, there is no evidence of an increased risk of breast cancer in women who meet the criterion of 'ever' (generally < 5 years) having used OCs. These studies mostly addressed OC use in the later reproductive years. In early reproductive years (under age 36), the estimated relative risk of breast cancer was 1.43 after 4–8 years' use and 1.74 for 8 years of total OC use irrespective of its relation with intake during specific reproductive milestones. The excess risk drops rapidly after the drug is stopped suggesting a late stage-promoting rather than an initiating effect.[20–24]

Many questions remain, especially regarding the risk of OC use prior to a first full-term pregnancy, prolonged use after age 40 and the possibility of a latent effect.[25] Little information is available on the effect of low-dose oestrogens and the new generation progestins that are currently employed.

Yet, any increase in risk of breast cancer with long-term OC use may be counterbalanced by a reduced risk of endometrial and ovarian cancer.[26]

As with combined OCs, the progestogen-only pills (POP) reduce the incidence of benign breast disease. A 35–40% lower breast cancer risk in long-term POP users was reported with a 15% reduction in the relative risk of breast cancer per year of use.[22]

In vitro evidence suggests that some synthetic progestins, especially the 19-nortestosterone derivatives, exert oestrogenic effects through the oestrogen receptor. This may increase the 'total oestrogenic' content of an OC. MPA did not stimulate cell proliferation.[27]

Hormone replacement therapy

Breast cancer is, for many, the main concern regarding the use of hormone replacement therapy (HRT).[28] It is now clear that risk is only marginally increased, and survival of breast cancer may be improved among current and past users of HRT.[29]

In Grady's meta-analysis of 39 studies, the risk of breast cancer with oestrogen-only hormone therapy ranged from 0.2 to 3.1 (and with added progestogens from 0.2 to 4.4).[30]

A different relationship between breast cancer and HRT was found among current or recent/past users of oestrogens as opposed to more remote use. 'Ever use' of oestrogen replacement therapy showed little breast cancer risk.[31] After 15 years of use the RR was 1.30. Steinberg et al[32] performed a meta-analysis of studies of the effect of oestrogens on risk of breast cancer, with controls being potential sources of heterogeneity. They found that conjugated equine oestrogens increased the risk of breast cancer after 10 years of oestrogen use by at least 15% and up to 29%. There was a suggestion of a modest increase in risk associated with synthethic oestrogens compared with conjugated equine oestrogens. Equine oestrogens may not be converted to catechol oestrogens, previously associated with breast cancer. Because adding a progestin to the oestrogen regimen is protective for endometrial cancer, it has been suggested that adding a progestin to the oestrogen regimen might also be protective for breast cancer. Bergkvist et al[33] first reported an elevated RR of breast cancer of 4.4 in long-term (> 6 years) users of combined HRT relative to the general Swedish female population presumed to be non-users. Several questions have been raised regarding selection bias, detection bias and the fact that Bergkvists' risk estimate was based on only 10 cases of breast cancer; these questions were of special interest to those who found that combined HRT users had a lower breast cancer incidence than those not using it.[34] Combined data from published reports specifically addressing the hypothesis of whether the addition of progestins to oestrogen therapy increases breast cancer risk concluded that the addition of progestins to oestrogen replacement was not protective and does not reduce risk of breast cancer. These data do not support additional use of progestins among hysterectomized women on oestrogens.

HRT may induce mammographic changes such as symmetric and asymetric increase in breast density, increase in size of fibroadenomas and development or increase in size of breast cysts.[35] Oestrogen alone promotes enlargment of breast cysts and fibroadenomas, whereas treatment with combined oestrogen and progesterone is more likely to be associated with diffuse increase in fibroglandular tissue. This may interfere with mammographic screening for breast cancer.

Other hormones

Several studies have suggested a slightly increased risk of breast cancer (RR 1.3) in women who took diethylstilbestrol (DES) in pregnancy. The risk of breast cancer increased with the length of time since the exposure. These women should be encouraged to perform monthly breast self-examination, have breast examinations by their physicians yearly and follow the established recommendations for mammography screening.[36] The British Study by Vessey et al,[37] with a smaller number of patients, failed to show an increased breast cancer risk among those who took DES.

Epidemiological data studying any link between long-acting injectable contraceptives and hormonal implants and breast cancer risk are scarce. There is some evidence that breast cancer risk is increased in women who used depot-medroxyprogesterone acetate (DMPA) when very young (before age 25 for ever-use). Initial concerns about possible carcinogenic effects of long-term DMPA use in other age groups have turned out to be unfounded. The WHO includes DMPA on its list of essential drugs.[38] There is no data concerning oestradiol or testosterone implants in relation to breast cancer risk.

Interaction among risk factors

It is evident that most reports evaluating risk factors have considered only the variable under study, providing no information on its interaction with other risk factors. Reproductive variables may add to the breast cancer risk in women with a family history.[39]

The effect of oral contraceptives on risk of familial breast cancer is controversial. One study[40] found no significant effect associated with early use of OCs while another[41] showed that use of oral contraceptives was more prevalent in such women who developed breast cancer.

The advisability of prescribing HRT to women with a family history of breast cancer has been of clinical concern. Most studies are not sufficiently powerful to detect possible weak effects in familial subgroups, and results showing whether there is an interaction between family history and use of HRT on breast cancer risk are inconsistent.[16] HRT should, therefore, not be prescribed to all postmenopausal women, because some have no symptoms and no increased risk of osteoporosis or cardiovascular disease. However, oestrogens should not be withheld in the woman with a family history of ovarian-breast cancer who, therefore, undergoes an oophorectomy at early age. Benign breast disease does not appear to modify the relationship between HRT and the risk of breast cancer.[42] Benign breast disease (atypical hyperplasia) becomes a more important breast cancer risk factor when a woman also has a family history of breast cancer.[43]

The Collaborative Group on Hormonal Factors in Breast Cancer was formed in 1992 to collate worldwide evidence on the role of these factors. Almost all groups that have carried out epidemiological studies of breast cancer are participating in this international collaborative reanalysis of data. The results, based on more than 40 000 women with breast cancer, should make it possible to estimate how much of the variation in breast cancer risk can be attributed to hormonal and reproductive factors.[44]

BREAST CANCER DURING OR SHORTLY AFTER PREGNANCY

Approximately 15% of all breast cancers are seen in women of childbearing age and the current trend in many populations to delay pregnancy until a late age may increase this proportion. Young age is a poor prognostic factor for breast cancer[45] and part of this may be explained by the deleterious effect of concurrent or recent pregnancy on breast cancer survival.[46] The shorter the time between a pregnancy and the diagnosis of breast cancer, the greater the risk of mortality. However, when the age of the patient at diagnosis and the stage of disease are comparable in pregnant and non-pregnant patients, pregnancy has little influence on prognosis.[47]

Yet, a woman diagnosed with breast cancer during pregnancy or lactation is likely to fare worse than a woman of a similar age who is not pregnant.[48] The high prevalence of advanced disease (more likely node positive) implies that there may be a delay in diagnosis, but others linked this with the immunosuppressive effect of pregnancy. Breast examination should be part of the prenatal examination, and appropriate diagnostic tests (including mammography with shielding of the fetus) should be performed if any abnormality is noted. Cancer of the breast, diagnosed during pregnancy, should be staged and treated promptly in the same manner as for non-pregnant patients. The need for radiotherapy, chemotherapy or hormone therapy after surgical resection of the breast tumour will depend on the stage and tumour biology. Most breast cancers during pregnancy and lactation are oestrogen-receptor negative and the effect of hormone therapy may be negligible. Therefore, therapeutic abortion, ovarian ablation and other forms of endocrine therapy are not routinely indicated. Abortion may be advised if adjuvant therapy is started in the first trimester, or in the occasional case of rapidly progressing advanced disease. The risk to the fetus from irradiation of the breast depends upon the dose of radiation, distance of fetus from the field (hence gestational age), field size and energy of the radiation. It is clear that radiotherapy should be avoided if at all possible in the first trimester, as should chemotherapy. When administered during the first trimester of pregnancy, chemotherapy carries an approximate 10% risk of fetal teratogenesis. Adverse effects of chemotherapy are related to dose of the drug, synergism with other drugs and radiotherapy, and the pharmacology of the individual drug; antimetabolites (such as methotrexate) and alkylating agents are abortifacient and teratogenic.

No cases of maternal breast cancer metastasizing to the fetus have been documented. Placental metastases are extremely rare but have been reported.

SCREENING, DIAGNOSIS AND MANAGEMENT

An NHS breast screening programme has been in operation in the UK since 1988. It aims to reduce mortality from breast cancer by 25% by screening all women aged 50–64 every 3 years using single oblique view mammography.[49] Women receiving HRT do not need to have more frequent screening, and a baseline mammogram before receiving HRT is not required by this programme. The gynaecologist should encourage women to attend screening and provide information, advice, and reassurance at all stages of the screening process.[50]

For individual women the issues are not so straightforward. Some who perceive themselves to be at an increased risk of breast cancer (e.g. if they have a strong family history of the disease) might argue that the findings in the general population do not apply to them. Many argue that women with a family history of breast cancer should be offered routine mammography before they are 50 even if mammography is not very sensitive in this group. Others say that what needs to be done is to ensure that such women are properly informed and leave it to them and their doctors to decide what is most appropriate.[51]

In order to improve breast cancer in an early stage, a careful breast examination should be part of a routine gynaecological/obstetrical examination, not only in the women with a cancer history. Conventional mammography, ultrasound and fine needle aspiration or biopsy are indicated when an abnormal breast lump is palpated. All these investigations may be inadequately sensitive to detect breast cancer, especially in young patients. The dense breasts and diffuse growth pattern of the tumours make breast lesions difficult to identify in premenopausal women, especially during pregnancy and lactation. When all investigations are negative and the mass is persistent or there is diagnostic concern, excision biopsy is the only way of obtaining a definitive diagnosis. Small but significant advances have been made in the management of breast cancer. Conservative breast surgery (lumpectomy with axillary dissection) in combination with radiotherapy is, in most cases, as effective as mastectomy for the local control of the cancer. There is some debate on whether circulating female hormones have an impact on the basic mechanisms of tumour invasion and metastasis. Veronesi et al[52] found that disease-free survival was enhanced for the node-positive woman where breast surgery was performed during the luteal phase of the menstrual cycle.

The acceptance that 'early' breast cancer is often a systemic disease at diagnosis has led to various types of systemic 'adjuvant' therapy. About four in every five new patients with breast cancer are menopausal and among such women several years of tamoxifen, an antioestrogen, has little toxicity. Tamoxifen prolongs the disease-free interval and it has a definite survival benefit in women of different ages, different stages, whether receiving concurrent chemotherapy or not and irrespective of oestrogen-receptor status.[53] The steroid receptor status of breast tissue is, however, the best marker for predicting response to endocrine therapy.

Among younger women, tamoxifen shows distinct risk reductions but these are less definite than in postmenopausal women. Cytotoxic chemotherapy and other forms of endocrine therapy (aromatase inhibitors, LHRH agonists and ovarian ablation) confer a survival benefit in premenopausal women with breast cancer. The prognostic significance of chemotherapy-induced-amenorrhea[54] raises the possibility that some of the benefits of cytotoxic chemotherapy in young women is attributable to endocrine effects on ovarian follicles. There is renewed interest in the use of ovarian ablation as a form of systemic adjuvant therapy in premenopausal women on the basis of the meta-analysis[53] showing a reduction in annual mortality of 25%, similar to that seen in younger women using polychemotherapy. Ovarian ablation has continuing and additional benefits when combined with chemotherapy.

Among the most important issues currently under study are: the role of dose intensity of chemotherapy with and without cytokine support, the effect of the combined use of chemotherapy with various endocrine therapies, the role of preoperative chemotherapy, and the efficacy of therapy in relation to various prognostic and predictive factors.[2]

THE WOMAN SURVIVING BREAST CANCER

Many patients with breast cancer who appear to be disease-free after treatment have micrometastases and will eventually relapse and die with overt metastases. Lifelong follow-up has many important functions even though distant spread cannot be cured. Attention has not only turned to improving length of survival but also quality of life.

Case notes should contain detailed information on a woman's breast history. Women with breast cancer may need care for problems such as sexual dysfunction, contraception, subsequent pregnancy and HRT. Physical and psychological effects of breast cancer, which include severe depression, may, without relief, worsen psychological morbidity and quality of life.[55]

Subsequent contraception, pregnancy and HRT

Ovulation and menstruation can be maintained or re-established after chemotherapy or endocrine therapy (tamoxifen, LHRH-agonists). Bianco et al[54] found that 94% of premenopausal women over 40 years of age became amenorrhoeic after CMF compared with 31% of women 40 years or younger. In 12%, normal menses resumed after temporary drug-induced amenorrhea. Biochemical parameters of menopause (elevated FSH) may temporarily be raised and a subsequent pregnancy is not excluded. Considering the potential risk of OCs in women who have been treated for breast cancer, they are not recommended and other effective alternatives should be considered.

The hormonal changes with pregnancy, subsequent to breast cancer, may stimulate growth of the remaining breast cancer cells. In the past, breast cancer patients were advised against subsequent pregnancies. However, in some studies pregnancy was found to improve survival but they did not allow the assessment of whether such results were related to the possible beneficial biological effect of pregnancy itself or to a selection bias (i.e. those who feel well have children and those who are affected by the disease do not). Some called it the 'healthy mother effect'.[56] Most studies have concluded that a subsequent pregnancy does not adversely affect and therapeutic abortion does not improve the prognosis of women previously treated for breast cancer. Adjuvant chemotherapy and radiotherapy have no ill effect upon a subsequent pregnancy or upon the fetus, whereas continuing tamoxifen while pregnant may have.

Most clinicians advise patients who have been treated for cancer of the breast to wait 2 years before becoming pregnant. In advising a breast cancer patient regarding subsequent pregnancies, careful consideration of the individual situation is recommended: both the biological factors and the social, psychological and economic implications of bearing children whose mother has a potentially limited lifespan. Little is known about the effect of lactation on breast cancer relapse but most emphasize that this should be discouraged.

Most systemic treatments for breast cancer produce varying degrees of menopausal symptoms in premenopausal women. Because oestrogen replacement therapy has well documented health benefits, some clinicians may consider it for women who appear to be disease-free. This decision must be based on the theoretical risk of recurrence as well as on the potential health benefits. Treatment with HRT and tamoxifen has been recommended if symptoms are severe. Tamoxifen alone may increase vaginal oestrogenicity, bone calcium content and cardiovascular health, but some women will continue to suffer from hot flushes. Women with a small breast cancer, node-free and relatively non-agressive, may also do well on HRT but they should have strict supervision so that breast cancer is more likely to be detected at a stage which is associated with a high survival rate after treatment. Little evidence on whether HRT may increase the rate of relapse or induce new cancer exists, and a trial is urgently needed to address this problem.[55] Women with known secondary spread but who are severely disadvantaged by their oestrogen deficiency symptoms should initially be offered high-dose progestogens and if their symptoms persist, oestrogen should be added to the regimen until the symptoms subside.

Monitoring adjuvant therapy

The toxicology of tamoxifen has proved to be a controversial issue. The gynaecologist should be aware of potential unwanted effects of tamoxifen and help women to recognize them.[57] Premenopausal women on tamoxifen may have permanent or temporary amenorrhea, menstrual irregularity and hot flushes; increased vaginal discharge has been reported in both pre- and post-menopausal women. Tamoxifen is able to induce ovarian cysts. The impact of many years of ovarian stimulation by tamoxifen in young women and the effect of supraphysiological serum levels of 17β-oestradiol must be evaluated further. It should also be emphasized that tamoxifen is potentially terato-genic[58] and premenopausal women must be informed that pregnancy can occur while taking tamoxifen; a safe contraceptive must be considered.

Tamoxifen may stimulate the endometrium towards hyperplasia and polyp formation. Endometriosis, uterine fibroids and endometrial cancers have all occured during treatment with tamoxifen. Vaginal bleeding should always be investigated by hysteroscopy and endometrial curettage to exclude an endometrial cancer. Routine screening using transvaginal ultrasound (TVS) or hysteroscopy and endometrial sampling is feasible but may not be recommended because of the low incidence of endometrial cancer on tamox-ifen, the high false positive rate of TVS and the lack of established benefit from screening. As in women with an intact uterus, on HRT, a balance with progestins may eliminate or protect against uterine stimulation by tamoxifen. However, polyps have been found on combined treatment and tamoxifen remains a mystery drug which has effects on the uterus not seen with HRT.

PRIMARY PREVENTION

The majority of breast cancer occurs in women with no particular risk factor. Therefore, it has been suggested that the ideal prevention of breast cancer should be an incidental activity of a contraceptive or a hormone replacement drug that reduces breast cancer risk.[59]

A contraceptive based on GnRH-agonists in combination with low dose oestro-progesterones may result in significant reductions in mammographic densities, a breast cancer risk factor (D V Spicer et al, personal communica-tion). Tamoxifen has antioestrogenic and oestrogenic qualities. Safety moni-toring has encouraged national trials in many nations to evaluate tamoxifen as a breast cancer chemopreventative.[60] Regular screening for pelvic pathology with tamoxifen is recommended in healthy women. A thick endometrium in

TVS needs careful evaluation with hysteroscopy and endometrial biopsy to exclude (pre)cancerous conditions requiring treatment.[61]

CONCLUSIONS

The cause of breast cancer is not known and the great majority of women with breast cancer do not have any of the known risk factors. A large effect of reproductive variables and hormone therapy on breast cancer risk is excluded, however, this does not rule out some risk associated with a patient's menstrual and obstetrical history and with current or long-term use of female sex hormones.

For any woman, with inherited cancer or not, the key to eliminating mortality is early detection (secondary prevention); breast examination is an integral part of the gynaecological examination. The value of primary prevention with tamoxifen is currently being evaluated.

The breast cancer patient may present a number of challenges for the obstetrician/gynaecologist when discussing risk factors and treatment alternatives related with subsequent pregnancy, contraception and HRT.

REFERENCES

1 DeWaard F. Preventive intervention in breast cancer, but when? Eur J Cancer Prev 1992; 1: 395–399
2 Harris J R, Lippman M E, Veronesi U, Willett W. Breast cancer. N Engl J Med 1992; 327: 319–328, 473–480
3 Kelsey J L, Gammon M D, John E M. Reproductive factors and breast cancer. Epidemiol Rev 1993; 15: 36–47
4 Olsson H, Ranstam J, Olsson M L. The number of menstrual cycles prior to the first full term pregnancy—an important risk factor of breast cancer? Acta Oncol 1987; 5: 387–389
5 Whelan E A, Sandler D P, Root J, Smith K R, Voda A M. Menstrual cycle pattern and risk of breast cancer. Am J Epidemiol 1992; 136: A 965
6 Ferguson D J P, Anderson T J. Morphological evaluation of cell turnover in relation to the menstrual cycle in the 'resting' human breast. Br J Cancer 1981; 44: 177–181
7 Wang D Y, Fentiman I S. Epidemiology and endocrinology of benign breast disease. Breast Cancer Res Treat 1985; 6: 6–36
8 Moore J W, Thomas B S, Wang D Y. Endocrine status and the epidemiology and clinical course of breast cancer. Cancer Surv 1986; 5: 537–559
9 Russo J, Tay L K, Russo I H. Differentiation of the mammary gland and susceptibility to carcinogens. Breast Cancer Res Treat 1982; 2: 5–73
10 Williams E M I, Jones L, Vessey M P, McPherson K. Short term increase in risk of breast cancer associated with full term pregnancy. Br Med J 1990; 300: 578–579
11 Cummings P, Stanford J L, Daling J R, Weiss N S, McKnight B. Risk of breast cancer in relation to the interval since last full term pregnancy. Br Med J 1994; 308: 1672–1674
12 Kalache A, Maguire A, Thompson S G. Age at last full-term pregnancy and risk of breast cancer. Lancet 1993; 341: 33–36
13 UK national case-control study group. Breast feeding and risk of breast cancer in young women. Br Med J 1993; 307: 17–20
14 WHO collaborative study of neoplasia and steroid contraceptives. Breast cancer and prolonged lactation. Int J Epidemiol 1993; 22: 619–626
15 Newcomb P A, Storer B E, Longnecker M P et al. Lactation and reduced risk of premenopausal breast cancer. N Engl J Med 1994; 330: 81–87
16 Evans D G R, Fentiman I S, McPherson K, Asbury D, Ponder B A J, Howell A. Familial breast cancer. Br Med J 1994; 308: 183–187

17 Narod S A, Feunteun J, Lynch H T et al. Familial breast-ovarian cancer locus on chromosome 17q12-q23. Lancet 1991; 338: 82–83

18 Slamon D J, Godolphin W, Jones L A et al. Studies of the HER/neu proto-oncogene in human breast and ovarian cancer. Science 1989; 244: 707–712

19 Malone K E, Daling J R, Weiss N S. Oral contraceptives in relation to breast cancer. Epidemiol Rev 1993; 15: 80–97

20 Miller D R, Rosenberg L, Kaufman D W, Stolley P, Warshauer M E, Shapiro S. Breast cancer before age 45 and oral contraceptive use: new findings. Am J Epidemiol 1989; 129: 269–280

21 Romieu I, Willett W C, Colditz G A et al. Prospective study of oral contraceptive use and the risk of breast cancer in women. J Natl Cancer Inst 1989; 81: 1313–1321

22 UK national case-control study group. Oral contraceptive use and breast cancer risk in young women. Lancet 1989; i: 973–982

23 WHO collaborative study of neoplasia and steroid contraceptives. Breast cancer and combined oral contraceptives: results from a multinational study. Br J Cancer 1990; 61: 110–119

24 Wingo P A, Lee N C, Ory H W, Beral V, Peterson H B, Rhodes P. Age-specific differences in the relationship between oral contraceptive use and breast cancer. Obstet Gynecol 1991; 78: 161–170

25 McPherson K. Latent effects in the interpretation of any association between oral contraceptives and breast cancer. In: Benign breast disease (Proceedings of the 4th international benign breast symposium, Manchester). Lancashire: The Parthenon Publishing Group, 1991: 165–175

26 Vessey M P. Oral contraception and cancer. In: Filshie M, Guillebaud J, eds. Contraception: science and practice. London: Butterworths, 1989: 52–69

27 Jordan V C, Jeng M H, Catherino W H, Parker C J. The oestrogenic activity of synthetic progestins used in oral contraceptives. Cancer 1993; 71: 1501–1505

28 Pilote L, Hlatky M. Hormone replacement therapy after menopause; importance of heart disease in women's decision making. J Am Coll Cardiol 1994; 23: 51A

29 Hunt K, Vessey M, McPherson K. Mortality in a cohort of long-term users of hormone replacement therapy: an updated analysis. Br J Obstet Gynaecol 1990; 97: 1080–1086

30 Grady D, Rubin S M, Pettiti D B et al. Hormone therapy to prevent disease and prolong life in postmenopausal women. Ann Intern Med 1992; 117: 1016–1037

31 Steinberg K K, Thacker S B, Smith S J, Zack M M, Flanders W D, Berkelman R L. A meta-analysis of the effect of oestrogen replacement therapy on the risk of breast cancer. JAMA 1991; 15: 1985–1990

32 Steinberg K K, Smith S J, Thacker S B, Stroup D F. Breast cancer risk and duration of oestrogen use: the role of study design in meta-analysis. Epidemiology 1994; 5: 415–421

33 Bergkvist L, Adami H O, Persson I, Hoover R, Schairer C. The risk of breast cancer after oestrogen and oestrogen-progestin replacement. N Engl J Med 1989; 321: 293–297

34 Editorial. Gambrell R D. Oestrogen therapy and breast cancer. Int J Fertil 1990; 35: 202–204

35 Cyrlak D, Wong C H. Mammographic changes in postmenopausal women undergoing hormonal replacement therapy. Am J Radiol 1993; 161: 1177–1183

36 Greenberg E R, Barnes A B, Resseguie L et al. Breast cancer in mothers given diethylstilbestrol in pregnancy. N Engl J Med 1984; 311: 1393–1398

37 Vessey M P, Fairweather D V I, Norman-Smith B, Buckley J. A randomised double-blind controlled trial of the value of stilbestrol therapy in pregnancy: Long-term follow-up of mothers and their offspring. Br J Obstet Gynaecol 1983; 90: 1007–1017

38 Depot-medroxyprogesterone acetate (DMPA) and cancer: Memorandum from a WHO meeting. Bull WHO 1993; 71: 669–676

39 Sellers T A, Lawrence H K, Potter J D et al. Effect of family history, body-fat distribution, and reproductive factors on the risk of postmenopausal breast cancer. N Engl J Med 1992; 326: 1323–1329

40 Olsson H, Moller T R, Ranstam J. Early oral contraceptive use and premenopausal breast cancer – final report from a study in southern Sweden. J Natl Cancer Inst 1989; 81: 1000–1004

41 Black M M, Barclay T H C, Polednak A, Kwon C S, Leis H P, Pilnik S. Family history, oral contraceptive usage and breast cancer. Cancer 1983; 51: 2147–2151

42 Colditz G A, Egan K M, Stampfer M J. Hormone replacement therapy and risk of breast

cancer: Results from epidemiologic studies. Am J Obstet Gynecol 1993; 168: 1473–1480
43 Dupont W D, Page D L. Risk factors for breast cancer in women with proliferative breast disease. N Engl J Med 1985; 312: 146–151
44 Beral V. Personal communication, 1994 'Have we lost our way' by looking for new causes of breast cancer? Lancet Conference 'The Challenge of breast cancer'
45 de La Rochefordiere A, Asselain B, Campana F et al. Age as prognostic factor in premenopausal breast carcinoma. Lancet 1993; 341: 1039–1043
46 Guinee V F, Olsson H, Möller T et al. Effect of pregnancy on prognosis for young women with breast cancer. Lancet 1994; 343: 1587–1589
47 Petrek J A, Dukoff R, Rogatko A. Prognosis of pregnancy-associated breast cancer. Cancer 1991; 67: 869–872
48 Saunders C M, Baum M. Breast cancer and pregnancy: a review. J Royal Soc Med 1994; 86: 162–165
49 Austoker J. Screening and self examination for breast cancer. Br Med J 1994; 309: 168–174
50 Marchant D J. Breast cancer. Challenge and responsibility. Cancer 1993; 71: 1518–1522
51 Beral V. Breast cancer. Mammographic screening. Lancet 1993; 341: 1509–1510
52 Veronesi U, Luini A, Mariani L et al. Effect of menstrual phase on surgical treatment of breast cancer. Lancet 1994; 343: 1545–1547
53 Early breast cancer trialists' collaborative group. Systemic treatment of early breast cancer by hormonal, cytotoxic or immune therapy. Lancet 1992; 339: 1–15, 71–85
54 Bianco A R, Del Mastro L, Gallo C, Perrone F, Matano E, Pagliarulo C, De Placido S. Prognostic role of amenorrhea induced by adjuvant chemotherapy in premenopausal patients with early breast cancer. Br J Cancer 1991; 63: 799–803
55 Baum M. Hormone replacement and breast cancer. Lancet 1994; 343: 53
56 Sankila R, Heinävaara S, Hakulinen T. Survival of breast cancer patients after subsequent term pregnancy: 'Healthy mother effect'. Am J Obstet Gynecol 1994; 170: 818–823
57 Neven P, Shephered J H, Lowe D G. Tamoxifen and the gynaecologist. Br J Obstet Gynaecol 1993; 100: 893–897
58 Cullins S L, Pridjian G, Sutherland C M. Goldenhar's syndrome associated with tamoxifen given to the mother during gestation. JAMA 1994; 271: 1905–1906
59 Editorial. Baum M, Ziv Y, Colletta A A. Can we prevent breast cancer? Br J Cancer 1991; 64: 205–207
60 Powles T J, Jones A L, Ashley S E et al. The Royal Marsden Hospital pilot tamoxifen chemoprevention trial. Breast Cancer Res Treat 1994; 31: 73–82
61 Kedar R P, Bourne T H, Powles T J, Collins W P, Ashley S E, Cosgrove D O, Campbell S Effects of tamoxifen on the uterus and ovaries involved in a randomised breast cancer prevention trial. Lancet 1994; 343: 1318–1321

22 Primary cancer of the fallopian tube

F. Lawton   C. Lees   C. Kelleher

Although a common site of metastatic spread, primary tumours of the fallopian tube are rare. A great variety of benign tumours arise in the fallopian tube, most found incidentally at surgery and of no clinical importance. Some benign tumours, however, deserve mention. The commonest is the adenomatoid tumour, also known as a reticulo-endothelioma, which is usually only diagnosed on microscopic examination of the myosalpinx but may occasionally project from the serosa and be apparent at laparotomy. These tumours may be confused with other benign neoplasms, for instance lymphangiomas and leiomyomas, but also, more importantly, may be confused with malignant neoplasms such as mesotheliomas and low-grade adenocarcinomas. Tubal leiomyomas resemble their uterine counterparts and may undergo similar degenerative changes. Cystic teratomas of the tube have been reported but, unlike their ovarian equivalent, no cases of malignant change arising within such a teratoma have been reported.

The majority of tubal malignancies are secondary from the uterus or ovary or arise from malignant disease within the gastrointestinal tract. Most commonly, the primary cancer is the ipsilateral ovary where spread is by direct invasion, or from the contralateral ovary via transcoelomic spread. Spread from advanced cervical or uterine cancer occurs occasionally. A classification of fallopian tube tumours is given in Table 22.1.

TUBAL CANCER

The first case of tubal carcinoma was reported by Renaud to a meeting of the Manchester Pathological Society in 1847, whilst the first published case report appeared in 1888. Since then about 1500 or so cases have been documented in the world literature, but most series contain only a handful of cases. The reported annual incidence is approximately 3 per 1000 genital tract cancers or 3.6 cases per million cancers.[1] Owing to the rarity of the disease, studies of more than 30 patients are uncommon, and the limited experience at any one centre means that the natural history of the cancer, prognostic factors and treatment options are much less well defined than for other female genital tract cancers.

Table 22.1 Classification of fallopian tube tumours

Benign tumours	Malignant tumours
Adenomatoid	*Primary*
Leiomyoma	Adenocarcinoma
Teratomas	papillary
cystic	papillary-alveolar
solid	alveolar-medullary
Fibroma	Sarcoma
Fibroadenoma	Choriocarcinoma
Papilloma	*Secondary*
Lipoma	
Haemangioma	
Lymphangioma	
Mesothelioma	
Mesonephroma	

Large single institution reports rely on prolonged retrospective recruitment; for instance the 71 patients from the MD Anderson Hospital were treated over a 33 year period, whilst the Mayo Clinic experience of 47 patients was gained over a 19 year period.[2,3] Consequently, it is difficult to conclude much from these reports because surgical techniques, staging criteria and treatment protocols tend to vary during the prolonged recruitment period. Therefore, comparisons of interinstitutional treatment results are fraught with problems.

DIAGNOSIS

It is important to distinguish invasive tubal cancer from atypical epithelial hyperplasia – florid examples of the latter can show papillary formation, nuclear pleomorphism and mitotic activity and the abnormal epithelium can penetrate the muscularis. These changes can occur in association with tuberculosis (TB) and other bacterial infections. The criteria of Hu et al are usually applied to the diagnosis of primary tubal cancer as opposed to secondary spread of other cancers to the tube.[4] These criteria specify that the tumour should arise from tubal epithelium with the majority of the cancer located in the tube, that the histological features resemble a tubal pattern, that there is a demonstrable area of transition between normal and malignant endosalpinx and that the uterus and ovaries are either normal or contain less tumour than the tube.

AETIOLOGY

The aetiology of tubal cancer is unknown but early reports suggested an association with chronic tubal damage citing the high incidence of a history of infertility in patients with tubal cancer. Infertility rates of up to 70% have been reported and a high frequency of other synchronous benign gynaecological pathology – endometriosis, salpingitis, ovarian cysts, fibroids – has been noted.[2,5,6,7] Tuberculous salpingitis has also been reported as a co-existing finding in tubal cancer, but it appears that the rate of pelvic TB is no higher than in the general population.[8] It is likely that these associations are merely those of a rare tumour with relatively common pelvic pathologies. It is, of course, important to distinguish the adenomatous reaction to tuberculous infection of the tube from low-grade tubal cancer.

Papillary adenocarcinoma is the commonest histological type but, rarely, other primary malignancies – medullary carcinoma, lymphosarcoma and mixed mesodermal tumours – have been reported.[9] Glandular structures like those within serous ovarian carcinomas and psammoma bodies are sometimes reported and most tumours are moderately or poorly differentiated. Other, rarer cancers include endometrioid adenocarcinomas, squamous cell, clear cell and transitional cell carcinomas. Sarcomas of the fallopian tube are extremely rare, with only 35 cases worldwide of the 'commonest' variant – malignant mixed mullerian tumours. As with their uterine counterparts, the prognosis is poor; they are relatively radioresistant and show usually only a limited response to chemotherapy.

Carcinoma in situ has been reported, usually as an incidental finding during histological examination of 'normal' tubes excised during hysterectomy.[10] The significance of such a finding is unclear.

CLINICAL FEATURES

Primary adenocarcinoma of the fallopian tube has a mean age at diagnosis of 55 years, but cases have been reported in women aged 20 to over 80 years. Presenting symptoms are variable and non-specific but are, most commonly, abnormal vaginal bleeding or discharge and pelvi-abdominal pain. Other symptoms such as abdominal distension, urinary symptoms or non-specific gastrointestinal complaints occur. The frequency of these presenting complaints in five studies comprising 192 patients are given in Table 22.2.

Rarely is a diagnosis of fallopian tube cancer entertained preoperatively or even suspected at laparotomy and failure of diagnosis is, consequently, most often related to a lack of a high index of suspicion. There is also frequently,

Table 22.2 Tubal cancer – presenting symptoms in 192 patients (reproduced with permission)[7,11,16,22,28]

Symptom	
Vaginal bleeding	34%
Vaginal discharge	20%
Pain	23%
Abdominal distension	9%
Other	8%
Urinary frequency	3%
None	3%

Table 22.3 Clinical presentations which might suggest tubal cancer

---

The presence of the triad of symptoms – pain, serosanguinous discharge and a pelvic mass – *hydrops tubae profluens*.

Persistent unexplained abnormal vaginal bleeding or vaginal discharge with negative D&C, particularly in women aged over 40.

Persistent unexplained pelvic, lower abdominal and/or low back pain.

Unexplained abnormal cervical cytology.

Presence of an adnexal mass.

---

and like ovarian cancer, a delay in diagnosis of many months between the onset of symptoms and surgical exploration, because the presenting complaints are so non-specific.[7,11] In one series of 71 patients, the correct preoperative diagnosis was made in only 2 patients.[2] The classical triad of symptoms – a vaginal discharge that is profuse, recurrent and amber to red in colour, pain, and an adnexal mass, so-called *hydrops tubae profluens* – and first described in 1916 by Latzko, is reported rarely.

The diagnosis may be suspected when malignant glandular cells are detected in a cervical smear in a woman with negative colposcopic findings and negative cervical and endometrial histology. In such patients it has been suggested that vaginal ultrasound and recourse to laparoscopy may be useful diagnostic tools.[12]

The tumour marker CA125 may be elevated in cases of tubal cancer.[13] In one paper the authors reported two patients enrolled in a large ovarian cancer screening programme who had elevated CA125 levels (43 and 57 U/ml, normal = < 35 U/ml) and normal pelvic ultrasound examinations. In the first patient a 7 cm left-sided pelvic mass, which at laparotomy was found to be a primary tubal cancer, was eventually detected by ultrasound 11 months later after further raised CA125 levels at 3,6 and 9 months. In the second patient the diagnosis was made 3 months after the initial CA125 estimation. CA125, however, cannot distinguish tubal cancers from other, commoner gynaecological cancers nor from benign pathology.[14] Table 22.3 lists the clinical circumstances in which a high index of suspicion of the diagnosis of fallopian tube cancer might be entertained.

The most common preoperative finding is a pelvi-abdominal mass but, not suprisingly, rarely is a diagnosis of tubal cancer considered. In a total of 262 patients with tubal cancer in six recent series, the true diagnosis was suspected in only 6 cases.[2,3,7,11,15,16]

At laparotomy, gross tubal enlargement may suggest hydro-or pyosalpinx, but because tubal cancer is, typically, unilateral the finding of a macroscopically normal contralateral tube should emphasize the possibility of the latter diagnosis. Small lesions may produce no visible tubal abnormality although the tube may feel abnormal. It is not an unreasonable maxim that

Table 22.4 Staging system for tubal cancer (modified Erez's classification)

Stage	Criteria
I	Tumour limited to the tube, either mucosal or with muscularis invasion.
IIA	Tumour has breached the serosa but there is no invasion of adjoining organs.
IIB	Tumour invading surrounding pelvic organs.
III	Metastatic lesions outside the pelvis but within the abdominal cavity.
IV	Extra-abdominal disease.

an abnormal tube at laparotomy should not be ignored. In more advanced cases, with large tumour masses encompassing the ovary and adjacent bowel and pelvic sidewall, the clinical distinction from ovarian or even uterine cancer may be impossible.

STAGING AND SPREAD OF THE DISEASE

The most frequently used staging system resembles the FIGO classification for ovarian cancer and defines the limits of stage I, II and III disease as the fallopian tubes, the pelvic organs and peritoneum and extrapelvic stuctures (bowel, omentum, lymph nodes), respectively. Like ovarian cancer staging, stage IV disease includes pleural effusions or intrahepatic metastases. This system is practical inasmuch as it will be familiar to most gynaecologists, but contains many subdivisions. Consequently, few institutions will have enough patients in any one stage to allow a meaningful analysis of prognostic factors or to compare results.

From a prognostic point of view, a better staging system, resembling the Dukes' system for colon cancer, was suggested by Erez et al in 1967 and is shown in Table 22.4.[17] This system acknowledges that the primary tumour arises in a hollow viscus and emphasizes that, in early stage disease, tubal penetration and therefore lymphatic spread is important, and that in later stage disease, gross spread, resembling that of ovarian cancer over peritoneal surfaces, assumes importance.

Approximately two-thirds of patients present with stage I or II disease according to the FIGO system, whereas the Erez system leads to an almost equal distribution of cases between the four stages.[18] This is not merely staging system semantics but has important prognostic and clinical implications. Peters et al demonstrated that in disease limited to the tube the depth of invasion of the wall correlated with the risk of treatment failure.[19] Overall, life table analysis showed only a 55% chance of 5 year survival for FIGO stage I disease but for those patients where there was no tubal wall penetration the chance of 5 year survival was 80%. This fell to 60% if the depth of invasion was less than 50% penetration, and to less than 20% if there was deeper invasion. Clearly, if the FIGO system is unable to distinguish between these subgroups of stage I disease, it will be of little help in evaluating risk of recurrence and, therefore, will be of limited prognostic significance.

The parenchymal lymphatic drainage of the fallopian tubes is extensive, which facilitates the spread of disease once the serosa had been breached. In a small series of 15 patients, para-aortic lymph node metastases were reported in one-third of patients with inguinal, mediastinal and supraclavicular deposits.[20]

The other major mechanism of spread is transcoelomic migration of malignant cells, either by spill of cells through the tubal ostium or by shedding of cells from the serosal surface once the tubal wall has been penetrated. Once this has occurred spread of fallopian tube cancer resembles that of ovarian cancer with spread to adjacent organs and to other sites within the peritoneal cavity.

SURGICAL FINDINGS AND MANAGEMENT

The tumour is bilateral in 10–20% of patients. The tube is usually swollen or distorted but, as mentioned previously, in some patients may look normal and even the intraoperative diagnosis may be wrong in 50% of cases.[8] In patients where the site of initial disease can be ascertained, the distal part of the tube seems to be involved much more often than the isthmus.[3,21]

Although total abdominal hysterectomy with bilateral salpingo-oophorectomy has been the most common surgical procedure, many reports have documented less complete surgery in the form of subtotal hysterectomy or unilateral salpingo-oophorectomy, presumably as a consequence of an unexpected diagnosis. The current recommendation is to carry out total abdominal hysterectomy, bilateral salpingo-oophorectomy and omentectomy. Retroperitoneal node sampling should be carried out, particularly for patients with disease confined clinically to the tubes, but it is unlikely that radical lymphadenectomy will have any impact on prognosis because the extensive tubal lymph drainage would necessitate complete pelvic, para-aortic and inguinal lymphadenectomy. In patients with advanced disease, tumour debulking should be attempted as the amount of tumour residuum, analogous to the situation with epithelial ovarian cancer, appears to be an important prognostic factor. In the study by Eddy et al the median survival for patients with no gross residual disease was 30 months, was 22 months when there was residual disease up to 2 cm in diameter and was 17 months for those with more extensive disease.[2] In the Mayo Clinic report the 5 year survival for patients with tumour residuum of 1 cm or less was 57%, whereas only 3 of 15 patients with more extensive disease were alive at 2 years.[3]

PROGNOSIS

The most important prognostic factor, again akin to ovarian cancer, is the stage or distribution of the disease at the time of diagnosis. In a recent report, combining survival figures from eight relatively large studies, Baeklandt et al reported the 5 year survival rate, for patients with disease confined to the tube at the time of diagnosis, to be about 60%, with survival for stage II disease at about 40%. Only about 10% of patients with advanced disease will survive 5 years.[12]

However, unlike ovarian cancer the prognostic significance of tumour grade seems minimal, with most reports showing little or no correlation between tumour differentiation and survival.[3,7,15,19] It should be remembered, however, that this may be a function of small patient numbers within each individual report. In addition, the fact that various histological patterns can be seen within individual cancers may further complicate the picture. Firm conclusions cannot be made as to whether the site of the cancer within the tube is of prognostic significance although it is logical to assume that those in the distal portion may have an increased propensity for early dissemination via the tubal lumen to the ovaries and other pelvic organs.

POSTSURGICAL THERAPY

Few reports contain enough patients, treated prospectively with standard regimens, to allow firm conclusions to be made about postsurgical therapy. However, using the analogy of ovarian cancer, treatment principles can be outlined. The morphological similarities between tubal epithelium and some serous ovarian cancers suggests that therapy effective in ovarian cancer might be appropriate in the management of tubal cancer. The poor survival rate for even patients with early stage cancer – the median survival for patients with FIGO stage I disease treated by surgery alone in one study was less than 3 years[2] – underlines the need for further postsurgical therapy in almost all stages of disease.

As with ovarian cancer radiotherapy delivered to the pelvis alone is inadequate, with Peters et al projecting 5 and 10 year survival rates after pelvic irradiation of only 29% and 15%, respectively.[19] Denham and Maclennan reported that 7 of 12 patients with stage I or II disease suffered relapses at extrapelvic sites following pelvic radiotherapy,[22] and McMurray et al reported that 50% of recurrences were in the upper abdomen, with 44% of their patients having evidence of extraperitoneal relapse.[15] In addition, Semrad et al documented that 10 of 14 patients had evidence of disease relapse outside the peritoneal cavity, of which 7 were within inguinal, mediastinal or supraclavicular nodes and three within the pleural cavity.[21] Clearly, local or loco-regional therapy is inadequate. Systemic therapy must be employed.

The use of chemotherapy in tubal cancer was described over 20 years ago with the conclusion that '. . . chemotherapy should be considered in the overall plan of management but requires further evaluation'.[23] Such evaluation, however, is difficult because most reports contain patients treated with a variety of adjuvant therapies – pelvic or whole abdominal radiotherapy, intraperitoneal radioisotopes and single or combination chemotherapy regimens – with few patient numbers in any therapeutic subgroup.

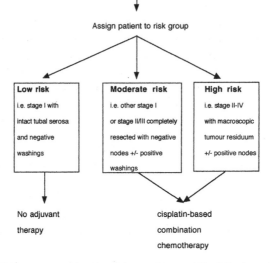

Fig. 22.1 Suggested management protocol for carcinoma of the fallopian tube.

An early report by Boronow indicated that disseminated tubal cancer was chemosensitive, documenting a complete response to alkylating agent therapy.[24] Deppe et al first reported the activity of cisplatinum in the disease with two surgically documented complete responses,[25] and further evidence of high activity has been provided subsequently by other groups. Maxson et al reported a clinical response rate of 92% in 12 patients, while Peters et al reported an 81% response.[19,26] However, the latter paper concluded that there was no clear advantage to any form of adjuvant therapy for patients with stage 1 disease but a significant improvement in median survival was shown for patients with extrapelvic disease treated with combination chemotherapy regimens compared with those receiving other forms of therapy (28 months versus 16 months; $P < 0.04$). In addition, all patients surviving more than 2 years received cisplatinum. From a number of reports it would seem that a response rate of more than 80% can be expected with the use of platinum-containing regimens, with a duration of reponse ranging from 12 months to more than 6 years.[3,15,27–29,30]

Hormonal therapy has yet to be evaluated in a significant number of patients although its use is, theoretically, attractive because normal tubal epithelium is clearly hormone sensitive in that it shows histological variation during the menstrual cycle.

In the absence of large, prospective studies it is not unreasonable to treat fallopian tube cancer by stage and risk category, as with ovarian cancer, using the strategy outlined in Fig. 22.1.

CONCLUSIONS

Advances in the diagnosis and management of this rare cancer have been made over the years and firm conclusions about certain aspects of the disease can be reached. The importance of a thorough staging laparotomy is apparent as is adequate debulking surgery. There can be little argument that adjuvant treatment should be offered to all patients with, perhaps, the exception of those having stage I disease with minimal mucosal penetration. Platinum-based combination regimens are the most active and most likely to lead to a prolonged disease-free interval.

Nevertheless, the limited experience of the disease at single institutions and the paucity of cases in the world literature has prevented the development of large randomized trials which might be able to compare various treatment regimens. Comparison between institutions is hampered by a lack of a uniform staging system. Further advances in this rare disease are unlikely to be made unless international collaborative studies are established.

In 1951 Stanley Way wrote that 'the paucity of reports of primary carcinoma of the fallopian tube demands that every case be reported in detail'. In the 1990s that plea is no less important.

REFERENCES

1 Hanton E M, Malkasian G D Jr, Dahlin D C, Pratt J H. Primary carcinoma of the fallopian tube. Am J Obstet Gynecol 1966; 94: 832–839
2 Eddy G L, Copeland L J, Gerhenson D M, Atkinson E N, Wharton J T, Rutledge F N. Fallopian tube carcinoma. Obstet Gynecol 1984; 64: 546–552
3 Podratz K C, Podczaski E S, Gaffey T A, O'Brien P C, Schray M F, Malkasian G D Jr. Primary carcinoma of the fallopian tube. Am J Obstet Gynecol 1986; 154: 1319–1326
4 Hu C Y, Taylor M L, Hertig A T. Carcinoma of the fallopian tube. Am J Obstet Gynecol 1950; 59: 58–67
5 Engstrom L. Primary carcinoma of the fallopian tube. Acta Obstet Gynecol Scand 1957; 36: 289–305
6 Boutselis G J, Thompson N J. Clinical aspects of primary carcinoma of the fallopian tube. A clinical study of 14 cases. Am J Obstet Gynecol 1971; 111: 98–101
7 Yoonessi M. Carcinoma of the fallopian tube. Obstet Gynecol Surv 1979; 34: 257–270
8 Sedlis A. Primary carcinoma of the fallopian tube. Obstet Gynecol Surv 1961; 16: 209–226
9 Park R C, Parmley T H. Fallopian tube cancer. In: McGowan L, ed. Gynecologic oncology. New York: Appleton Century Crofts, 1978: pp 274–280
10 Bannatyne P, Russell P. Early adenocarcinoma of the fallopian tubes. A case for multifocal tumorigenesis. Diag Gynecol Obstet 1981; 3: 49–60
11 Hee P, Pagel J D. Primary carcinoma of the fallopian tube. Eur J Obstet Gynecol Reprod Biol 1987; 25: 131–138
12 Baeklandt M, Kockx M, Wesling F, Gerris J. Primary adenocarcinoma of the fallopian tube. Review of the literature. Int J Gynecol Cancer 1993; 3: 65–70

13 Prys Davies A, Fish A, Woolas R, Oram D. Raised serum CA125 preceding the diagnosis of carcinoma of the fallopian tube. Br J Obstet Gynaecol 1991; 98: 602–603

14 Niloff J M, Klug T L, Schaetzl E, Zurawski V R, Knapp R C, Bast R C. Elevation of serum CA 125 in carcinomas of the fallopian tube, endometrium and endocervix. Am J Obstet Gynecol 1984; 148: 1057–1058

15 McMurray E H, Jacobs A J, Perez C A, Camel H M, Kao M S, Galakatos A. Carcinoma of the fallopian tube. Cancer 1986; 58: 2070–2075

16 Asmussen M, Kaern J, Kjoerstad K, Wright P B, Abeler V. Primary adenocarcinoma localized to the fallopian tubes: report on 33 cases. Gynecol Oncol 1988; 30: 183–186

17 Erez S, Kaplan A L, Wall J A. Clinical staging of carcinoma of the uterine tube. Obstet Gynecol 1967; 30: 547–550

18 Benedet J L, Miller D M. Tumors of fallopian tube: clinical features, staging and management. In: Coppleson M, ed. Gynecologic oncology, 2nd edn. Edinburgh: Churchill Livingstone, 1992: pp 853–860

19 Peters W A, Andersen W A, Hopkins M P, Kumar N B, Morley G W. Prognostic features of carcinoma of the fallopian tube. Obstet Gynecol 1988; 71: 757–762

20 Tamimi H K, Figge D C. Adenocarcinoma of the uterine tube: potential for lymph node metastases. Am J Obstet Gynecol 1981; 141: 132–137

21 Semrad N, Watring W, Fu Y-S, Hallat J, Ryoo M, Lagasse L. Fallopian tube adenocarcinoma: common extraperitoneal recurrence. Gynecol Oncol 1986; 24: 230–235

22 Denham J W, Maclennan K A. The management of primary carcinoma of the fallopian tube. Experience of 40 cases. Cancer 1984; 53: 166–172

23 Dodson M G, Ford J H, Averette H E. Clinical aspects of fallopian tube carcinoma. Obstet Gynecol 1970; 36: 935–939

24 Boronow R C. Chemotherapy for disseminated tubal cancer. Obstet Gynecol 1973; 42: 62–66

25 Deppe G, Bruckner H W, Cohen C J. Combination chemotherapy for advanced carcinoma of the fallopian tube. Obstet Gynecol 1980; 56: 530–532

26 Maxson W Z, Stehman F B, Ulbright T M, Sutton G P, Ehrlich C E. Primary carcinoma of the fallopian tube: evidence for activity of cisplatin combination therapy. Gynecol Oncol 1987; 26: 305–313

27 Jacobs A J, McMurray E H, Parham J, Kao M S, Galakatos A E, Perez C A, Camel M H. Treatment of carcinoma of the fallopian tube using cisplatin, doxorubicin and cyclophosphamide. Am J Clin Oncol [CCT] 1986; 9: 436–439

28 Raju K S, Barker G H, Wiltshaw E. Primary Carcinoma of the fallopian tube. Report of 22 cases. Br J Obstet Gynaecol 1981; 88: 1124–1129

29 Rose P G, Piver M S, Tsukada Y. Fallopian tube cancer. Cancer 1990; 66: 2661–2667

30 Gurney H, Murphy D, Crowther D. The management of primary fallopian tube carcinoma. Br J Obstet Gynaecol 1990; 97: 822–826

23 The role of viruses in gynaecological oncology

A. B. MacLean   J. C. M. Macnab

INTRODUCTION

Superficially, there would appear to be little doubt that viruses, and in particular human papilloma virus (HPV), cause cervical cancer. However, it would be wrong for the trainee in gynaecology to believe that the aetiology of cervical carcinoma is completely known and understood. Much has been written in the last 10 years associating HPV with cervical intraepithelial neoplasia (CIN) and cervical carcinoma. The molecular aspects which explain carcinogenesis are becoming clearer, but epidemiological studies continue to produce what appears to be conflicting evidence. This chapter will focus on cervical and vulval carcinoma because there is no significant body of evidence at present to link viruses with endometrial or epithelial ovarian carcinoma.[1]

EVIDENCE FOR A TRANSMISSIBLE AGENT IN CERVICAL CANCER

In 1842 Rigoni-Stern[2] reported from Padua that death due to uterine cancer occurred more frequently in married than in unmarried women. Women who have never had intercourse are unlikely to develop cervical cancer stated Gagnon[3] studying French Canadian Catholic nuns. Prostitutes, on the other hand, had an increased risk of developing cervical cancer,[4,5] as did those women who had first intercourse at a young age[6], or who had a history of sexually transmitted disease.[7] Kessler[8] suggested that a male transmissible factor was responsible, as the second partners of men whose first wives had developed cervical carcinoma had an increased risk of cervical neoplasia.

Over the last 30 years there has been accumulating evidence that cervical carcinoma is associated with a sexually transmitted virus. Initial studies focused on herpes simplex virus (HSV) but more recently studies show that HPV is the most likely aetiological agent (reviewed[9-11]).

VIRUSES WHICH CAUSE TUMOURS

Evidence that viruses can cause cancer has been available since the beginning of this century. Ellerman and Bang[12] in 1908 showed that a filterable agent [later named avian erythroblastosis virus (AEV)] was responsible for inducing chicken leukaemia, while Rous[13] in 1911 showed Rous sarcoma virus (RSV) caused sarcomas in chickens.[14] It is now known that these viruses are retroviruses and conclusive evidence now exists that retroviruses can cause leukaemia in mice and cats, and mammary carcinoma in certain genetic strains of mice. Viruses of the papova group (polyoma virus, simian virus 40 (SV40) and papilloma virus) have been implicated in a variety of animal tumours. Papilloma virus of rabbits (Shope virus) is associated with malignant lesions in cotton-tail rabbits; the difference in behaviour of the virus in rabbits in the wild (virus causes warts only) compared with laboratory rabbits (virus causes carcinoma) suggest some co-factor is involved. Jarrett et al[15] and Campo et al[16] demonstrated that bovine papilloma virus is responsible for inducing papillomas in the alimentary tract of cattle. These papillomas frequently progress to tumours in areas where bracken is eaten; the bracken fern complicates grazing in the west of Scotland. Bracken is thought to be a co-factor because it contains quercetin, a potential carcinogen; but bracken also contains immunosuppressants which may be important. Viruses of the Herpes genus can on injection into animals cause tumours: e.g. Marek's Disease herpes virus (MDHV) in chickens causing lymphomatosis, Lucke herpes virus (LHV) causing renal carcinoma in the frog, and herpes virus saimiri (HVS) and herpes virus ateles (HVA) the latter two causing T-cell lymphomas in monkeys.

Various human tumours including Burkitt's lymphoma, nasopharyngeal carcinoma, hepatocellular carcinoma, Kaposi's sarcoma, T-cell leukaemia, epidermodysplasia verruciformis as well as cervical and vulval carcinoma have been associated with the continuous presence of viruses.[17-20] However, it has been exceedingly difficult to prove that one or other of these human tumours is actually caused by the associated virus. For example, Epstein-Barr virus (EBV) immortalises B lymphocytes which can become tumorigenic if c-myc is translocated from its normal position in chromosome 8 to chromosome 14 where it is increased in expression by the upstream immunoglobulin promoter. However, it is proposed that it requires an alteration of cell surveillance, e.g. by Falciparum malaria to allow unrestricted growth of EBV-carrying B cells, and increase the risk of chromosomal translocation which, in turn, results in the development of Burkitt's lymphoma[19]. Similarly, although integration of hepatitis B virus appears to be associated with hepatocellular carcinoma the mechanisms of integration or its effect on genetic expression are not well understood.[20]

PROOF OF CAUSATION OF CANCER BY VIRUSES

Traditionally Koch's postulates, defined 100 years ago, have been used to show cause and effect of infectious agents. Additional criteria relevant to viral infection have been added more recently. Evans[21] has defined epidemiological, serological, and biological criteria that should be fulfilled to relate viruses

Table 23.1 Criteria showing a causal link between herpes simplex virus and cervical carcinoma

1. Presence of viral DNA in the tumour or cell lines derived from the tumour.
2. Presence of viral RNA.
3. Presence and function of viral proteins.
4. Continuous spectrum of progression from virus infection to cancer.
5. Occurrence in the same tissue of different virus types in lesions which differ in their progression.
6. Occurrence of particular virus types in tumours from different tissues.
7. In vitro transformation of cell lines and tumourigenesis of animals by virus.
8. In vitro transformation of cell lines and in vivo tumourigenesis of animals by viral DNA.
9. Epidemiology.
10. Serology.
11. Vaccination.

to cancer. Evans identified obstacles in establishing a possible aetiological role, including:

1 The long incubation period between exposure to the suspected agent and the development of the disease.
2 The relatively low incidence of most cancers which makes prospective studies almost impossible because of the large number of persons who must be kept under observation.
3 The possibility that cancer may result from virus reactivation occurring years after the initial primary infection.
4 The widespread and ubiquitous nature of the viruses under greatest suspicion of oncogenicity.
5 The probable role of infectious, environmental and/or genetic co-factors in producing cancer.
6 The difficulty in fully reproducing the disease in animals.
7 The impossibility of human experimentation with potentially oncogenic agents.

Evans' criteria were used by Aurelian et al[22] to show a causal association between herpes simplex virus and cervical carcinoma. These are similar to more recent ones described by Fey and Larsen[19] (see Table 23.1).

Links between human papilloma virus and cancer

HPV is one of various DNA viruses found in the genital tract. It can be sexually transmitted, as found by the wives of servicemen who developed genital warts after their husbands' return from the Korean war,[23] and the presence of HPV-associated lesions of the cervix in consorts of men with penile condyloma acuminata.[24] However, transmission may occur from other skin surfaces and contacts. There are more than 60 types of HPV, characterised by differences within the DNA sequences as detected by stringent DNA/DNA hybridisation. Several types are associated with genital malignancies or premalignancies. HPV 6 and HPV 11 are associated predominantly with low grade CIN or condylomata and are called low risk types as low grade lesions rarely progress to high grade CIN or invasive cancer. HPV types 16, 18, 31, 33 and 35, on the other hand, are termed high risk types as they are most frequently associated with high grade CIN or with invasive carcinoma.

The initial links between HPV and cervical neoplasia followed the description of condylomatous wart lesions of the cervix and their association with abnormal cytology.[25,26] The postulate was that HPV caused the cervical epithelium to undergo change through a spectrum of inflammation, atypia and eventually neoplasia. Furthermore, when high grade CIN and carcinoma were examined using hybridisation technology, HPV DNA could be found amongst the cellular DNA in 80–95% of samples and often integrated with it.[27-29] Integration appeared to be associated with progression from CIN to carcinoma. The use of DNA/DNA hybridisation (Southern blotting) showed that carcinoma and CIN 3 were frequently associated with HPV 16 and HPV 18 DNA, but not with HPV 6 and HPV 11. However, Southern blotting is a complex and time consuming technique and limited numbers of specimens can be assessed this way.

When further specimens were examined, two sets of observations were made which showed that HPV DNA was not unique to the cancerous lesions. Macnab et al[30] found that 84% of cervical and vulval carcinoma contained HPV 16 DNA, but also found the virus DNA in 73% of histologically normal control tissue adjacent to the lesion. This control tissue was taken from the uterus at radical hysterectomy or from a strip of abdominal wall skin superior to the transverse abdominal incision at radical vulvectomy and at least 2 cm from the nearest tumour edge. When specimens of ectocervical epithelium taken at hysterectomy performed for non-neoplastic conditions were examined, only 11% contained HPV 16 DNA. Meanwell et al[31] found HPV 16 DNA in 35% of women with normal cervical smears. They, however found no evidence of virus DNA integration, whereas Macnab's group[32] detected HPV DNA integrated within the host chromosome and surprisingly, sometimes present in higher viral copy numbers in normal tissue than in the neoplastic tissue. Therefore, if HPV was associated with neoplasia, what was one to make of its presence in adjacent tissue? Was this responsible for the risk of recurrent tumour, and were those women with negative smears but HPV in their cervix already progressing towards genital tract lesions?

The introduction of polymerase chain reaction (PCR) provided a technique that was no less complex, but certainly quicker and more sensitive than DNA detection by Southern blotting and PCR is capable of detecting a single virus particle among a million cells. Young et al[33] reported that of 38 women with an abnormal smear 36 had HPV 16 and 22 had both HPV 16 and HPV 11. However, 7 of 10 women with a normal smear also tested positive for HPV 16 or HPV 11 DNA. Tidy et al[34] reported that 67% of dyskaryotic smears contained HPV 16, and, if carcinoma was present the figure rose to 100%. Again, 117 of 140 (84%) of the normal smears were also positive. The technique of PCR is so sensitive that cross-contamination is a major threat to the accuracy of results. Concerns have been expressed about variations in prevalence among normal and abnormal tissue and in the reproducibility of results. Some of the differences are due to the use of different primer sets, or perhaps deletions in the virus DNA which is integrated.[35]

MOLECULAR EVIDENCE LINKING VIRUSES WITH CERVICAL CANCER

Human papilloma virus

The inability to culture papilloma viruses in vitro in regular tissue culture systems has frustrated both the isolation of the virus and the subsequent study of its biological properties. Dramatic advances in molecular biology in recent years have led to the cloning and expression of many HPV types. The construction of clones expressing HPV proteins resulted in the generation of knowledge of the molecular biology of HPV being far in advance of the knowledge and understanding of biological function. HPVs are double stranded circular molecules which encode seven early gene products (E1–E7) and two late gene products (L1 and L2), the latter involved in capsid assembly. In benign tissues (e.g. genital warts) the HPVs are replicated as circular episomes. In carcinoma tissue the virus DNA generally becomes integrated into the cell DNA but those DNA sequences coding for the E2-E5 proteins as well as the two late, L1 and L2, proteins are deleted out on integration. Expression of E6 and E7 are important for the phenotype of the tumour cell and the molecular mechanisms by which E6 and E7 function are believed to be as follows.

Transformation assays, carried out by transfecting cloned HPV genes into human keratinocytes cultured in vitro, have shown that E6 and E7 are sufficient and necessary to immortalise cells.[36,37] Immortal cells, however, are not tumorigenic in nude mice. Nonetheless, both E6 and E7 are expressed in immortalised cells and also in human cervical tumours. The function of E6 and E7 gene products has been studied in detail in the high risk types HPV 16 and HPV 18. Both E6 and E7 proteins bind to a class of cell coded genes called a tumour suppressor gene or sometimes, an anti-oncogene (reviewed[38]). Tumour suppressor genes function by maintaining the normal state of a cell (reviewed[39]) and deletions or mutations in these suppressor genes disable the gene function and lead to the development of cancers. This is in contrast to oncogenes which can code for a dominant transforming gene product which controls the cell phenotype. Two of the most studied tumour suppressor gene products, p53 and Rb, are the targets to which E6 and E7 bind respectively. Binding may be equated with disruption of the normal cell phenotype and E6 effectively degrades the ubiquitinated form of p53 protein by ATP dependent hydrolysis.[40] Mutational analysis of HPV 16 E6 demonstrates that p53 degradation is necessary for the immortalization of mammary epithelial cells[41]. Low risk HPV 6 and HPV 11 do not bind p53.

Interestingly in those cervical cancers where HPV is not detected, p53 is usually present in a mutated form in which it can act like an oncogene.[42]

In HPV 16 and HPV 18 the E7 protein binds to Rb, a recessive tumour suppressor gene, first detected in retinoblastoma where it is usually associated either with a deletion of both alleles or deletion of one allele and mutation of the other. Binding to Rb, however, is regulated by phosphorylation of the Rb protein and its phosphorylation status is in turn regulated by cell cycle control.[43] E7 binds to the underphosphorylated Rb which is found in resting cells (Go), whereas Rb, when phosphorylated at multiple sites, is associated with DNA replication (S) and mitosis (M). In resting cells, Rb is bound to the transcription factor E2F. If E7 is expressed in cells it binds to Rb in a complex. This frees E2F which, on release, gives rise to a new activity which promotes cell division.[44] Cyclin A is also believed to have a role in DNA replication in this complex. Thus expression of E6 and E7 result in loss of control at a checkpoint in the cell cycle. It is currently thought that cell cycle kinase complexes require to form with E6 and E7 before neoplastic transformation occurs. The quaternary cyclin/cyclin-dependent kinase (CDK), present in normal cells, dissociates from p21 and proliferating cell nuclear antigen (PCNA) on complexing with E6 and E7. This is a necessary prelude to neoplastic transformation.[45]

Low risk types HPV 6 and HPV 11 bind Rb much less tightly than do HPV 16 and HPV 18.

E5 has an additional function in transformation. Its expression in cells induces anchorage independence as measured by the efficiency of colony formation in semi-solid medium which is increased by epidermal growth factor.[46] E5 affects EGF-mediated signal transduction to the nucleus, possibly by stimulating MAP kinase.[47] E5 stimulates MAP kinase in both the presence and absence of EGF so E5 may enhance the response to growth factor stimulation. Does the foregoing information mean that many unrelated hypothesis are attributed to HPV function? No! On the contrary, it shows that HPV is now known to fit into several of the well understood molecular pathways leading to carcinogenesis, which is recognized to be a multistage process.

Not all tumours contain viruses but the mechanisms by which tumour cells preferentially grow via the disruption of tumour-suppressor genes are similar in all tumours. Absence of DNA transforming viruses in tumours where alterations in the tumour-suppressor gene can be detected strongly suggest not only that there are cellular equivalents of the virus coded proteins in cancer cells but also that these cellular equivalents probably function by mechanisms similar to those already elucidated and discussed here for the virus gene products (oncoproteins).

However, histologically normal tissues can and do contain HPV 16 and HPV 18, which is sometimes even integrated, as described earlier.[30-32] To study the effects of these HPV DNA sequences in normal tissue on the recurrence of a tumour or the progression of disease after resection, Walkinshaw et al[48] followed up several women over a 3–4 year period and found no increased evidence of tumour recurrence in patients with HPV 16 in the control tissues. Thus HPV 16 alone is clearly not sufficient to cause tumourigenicity even in a host which has already shown cancer susceptibility involved with papillomavirus.

This further emphasises that HPV DNA present in cervical cells in vivo needs other cofactors to progress to oncogenesis and demonstrates the multi-factorial nature of carcinogenesis. As stated E6 and E7 have been shown to immortalise cells in vitro. These cells are not oncogenic and require other co-factors to become oncogenic. Other co-factors in the form of oncogenes or virus functions, e.g. a clone encoding the small subunit of the HSV ribonu-cleotide reductase, can, on transfection into cells immortalised by HPV, induce tumours in nude mice.[49]

Herpes simplex virus

Herpes simplex type 2 (HSV-2) was historically associated with cervical car-cinoma and, prior to the discovery of genital strains of papillomavirus, HSV-2 was much studied as a causative agent. The HSV-2 coded ribonucleotide reductase (RR) was implicated in inducing transformation of cultured cells in vitro, and one proposal for RR function is the destabilisation of nucleotide pools. This enzyme has two sub-units and the larger codes for a protein kinase enzyme activity which in other situations e.g. retroviruses is crucial to the expression of transformed cells. HSV-2 DNA was seldom retained in cells transformed in vitro but was detected in 10–15% of cervical tumours.[50,50a,51] It seems that if HSV-2 has a role in the development of cervi-cal cancer it functions by a mechanism different from other DNA transform-ing viruses which usually integrate their DNA and code for a dominant transforming oncogene (oncoprotein). Infection with HSV can change cells causing them to behave in a number of ways similar to tumour cells (reviewed[51]). These changes include the amplification of cell coded genes, chromosome breakage, mutagenesis, induction of endogenous retroviruses and also the induction of cell coded proteins which could control carcino-genic pathways or regulate second messengers. Chromosome breakage due to HSV infection was initially known as early as 1961 and recently the HSV virion itself has been shown to be mutagenic[52] in the absence of expression of any virus coded protein.

Recent studies have centred on a set of cell coded proteins characteristic of tumour cells and induced by HSV infection. One such tumour-specific protein is a form of the mitochondrial aspartate aminotransaminase (mAAT).[53] This protein can be detected in tumour but not control cells. It is induced fourfold by HSV infection but its specialised function in tumour cells is, as yet, unknown. In cells mAAT is a key enzyme in intermediate metabolism and provides energy. Tumour cells have greatly increased levels of aerobic glycolysis, energy being preferentially provided by glutamine rather than glucose (reviewed[54]).This is exemplified by Hela cells, derived from a cancer of the cervix and expressing HPV 18.[55] Glutamine in cells is converted to glutamate by glutaminase but to enter the energy system it requires to be converted by mAAT in the presence of oxaloacetate to alpha ketoglutarate and aspartate. Thus HSV induces an enzyme of particular importance in cancer cell metabolism which may confer a growth advantage on a small number of abnormal cells immortalised by HPV, and containing genetic abnormalities. Chemotherapeutic agents successfully used in the control of leukaemic cell growth [e.g. L-glutamic acid gamma hydroxamate (GAH)] specifically target mAAT both in vivo and in vitro,[56] further suggesting that mAAT may have an important role in tumour cell growth.

Human cytomegalovirus

Another virus which has been associated with cervical neoplasia is human cytomegalovirus (HCMV), the DNA of which has been identified in malignant and premalignant disease (reviewed[57]). However, a role for HCMV DNA in cervical neoplasia has not been established and a more credible role for HCMV could be that described by Albrecht's group who demonstrated the induction of proto-oncogenes, e.g. c-fos and c-myc by HCMV infection, thus potentiating cell division.[58] This role has potential for further investigation as have later studies from this group which show that HCMV can induce functions involved in cell signalling and second messenger induction.

IMMUNOLOGICAL EFFECTS OF VIRUSES

Immune modulation by herpes simplex virus and human cytomegalovirus

Both HSV and HCMV are well recognized common infectious agents of the female genital tract. Both viruses can modulate the immune response and are also modulated by the host in which both viruses can become latent and escape immune surveillance. HSV infection itself greatly alters the host immune response involving a number of different pathways which include: reducing antibody dependent cell mediated cytotoxicity (ADCC), decreasing phagocytic activity, increasing both interferon and the numbers of natural killer cells (NKC). In addition, HSV codes for the glycoprotein gC which binds complement and has an Fc receptor (which binds antibodies).

Unfortunately, most HSV and HCMV studies concentrated on a role for the virus in initiating oncogenic disease and studying the effects of virus DNA retention on the cell. Any role HSV and HCMV have might be more appropriate to later stages in the multistage process of carcinogenesis. An in vitro study by Matz' group has shown, for example, that immortalised cells plated immediately after HSV-2 infection can form colonies in semi-solid medium if they are not allowed to grow together with normal cells.[59] Loss of anchorage dependence is a function most closely associated with tumourigenesis in vivo.

Some interesting studies reveal that exposure to HSV (and not detection of HSV DNA) in patients with evidence of HPV 16 or HPV 18 infection is an added risk factor in developing invasive cervical cancer, increasing the risk by 9 fold.60 In this role HSV may be considered an important co-factor.

Immunological effects of human papilloma virus infection

Immunologically HPVs are of interest because they almost certainly depress the immune system perhaps in concert with co-factors. This is a reasonable assumption because in the bovine model papillomavirus type 4 DNA is not retained in tumours of the alimentary tract, being only required for proliferation of benign papillomas. However, the immune system in cattle cannot depress the growth of tumour cells which are initiated by papillomatosis. Moreover immunization against the bovine papillomavirus prevents progression of papillomas to carcinomas. Langerhans cells are decreased in the presence of HPV DNA, a finding which adds credence to the involvement of immune response in HPV carcinogenesis.[61] Therefore response to HPV infection may depend on the genetic make up of the host which the virus infects and how the virus behaves immunologically in different genetic hosts. Interestingly recent work shows that tumours associated with HPVs establish because they escape NKC surveillance.[62]

Apoptosis and its function in tumourigenesis

It would be premature to end this discussion without touching on a subject of current great interest, namely apoptosis or programmed cell death. To interfere with programmed cell death leads to the continued growth of a population of cells not intended to survive because their function in development, differentiation or growth regulation is required only at a certain defined stage and not thereafter. A gene which promotes cell death is p53, required for apoptosis of thymocytes treated with ionising radiation or with drugs which target the cell topoisomerase type 2, e.g. etoposide.[63,64] Transgenic mice, null mutant for p53, have thymocytes resistant to apoptosis. Thus p53 acts like a cell policeman to screen out cells which have sustained DNA damage and prevent the growth of cells which could become tumourigenic.[65] The cervix is an area of cell differentiation and development. The presence of HPV 16 E6 able to degrade p53 could have an involvement in altering cell growth and regulation which in turn would allow abnormal cells, possibly DNA damaged, to proliferate. No doubt this area of cell death has a very lively future and will yield further clues to the complex question of multistage carcinogenesis.[66] Very recent data suggest that inactivation of p53 increases sensitivity to multiple chemotherapeutic agents, including cisplatin, by delaying progression through S phase of the cell cycle. This implies that p53 has a role in DNA repair.[67]

Epidemiological evidence linking human papilloma virus with cervical neoplasia

Epidemiologists have sought to confirm that HPV is the transmissible cause of cervical neoplasia, using case-control studies and prospective investigations.

In a study of women with invasive cervical cancer, and matched controls, from four high risk areas in Panama, Mexico, Costa Rica and Columbia HPV 16 or HPV 18 was detected in 62% of 759 case patients and 32% of 1430 controls. The relative risk increased with increasing HPV DNA copy number.[68] Such case-control studies are complicated by a series of variables, not the least of which is the number of sexual partners. Women who have never had intercourse are unlikely to have HPV present in the genital tract.[69] Correlation between HPV presence and coital factors was disputed by Hording et al[70] who compared Greenlandic and Danish women. Greenland has one of the highest incidences of cervical cancer in the world, more than five times higher than Denmark (to which Greenland belongs). Greenlandic women commence sexual activity at a significantly younger age and are more likely to have more than 20 lifetime partners (53%) when compared with their Danish counterparts (4%). Despite these behavioural differences, HPV 16 DNA was found in a similar incidence (55% vs 45%) in Greenlandic and Danish women with cervical cancer. However, marked differences are found in the prevalence of HSV-2 antibodies (i.e. evidence of HSV infection) between these two populations.[71]

Munoz et al[72] and Schiffman[73] have reviewed other case-control studies and criticised the small sample sizes, potentially biased selection of study and control subjects, and expressed concern about the widely different prevalence of HPV DNA reported among cancer patients, and among controls or normal women. It appears likely that HPV detection by less sensitive techniques, e.g. filter in situ hybridisation, underestimates the real rate of HPV infection.[74] Although more recent studies have used PCR, there is no agreement on exact methods, e.g. what primers, should be used as the 'gold standard'.[73]

A further source of variation can be attributed to the different techniques used to obtain samples which include swab, scrape, cytobrush, lavage or biopsy.[73] Sherlock et al[74a] showed that biopsy material was more likely to contain HPV than scrape specimens of carcinoma in situ lesions, but conversely in low grade lesions, scrapes were more likely to be positive for HPV than biopsies. These differences may merely reflect sample size.

Studies on disease progression have focused on the likelihood of more advanced disease occurring in the presence of HPV. Thus Campion et al[24] reviewed 26 women who progressed to CIN 3 after initial evidence of mild atypia or dyskaryosis; 85% of those progressing had HPV 16 DNA, compared to 29% incidence in the original group. Syrjanen et al[75] found progression to CIN 3 in 66 of 508 women (12.9%) during a mean follow up period of 35 months, where HPV 6 and HPV 11 were found as frequently as HPV 16 and HPV 18.

Lorincz et al[76] reported on 398 women, seen in a private gynaecology clinic, who had HPV presence assessed by Southern blot hybridisation of cervical samples obtained from swabs. Women with normal smears were followed up for an average of 2 to 3 years by further smears; among those who originally had HPV 15% developed cytological changes consistent with cervical intraepithelial neoplasia compared with 5% who were HPV negative. Similarly Koutsky et al[77] followed a cohort of 241 women with normal smears using dot-filter hybridisation at 4 monthly intervals; the 2 year cumulative incidence of CIN 2-3 from the time of first positive test for HPV DNA was 28% compared with 3% if the smear remained HPV negative.

However, surprisingly, not all studies show disease progression in the presence of HPV. Carmichael and Maskens[78] reported on 235 women with mild to moderate cervical dysplasia; they found that those who had associated HPV infection, as identified by cytology, colposcopy or histology were more likely to regress spontaneously. Hirschowitz et al[79] found that women with borderline smears were less likely to develop subsequent high grade dyskaryosis if HPV infection was present than those where HPV was not present.

A study from the Royal Free Hospital[80] showed that the quantitation of viral (HPV16) load (using semi-quantitative PCR) rather than qualitative detection of viral presence was more important in predicting an association with high-grade CIN. However, in a longitudinal analysis of progression in these patients, those with HPV 16 DNA had a lower frequency of developing high grade CIN at 5 years than women without HPV 16 DNA.[81]

Differences in the results of these studies may be due to differences in the detection methods used. Kitchener et al[82] studied a series of sexually active women, recruited at a Family Planning Clinic, with a routine cervical smear in which koilocytosis suggested the presence of HPV infection but the absence of dyskaryosis. 10% of the women had HPV 16 DNA in tissue taken from the transformation zone, and some had HPV 16 in the apparently normal adjacent squamous epithelium. When DNA detection was performed on serial biopsies at 0, 9 and 18 months from the cohort of women who were originally HPV positive, HPV DNA was not necessarily detected consistently. There was no clear correlation between cytology, histology and HPV detection by hybridisation or PCR techniques.

In conclusion HPV has a strong correlation with the development of cervical cancer but other variable co-factors are involved.

The role of viruses in vulval cancer

Human papillomavirus

Vulval carcinoma has an incidence one-sixth to one-eighth that of cervical carcinoma, is usually found in older women and is rare under the age of 30 years. Its prevalence is higher in certain ethnic groups, e.g. in the West Indies and among American black women, where it has been linked to sexually transmitted infections including syphilis, lymphogranuloma venereum and granuloma inguinale. 20% or more of those with vulval carcinoma will have concurrent or previous cervical neoplasia. Women with vulval intraepithelial neoplasia (VIN) often have a history of previous genital warts.[83]

However, there may be two forms or subsets of vulval carcinoma.[83-86] The Vulval Invasion and Premalignancy Project (VIPP) conducted by members of the British Gynaecological Cancer Society found that among 171 vulval cancers, VIN was adjacent to 32% of cancers, non-neoplastic epithelial disorder (NNED) of the vulva to 36%, and both changes to a further 13%.[86] There were differences in the mean ages and likelihood of node involvement for those with VIN and with NNED. Andersen et al[84] have shown that those with adjacent VIN are more likely to have HPV present, as demonstrated by in situ hybridisation, (67% vs 13% other adjacent changes) and to have a history of smoking. Similarly Neill et al[87] found HPV DNA in 64% of carcinoma with coexisting VIN, but were unable to find HPV in carcinoma associated with NNED. Macnab et al[30] used DNA hybridisation to find HPV 16 in 9 of 11 vulval carcinomas (age range 29 to 87).

Herpes simplex virus

The role of herpes simplex in vulval cancer was investigated by Kaufman et al[87a] who showed HSV antigens in VIN. Macnab et al[30] could find HSV DNA sequences in only one of 11 vulval cancers tested by DNA hybridisation.

Immune responses and vulval carcinoma

As for the cervix, immunosuppression may have a role in the development of vulval cancer. Among 106 women with VIN, four developed cancer; two were under 40 years of age and were immune suppressed while the other two were elderly.[88] Friedrich et al[89] found features of immunosuppression in 50 women with VIN; one of these, a 21 year old, progressed to invasive carcinoma. In a New Zealand report[90] 4 women with VIN who had no treatment after biopsy developed invasive carcinoma 2–8 years later, and a fifth patient who was left under observation for 4 years before undergoing simple vulvectomy developed invasive carcinoma within one year: all five patients had associated squamous cell carcinoma of the cervix or CIN. The role of virus(es) in modifying immune surveillance in the vulva, and the risk of progression of VIN remains uncertain, but is currently being investigated in several centres studying HIV-positive women. However, unlike the cervix where viruses are associated with the great majority of carcinomas, there appears to be an association with virus found only in those vulval carcinomas with adjacent VIN.

Other considerations

Prevention of disease

So what are the prospects for decreasing the incidence of cervical or vulval neoplasia or preventing disease? Apart from the well publicised aims of barrier contraception to avoid virus spread, interest has centred around HPV vaccines and the ability to produce HPV particles by transfection of L1 and L2 capsid genes into cells. These particles might be used as a potential vaccine and, if indeed HPV does initiate cervical neoplastic disease, then the immunization of presexually active females should reduce the incidence of cervical premalignancy and neoplasia.

Recent advances in molecular biology and a history of expecting virus coded oncogenes to transform cells has discouraged experimental tumourigenesis with other viruses. The role of cell signalling and altered host immune response as a result of virus infection deserve further study in depth.

Problems of a limited perspective of the disease process

In 1846 W H Walshe,[91] Professor of Pathological Anatomy at University College London wrote 'The reader may well be spared an inquiry into speculations ascribing cancer to . . . the presence and action of a virus composed of an ammoniacal fluid containing oxide of nitrogen in excess'. Our understanding of viruses and viral carcinogenesis has progressed since those days. Nevertheless, our understanding of the cause of cervical cancer must encompass other factors including ageing, diet, smoking, immune deficiency and hormonal influences. Issac Berenblum, who in the 1940's described the precarcinogenic, epicarcinogenic and metacarcinogenic actions of certain chemicals including croton resin and benzpyrene[92] was later critical of the narrow approaches of some researchers.

'The association of viruses with tumour development has been particularly dramatic and has to a large extent vindicated some of the pioneers in the field who believed that the role of viruses in cancer was greater than most people imagined . . . progress was held back by the tendency of virologists to depreciate the importance of chemical carcinogenesis while those engaged in the latter branch of research tended to ignore altogether the role of viruses in cancer'.[93]

In conclusion the final word on viruses and cervical or vulval cancer remains still to be written.

REFERENCES

1 Beckmann A M, Sherman K J, Saran L, Weiss N S. Genital type human papillomavirus infection is not associated with surface epithelial ovarian carcinoma. Gynecol Oncol 1991; 43: 247–251.
2 Rigoni Stern D. Fatti statistici relativi alle malattie cancerose che servirono di base alle

poche cose dette dal dott. Giornale Servire Progressi Della Patalogia Della Terapeutica. 1842; 2: 507–514

3 Gagnon F. Contribution to the study of the etiology and prevention of cancer of the cervix of the uterus. Am J Obstet Gynaecol 1950; 60: 516–522

4 Moghissi K S, Mack H C, Porzak J P. Epidemiology of cervical cancer; study of a prison population. Am J Obstet Gynecol 1968; 100: 607–614.

5 Keighley E. Carcinoma of the cervix among prostitutes in a woman's prison. Br J Venereal Dis 1968; 44: 254–255

6 Berget A. 1978 Relation of dysplasia and carcinoma of the uterine cervix to age at onset of sexual life and number of coital partners. Danish Medical Bulletin. 25: 172–176.

7 Beral V. Cancer of the cervix: a sexually transmitted infection? Lancet 1974; i: 1037

8 Kessler II. Venereal factors in human cervical cancer: evidence from marital clusters. Cancer 1977; 39: 1912–1919

9 Kitchener H C. Genital virus infection and cervical neoplasia. Br J Obstet Gynaecol 1988; 95: 182–191

10 Kitchener H C. Does HPV cause cervical cancer? Commentary. Br J Obstet Gynaecol 1988; 95: 1089–1091.

11 Kitchener H C. Infection as an aetiological agent in carcinoma of the lower genital tract. In: MacLean A B (ed). Clinical Infection in Obstetrics and Gynaecology. Oxford:Blackwell, 1990, pp 339–356.

12 Ellerman N V, Bang O. Experimentelle leukämie bei hühnern. Centrabl bei Bakt 1908; 46: 595–609

13 Rous P. A sarcoma of fowl transmississble by an agent from the tumour cells. J Exp Med 1911; 13: 397–411

14 Walter J B, Israel M S. General Pathology. London: Churchill, 1967

15 Jarrett W FH, McNeil P E, Grimshaw W T R et al. High incidence area of cattle cancers with a possible interaction between an environmental carcinogen and a papilloma virus. Nature 1978; 274: 215–217

16 Campo M S, Moar M H, Jarrett W F H, Laird H M. A new papillomavirus associated with alimentary cancer in cattle. Nature 1980; 286: 180–182

17 Giraldo G, Beth E. The Role of Viruses in Human Cancer. Vol. 1. New York: Elsevier, 1980

18 Waterson AP. Human cancers and human viruses. BMJ 1982; 284: 446–448

19 Fey S J, Larsen P M. DNA viruses and human cancer. Cancer Lett 1988; 41: 1–18

20 Lancaster W D. Viral role in cervical and liver cancer. Cancer 1992; 70: 1794–1798

21 Evans A S. Introduction, epidemiological concepts and methods. In: Viral infections of humans, epidemiology and control. Evans A S, ed. Plenum Press, New York, 1976

22 Aurelian L, Manak M M, Mckinlay M et al. The herpes virus hypothesis – are Koch's postulates satisfied. Gynecol Oncol 1981; 12: S56–S87

23 Barrett T J, Silbar J D, McGinley J P. Genital warts – a venereal disease. J Am Med Assoc 1954; 154: 333–334

24 Campion M J, Singer A, Clarkson P K, McCance D J. Increased risk of cervical neoplasia in consorts of men with penile condylomata acuminata. Lancet 1985; i: 943–946

25 Meisels A, Fortin R, Roy M. Condylomatous lesions of the cervix and vagina II, Cytologic, and histopathologic study. Acta Cytologica 1977; 21: 379–384

26 Parola E, Savia E. Cytology of gynecologic condyloma acuminata. Acta Cytologica 1977; 21: 26–31.

27 Durst M, Gissman L, Ikenburg H, zur Hausen H. A papilloma virus DNA from a cervical carcinoma and its prevalence in cancer biopsy samples from different geographic regions. Proc Natl Acad Sci USA 1988; 80: 3812–3815

28 McCance D J, Walker P G, Dyson J L et al. Presence of human papillomavirus DNA sequences in cervical intraepithelial neoplasia. BMJ 1983; 287: 784–788

29 Schwarz E, Freese U K, Gissman L et al. Structure and transcription of human papillomavirus sequences in cervical carcinoma cells. Nature 1985; 314: 111–114

30 Macnab J C M, Walkinshaw S A, Cordiner J W, Clements J B. Human papillomavirus in clinically and histologically normal tissue of patients with genital cancer. N Engl J Med 1986; 315: 1052–1058

31 Meanwell C A, Cox M F, Blackledge G, Maitland NJ. HPV16 DNA in normal and malignant cervical epithelium : implications for the aetiology and behaviour of cervical neoplasia. Lancet 1987; i: 703–707

32 Murdoch J B, Cassidy LJ, Fletcher K, Cordiner J W, Macnab J C M. Histological and

cytological evidence of viral infection and human papillomavirus type 16 DNA sequences in cervical intraepithelial neoplasia and normal tissue in the west of Scotland: evaluation of treatment policy. BMJ 1988; 296: 381–385

33 Young L S, Bevan I S, Johnson M A et al. The London polymerase chain reaction : a new epidemiology tool for investigating cervial human papillomavirus infection. BMJ 1989; 298: 14–18

34 Tidy J A, Parru G C N, Ward P et al. High rate of human papillomavrius type 16 infection in cytologically normal cervices. Lancet 1989; 1: 434

35 Young L S, Tierney R J, Ellis J R M et al. PCR for the detection of genital human papillomavirus infection: a mixed blessing. Ann Med 1992; 24: 215–219

36 Schlegel R, Phelps W C, Zhang Y L, Barbosa M. Quantitative keratinocyte assay detects two biological activities of human papillomavirus DNA and identifies viral types associated with cervical carcinoma. EMBO J 1988; 7: 3181–3187

37 Sedman S A, Barbosa M S, Hubbert N L, Haas J A, Lowy D R, Schiller J T. The full-length E6 proteins of human papillomavirus type 16 has transforming and trans-activating activities and cooperates with E7 to immortalise keratinocytes in culture. J Virol 1991; 65: 4860–4866

38 Marx J. Learning how to suppress cancer. Science 1993; 269: 1385–1387

39 Levine A J. The tumour suppressor genes. Annu Rev Biochem 1993; 62: 623–651

40 Scheffner M, Werness B A, Huibregtse J M, Levine A J, Howley P M. The E6 oncoprotein encoded by human papillomavirus types 16 and 18 promotes the degradation of p53. Cell 1990; 63: 1129–1136

41 Dalal S, Gao Q, Androphy E J, Band V. Mutational analysis of HPV16 E6 demonstrates that p53 degradation is necessary for immortalization of mammary epithelial cells. J Virol 1996; 70: 683–688

42 Crook T, Fisher C, Vousden K. H. Modulation of immortalizing properties of human papilloma virus type 16 E7 by P53 expression. J Virol 1991; 65: 505–511.

43 Chen P L, Scully P, Shew J Y et al. Phosphorylation of the retinoblastoma gene product is modulated during the cell cycle and cellular differentiation. Cell 1989; 58: 1193–1198

44 Munger K, Werness B A, Dyson N, Phelps W C, Howley P M. Complex formation of human papillomavirus E7 proteins with the retinoblastoma tumour suppressor gene product. EMBO J 1989; 8: 4099–4105

45 Xiong Y, Kuppuswamy, Li Y et al. Mutational analysis of HPV 16 E6 demonstrates that p53 degradation is necessary for immortalization of mammalian epithelial cells. J Virol 1996; 70: 683–688

46 Straight S W, Hinkle P M, Jewers R J, McCance D J. The E5 oncoprotein of human papillomavirus type 16 transforms fibroblasts and effects the downregulation of the epidermal growth factor receptor in keratinocytes. J Virol 1993; 67: 4521–4532

47 Gu Z, Matlashewski G. Effect of human papillomavirus type 16 oncogenes on MAP Kinase activity. J Virol 1995; 69: 8051–8056

48 Walkinshaw SA, Cordiner JW, Clements JB, Macnab JCM. Prognosis of women with human papilloma virus DNA in normal tissue distal to invasive cervical and vulva cancer. Lancet 1987; i: 563

49 DiPaolo J A, Woodworth C D, Popescu N C, Koval D L, Lopez J V, Doniger J. HSV-2-induced tumorigenicity in HPV16-immortalized human genital keratinocytes. Virology 1990; 177: 777–779

50 Galloway D A, McDougall J K. The oncogenic potential of herpes simplex viruses: evidence for a 'hit and run' mechanism. Nature 1983; 302: 21–24

50a Cameron I R, Park M, Dutia B M, Orr A, Macnab J C M. Herpes simplex virus sequences involved in the initiation of oncogenic morphological transformation of rat cells are not required for maintenance of the transformed state. J Gen Virol 1987; 66: 517–527

51 Macnab J C M. Herpes simplex virus and human cytomegalovirus: their role in morphological transformation and genital cancers. J Gen Virol 1987; 68: 2525–2550

52 Clarke P, Clements J B. Mutagenesis occurring following infection with herpes simplex virus does not require virus replication. Virology 1991; 182: 597–606

53 Lucasson J F, McNab D, Collins T C et al. HSV-2 increases the mitochondrial asparate aminotransferase characteristic of tumour cells. Virology 1993; 205: 393–405

54 Baggetto LG. Deviant energetic metabolism of glycolytic cancer cells. Biochimie 1992; 74: 959–974

55 Reitzer L J, Wice B M, Kennell D. Evidence that glutamine, not sugar is the major energy source for cultured Hela cells. J Biol Chem 1979; 254: 2669–2676

56 Thomasset N, Goetsch L, Hamedi-Sangsari F et al. Inhibition of malate-aspartate shuttle by the anti-tumour drug L-glutamic acid monohydroxamate in L1210 leukaemia cells. Int J Cancer 1992; 51: 329–332

57 Stevenson K, Macnab J C M. Cervical carcinoma and human cytomegalovirus. Biomed Pharmacother 1989; 43: 173–176

58 Boldough I, Abubakar S, Albrecht T. Activation of proto-oncogenes: an immediate early event in human cytomegalovirus infection. Science 1990; 247: 561–564

59 Bauer G, Kahl S, Sawhney I S, Hofler P, Gerspach R, Matz B. Transformation of rodent fibroblasts by herpes simplex virus: Presence of morphological transforming region I (MTR1) is not required for the maintenance of the transformed state. Int J Cancer 1992; 51: 754–760

60 Hildesheim A, Mann V, Brinton L A et al. Herpes simplex virus type 2: a possible interaction with human papillomavirus types 16/18 in the development of invasive cervical cancer. Int J Cancer 1991; 49: 335–340

61 Hawthorn R J S, Murdoch J B, MacLean A B, Mackie R M. Langerhans cells and subtypes of human papillomavirus in cervical intraepithelial neoplasia. BMJ 1988; 297: 643–646

62 Routes J M, Ryan S. Oncogenicity of human papillomavirus or adenovirus transformed cells correlates with resistance to lysis by natural killer cells. J Virol 1995; 69: 7639–7647

63 Clarke A R, Purdie C A, Harrison D J et al. Thymocyte apoptosis induced by p53-dependent and independent pathways. Nature 1993; 362: 849–852

64 Lowe S W, Schmitt E M, Smith S , Osborne B A, Jacks T. p53 is required for radiation-induced apoptosis in mouse thymocytes. Nature 1993; 362: 847–849

65 Lane D P. A death in the life of p53. Nature 1993; 362: 786–787

66 Marx J. Cell death studies yield cancer clues. Science 1993; 269: 760–761

67 Hawkins D S, Demers G W, Galloway D A. Inactivation of p53 enhances sensitivity to multiple chemotherapeutic agents. Cancer Res 1996; 56: 892–898

68 Reeves W C, Brinton L A, Garcia M et al. Human papillomavirus infection and cervical cancer in Latin America. N Engl J Med 1989; 320: 1437–1441.

69 Fairley C K, Chen S, Trabrizi N, Leeton K, Quinn M A, Garland S M. The absence of genital human papillomavirus DNA in virginal women. International Journal of STD and AIDS 1992; 3: 414–417

70 Hording U, Daugaard S, Bock J E. Human papillomavirus, Epstein-Barr virus, and cervical carcinoma in Greenland. Int J Gynecol Cancer 1992; 2: 314–317

71 Kjaer S K, de Villiers E M, Hangaard B J et al. Human papillomavirus, herpes simplex virus and cervical cancer incidence in Greenland and Denmark. A population-based cross sectional study. Int J Cancer 1988; 41: 518–524

72 Munoz N, Bosch X, Kaldor J M. Does human papillomavirus cause cervical cancer. The state of the epidemiological evidence. Br J Cancer 1988; 57: 1–5

73 Schiffman M H. Recent progress in defining the epidemiology of human papillomavirus infection and cervical neoplasia. J Natl Cancer Inst 1992; 84: 396–398

74 De Villiers E M, Wagner D, Schneider A et al. Human papilloma infections in women with and without abnormal cervical cytology. Lancet 1987; ii: 703–706

74a Sherlock C H, Anderson G H, Benedet J L et al. Human papillomavirus infection of the uterine cervix. Tissue sampling and laboratory methods effect correlations between infection rates and dysplasia. Am J Clin Pathol 1992; 97: 692–698

75 Syrjanen K, Mantyjarvi R, Saarikoski S et al. Factors associated with progression of cervical human papillomavirus (HPV) infections into carcinoma in situ during a long term prosepctive follow-up. Br J Obstet Gynaecol 1988; 95: 1096–1102

76 Lorincz A T, Schiffman M H, Jaffur W J et al. Temporal association of human papillomavirus infection with cervical cytologic abnormalities. Am J Obstet Gynecol 1990; 162: 645–651

77 Koutsky L A, Holmes K K, Critchlow C W et al. Cohort study of the risk of cervical intrapithelial neoplasia grade 2 or 3 in relation to papillomavirus infection. N Engl J Med 1992; 327: 1272–1278

78 Carmichael J A, Maskens P D. Cervical dysplasia and human papillomavirus. Am J Obstet Gynecol 1989; 160: 916–918

79 Hirshowitz L, Raffle A E, Mackenzie E F D, Hughes A O. Long term follow up of women with borderline cervical smear results: effects of age and viral infection on progression to high grade dyskaryosis. BMJ 1992; 304: 1209–1212

80 Bavin P J, Giles J A, Deery A et al. Use of semi-quantitative PCR for human papillomavirus

DNA type 16 to identify women with high grade cervical disease in a population presenting with a mildly dyskaryotic smear report. Br J Cancer 1993; 67: 602–605

81 Downey G P, Bavin P J, Deery A R S et al. The relationship between human papillomavirus type 16 and the potential for progression of minor cervical disease. Lancet 1994; 344: 432–435

82 Kitchener H C, Neilson L, Burnett R A, Young L, Macnab J C M. Prospective serial study of viral change in the cervix and correlation with human papillomavirus genome status. Br J Obstet Gynaecol 1991; 98: 1042–1048.

83 Crum C R. Carcinoma of the vulva: epidemiology and pathogeneis. Obstet Gynaecol 1992; 79: 448–454

84 Andersen W A, Franquemont D W, Williams J et al. Vulvar squamous cell carcinoma and papillomaviruses: two separate entities. Am J Obstet Gynecol 1991; 165: 329–336

85 Kurman R J, Trimble C L, Shah K V. Human papillomavirus and the pathogenesis of vulvar carcinoma. Curr Opin Obstet Gynaecol 1992; 4: 582–585

86 MacLean A B. Precursors of vulval cancers. Curr Obstet Gynaecol 1993; 3: 149–156

87 Neill S M, Lessana-Leibowitch M, Pelisse M et al. Lichen sclerosus, invasive squamous cell carcinoma and human papilloma virus. Am J Obstet Gynecol 1990; 162: 1633–1634

87a Kaufmann R H, Dreesman G R, Burek J et al. Herpesvirus induced antigens in squamous cell carcinoma in situ of the vulva. New Engl J Med 1981; 305: 483–488

88 Buscema J, Woodruff J D, Parmley T H, Genadry R. Carcinoma in situ of the vulva. Obstet Gynaecol 1980; 55: 225–230

89 Friedrich E G, Wilkinson E J, Fu Y S. Carcinoma in situ of the vulva: a continuing challenge. Am J Obstet Gynecol 1980; 136: 830–838

90 Jones R W, McLean M R. Carcinoma in situ of the vulva: a review of 31 treated and 5 untreated cases. Obstet Gynaecol 1986; 68: 499–503

91 Walshe W H. The Nature and Treatment of Cancer. London: Taylor and Walton, 1846

92 Berenblum I. The mechanisms of carcinogenesis: a study of the significance of carcinogenic action and related phenomena. Cancer Res 1941; 1: 807–814

93 Berenblum I. Cancer research in historical perspective. Cancer Res 1977; 37: 1–7

24 The impact of molecular genetics in gynaecological cancer

I. Jacobs

Progress in understanding the molecular basis of disease has occurred at a rapid pace since the mid-1980s. The resultant information explosion has had as great an impact in the field of cancer as in any other branch of medicine and has transformed our understanding of the process of carcinogenesis. Although molecular information has not yet had a major impact in clinical oncology the potential impact is clear and is likely to emerge in the near future. The understanding of the process of carcinogenesis achieved using molecular technology provides exciting opportunities for the prevention, early detection and treatment of cancer. Despite the massive potential impact of molecular genetics in oncology the topic is often a daunting one for clinicians. It appears as a complex mass of facts, derived using unfamiliar technology and disguised in technical terms and nomenclature. The aim of this chapter is threefold: first, to provide a coherent and comprehensible framework of the general principles of carcinogenesis; second, to describe how the important events, which have been identified in the development of gynaecological malignancies, fit into this general framework; and third, to provide an overview of the potential impact of molecular genetics in the clinical management of gynaecological malignancy.

THE MOLECULAR BASIS OF CARCINOGENESIS

Cancer is a genetic disease

Cancer cells do not follow the normal restraints controlling cell division, cell-to-cell interaction and cellular mobility. This abnormal behaviour is inherited by the progeny of cancer cells, which behave in the same uncontrolled fashion. The fact that the division of cancer cells virtually never produces normal cells has long been regarded as evidence for a genetic basis for carcinogenesis. Further evidence for the genetic basis of cancer is the observation that agents which cause damage to DNA (chemical mutagens, ionizing radiation and some viruses) also increase susceptibility to cancer.[1,2] A genetic origin of cancer is also supported by studies of the clonal origin of tumours.[3,4] The vast majority of neoplasms appear to arise from a single cell which through subsequent division passes on its abnormality to daughter cells.

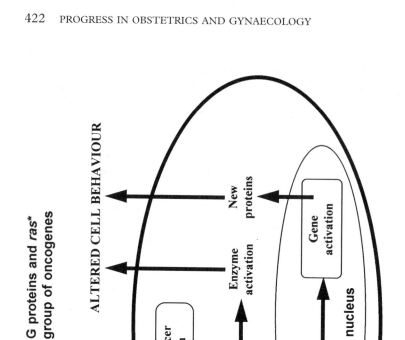

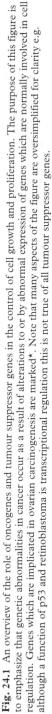

Fig. 24.1 An overview of the role of oncogenes and tumour suppressor genes in the control of cell growth and proliferation. The purpose of this figure is to emphasize that genetic abnormalities in cancer occur as a result of alterations to or by abnormal expression of genes which are normally involved in cell regulation. Genes which are implicated in ovarian carcinogenesis are marked*. Note that many aspects of the figure are oversimplified for clarity e.g. although a function of p53 and retinoblastoma is transcriptional regulation this is not true of all tumour suppressor genes.

From this perspective cancer can be regarded as an evolutionary process occurring at a cellular level. An initial genetic alteration provides a selective advantage for proliferation of a clone of cells. Further genetic alterations within this expanded clone of cells increases the proliferative advantage encouraging further expansion and eventually the formation of a clinically recognizable tumour.

The genetic changes in cancer involve genes which control normal cell growth and proliferation

As cancer is a consequence of genetic abnormalities disrupting normal cellular controls, normal cellular regulation is a logical starting point for understanding carcinogenesis. Cells communicate via a complex interacting set of signalling pathways, which are not yet entirely understood. Many of the essential principles of the signalling process are, however, well established[5] and are summarized in Fig. 24.1. The best understood mechanism of communication between cells is via the release of molecules that interact as agonists with receptors, either within the cell or, more frequently, in the cell membrane. This interaction results in a further signal within the cell which, via transducer proteins and secondary mechanisms, results in modified cell behaviour either by activating already synthesized target enzymes directly or by initiating transcription of genes and synthesis of their protein product. It should be recognized that Fig. 24.1 is an extremely simplified 'cartoon' of cellular control. Each of the various groups of molecules (i.e. agonist, receptor, transducer, etc.) has many different members and many of these can interact together resulting in a complex system of control which is difficult to analyse. The relevance of the simplification of cell signalling in Fig. 24.1 is that the genetic abnormalities observed in cancer are known to affect genes coding for all of the groups of molecules shown.

Oncogenes are altered forms of normal cellular genes (proto-oncogenes)

The first group of genes implicated in carcinogenesis were the oncogenes. The identification of these genes and their nomenclature are historically related to in vitro and animal work with virus-induced cancers. Although most retroviruses are harmless to an infected cell some acquire host cell genes which, when expressed by the virus without normal regulatory constraints, result in transformation of infected host cells. An important example of such a virus is RSV (Rous Sarcoma Virus).[6] As the viral genome is relatively small it was possible to identify the specific genes (viral oncogenes) involved in the transforming activity of retroviruses such as RSV. It was then possible to prepare DNA probes to look for homologous genes in normal cells.[7-10] Numerous viral oncogenes identified by this approach were found to have normal cellular homologues known as proto-oncogenes. Other workers

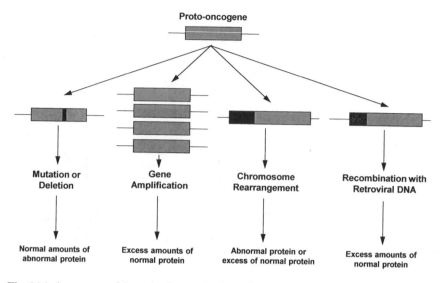

Fig. 24.2 A summary of the activation mechanisms of oncogenes.

identified oncogenes by transfecting cell lines with DNA from human cancer cell lines[11,12] and found that some of the transforming oncogenes identified were mutated versions of the proto-oncogenes identified by the retroviral approach.[13–17] The subject was further unified by the demonstration that chromosome translocations such as the Philadelphia Chromosome in chronic myeloid leukaemia[18] involved known oncogenes.[19] Approximately 100 proto-oncogenes have been identified and many can be assigned to the groups of functions summarized in Fig. 24.1. The mutation resulting in conversion of a proto-oncogene into an oncogene may occur in several different ways (Fig. 24.2) and may result in an abnormal protein produced at normal levels, overproduction of a normal protein or a normal protein produced inappropriately because of loss or alteration of control regions of the gene.

Tumour suppressor genes are of major importance in carcinogenesis

The second major group of genes implicated in carcinogenesis are the tumour suppressor genes. Initial evidence for the existence of this group of genes was provided by cell fusion studies. These studies showed that fusion of a transformed cell with a non-transformed cell frequently resulted in a non-transformed hybrid cell unless a specific chromosome was lost from the hybrid.[20–22] These findings suggested that the critical chromosome may contain a gene which suppresses transformation i.e. a tumour suppressor gene. The subsequent identification of the first tumour suppressor gene followed from the study of hereditary and sporadic retinoblastoma. Retinoblastoma is

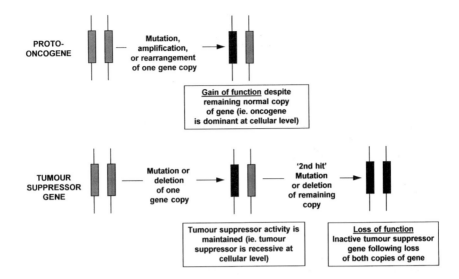

Fig. 24.3 A summary of the fundamental difference between oncogenes and tumour suppressor genes. Oncogenes are dominant at a cellular level and mutation of only one of the two gene copies is required for activation. Tumour suppressor genes are recessive at a cellular level. Both copies of the gene must usually be inactivated for loss of suppressor activity. An important exception to these general principles occurs when the product of a mutant copy of a tumour suppressor gene can interfere with the function of the product of the remaining wild-type copy of the gene. If this occurs both copies of the gene will be functionally inactive even though a normal wild-type copy of the gene remains. This is known as a dominant-negative effect, and an example is the p53 gene. The p53 protein functions as a dimer and dimers formed by wild-type and mutant protein are inactive. Loss of p53 tumour suppressor activity therefore seems to occur in some tumours following mutation of just one copy of the gene.

a rare childhood cancer in which hereditary disease is associated with multiple tumours affecting both eyes, whilst sporadic (non-hereditary) tumours occur at a slightly older age and involve a single tumour. On the basis of epidemiological and statistical analysis, Knudson[23] suggested that development of the cancer required two events. He postulated that in the hereditary form the first event was a germ line mutation present in every cell of the individual and that a second event in any of the many million retinoblasts could result in tumour formation. The rarity, later onset and unilateral nature of the sporadic form could be attributed to the need for two events in a single retinal cell in the absence of a germ line mutation. When the Rb (retinoblastoma) gene was mapped to chromosome 13q[24,25] and cloned[26-28] it was confirmed that in both familial and sporadic retinoblastoma the two copies of the gene were inactivated in tumour cells, consistent with Knudson's 'two hit' hypothesis.[29,30] Subsequently, a number of other tumour suppressor genes have been identified including p53,[31] APC[32,33] and DCC.[34] At a cellular level there is a fundamental difference in the mode of action of tumour suppressor genes and oncogenes (Fig. 24.3). Mutations creating oncogenes result in a gain of

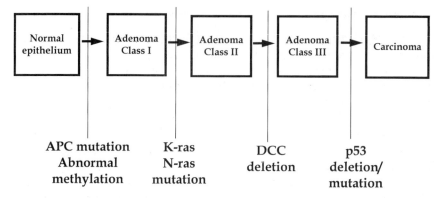

Fig. 24.4 The multistep model of carcinognesis in colorectal cancer. Modified from Vogelstein and Kinzler.[41]

function and will have an effect even in the presence of a remaining normal copy of the gene i.e. they are dominant at a cellular level. In contrast, tumour suppressor genes involve a loss of function and act recessively at a cellular level. In general, both copies of a tumour suppressor gene must be lost or inactivated for an effect on cellular regulation to occur.

Carcinogenesis is usually a multistep process

Although the spontaneous mutation rate of a gene is low (approximately 10^{-6} per gene per cell division) the total number of cell divisions in the lifetime of an individual is high (approximately 10^{16}) and consequently each gene is likely to have undergone at least 10^{10} spontaneous mutations.[35] Mutations affecting genes involved in carcinogenesis are therefore likely to be many fold more frequent than the observed rates of malignancy. Clearly, a single mutation of a single gene cannot generally be sufficient to cause cancer. Several lines of evidence support the concept of carcinogenesis as a multistep process. First, the relationship of cancer incidence and age is logarithmic and consistent with a requirement of 4–7 separate steps.[36] Second, in vitro studies of fibroblasts and studies of transgenic mice indicate that transformation requires at least two complementing oncogenes e.g. ras and myc.[37,38] Third, animal studies of chemical induction of tumours have revealed three stages in carcinogenesis; initiation which is irreversible, promotion which is reversible and progression. Most recently, direct evidence has been obtained for some cancers of the specific set of genetic alterations involved in carcinogenesis. One of the best examples of multistep carcinogenesis involving a common cancer is colorectal cancer,[39,40] which is illustrated in Fig. 24.4.

The genetic changes in cancer can be germ line or somatic events

An important distinction must be made between germ line and somatic mutations. Somatic mutations are found in the tumour cells but not the normal cells of an individual with cancer and cannot therefore be passed on to descendants of the patient. Germ line mutations predisposing to cancer involve all cells of the individual as well as the tumour, can be passed on to descendants of the individual and can be identified in DNA obtained from normal cells, such as a peripheral blood sample. The same genetic abnormalities frequently occur as both germ line and somatic mutations in different individuals. For example, mutations of the p53 gene are one of the commonest genetic changes found in human cancer.[42] In most cancers, mutation of p53 occurs as a somatic event but germ line p53 mutations have been identified in some families with the rare Li-Fraumeni syndrome[43] characterized by sarcomas, breast cancer and other malignancies occurring at a young age. Another example is germ line mutations of the APC gene which are responsible for familial adenomatous polyposis (FAP).[32,33] Somatic mutations of APC have been detected in over 80% of sporadic colorectal cancers[44,45] and appear to be one of the earliest events in colorectal carcinogenesis. Most of the familial cancer syndromes identified to date have an autosomal dominant pattern of inheritance. Individuals inheriting the germ line abnormality are at high risk of developing malignancy as the penetrance of most of these genes is of the order of 80%. It is possible that another class of genetic predispositions to cancer will be identified, which increase susceptibility to cancer but with a low penetrance (i.e. a relatively small proportion of individuals with the genetic abnormality develop cancer). Such individuals would not be easy to identify by familial studies because of the low penetrance but may account for a significant proportion of cancer cases.

GENETIC EVENTS IN GYNAECOLOGICAL CANCERS

Gynaecological cancers illustrate many of the important principles of molecular carcinogenesis

Gynaecological cancers provide examples of contrasting mechanisms of carcinogenesis. First, ovarian and endometrial cancer can occur as components of two important familial cancer syndromes (familial breast/ovarian cancer and Lynch II syndrome) because of germ line inheritance of predisposing genetic abnormalities. Second, in cervical cancer the initial genetic alteration is thought to be directly initiated by an environmental factor – papillomavirus. Third, in sporadic ovarian cancer the environmental factors associated with carcinogenesis are thought to operate indirectly by increasing the opportunity for spontaneous mutation in a number of critical genes. These different pathways of carcinogenesis are summarized in Fig. 24.5 and are described in more detail below.

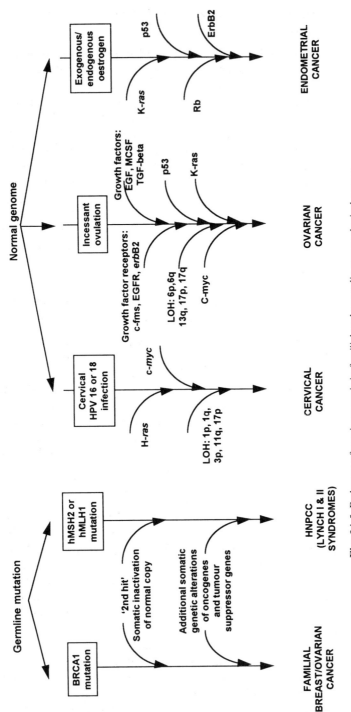

Fig. 24.5 Pathways of carcinogenesis in familial and sporadic gynaecological cancer.

A small proportion of ovarian and endometrial cancers are caused by familial syndromes

Pedigree studies of families with a high incidence of cancer have revealed three main syndromes associated with ovarian cancer.[46] Hereditary site-specific ovarian cancer without an excess of breast or colorectal cancer is the least common familial ovarian cancer syndrome. The most common hereditary form of ovarian cancer occurs in association with breast cancer. A large number of hereditary breast/ovarian cancer families have now been described in which there is a high frequency of both cancers and an association with an early age of onset. Less commonly, ovarian cancer occurs as part of the Lynch II syndrome. Women in Lynch II syndrome families most commonly develop colorectal or endometrial cancer. Some families have recently been described with an apparently high risk of site-specific endometrial cancer. It is important to recognize that all of these families combined probably account for less than 5% of cases of ovarian cancer and a smaller proportion of cases of endometrial cancer.

The gene responsible for familial breast/ovarian cancer is located on chromosome 17q and is probably a tumour suppressor gene

Identification of high risk families, together with the development of polymorphic DNA markers, made it possible to perform detailed linkage analysis with the aim of locating genes involved in familial cancer. A major step forward was the report by Hall et al[47] of linkage of early onset breast cancer to the polymorphic marker CMM86 located on chromosome 17q. Subsequently, Narod et al[48] described linkage to the same marker in breast/ovarian cancer families. Most recently, linkage to 17q was confirmed by a consortium of 13 research groups from Europe and the USA, which analysed linkage data on six genetic markers on 17q in 214 families.[49] Almost all breast/ovarian cancer families and 40% of the families with breast cancer alone have linkage to the BRCA1 (*B*reast *Ca*ncer *1*) gene on chromosome 17q. Intensive efforts are currently being made in a number of research units in Europe and the USA to further localize and ultimately clone the BRCA1 gene. Linkage analysis has identified a 1.5cM region on 17q which contains the BRCA1 gene (Fig. 24.6).[50-53] Mutational analysis of previously described genes located in this region of 17q has not revealed any abnormalities[50,54] and it seems likely that BRCA1 will prove to be a new gene. Analysis of loss of heterozygosity in tumours from familial breast/ovarian cancer families suggests that the BRCA1 gene is a tumour suppressor gene.[55] The identification of additional critical recombinant cases may further localize the BRCA1 gene and it is likely that a number of groups have now narrowed the region to <1cM. Most of the region of interest has now been cloned into vectors; this allows screening of cDNA libraries for expressed sequences that may represent new candidate genes. The size of this region suggests that it will contain

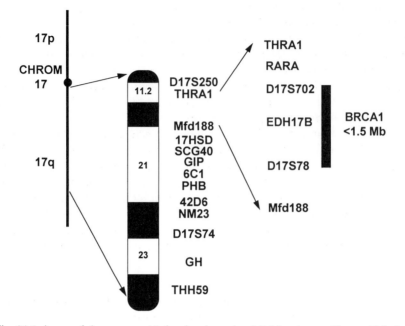

Fig. 24.6 A map of chromosome 17 showing the region 1.5cM region on 17q to which the BRCA1 gene has been mapped.[50-53] The letters/numbers identify markers which have been used in linkage analysis. The marker D17S74 (CMM86) to which linkage was initially demonstrated[47] is 17cM telomeric to the current region of interest.

approximately 30–50 genes. Ongoing work to locate BRCA1 will involve systematic identification, characterization and sequencing of candidate genes. The cloning of BRCA1 could therefore be reported before this chapter is published or may still be awaited in 5 years time!

The genetic basis of Lynch II syndrome is an abnormality of DNA repair

The identification of the genetic basis of Lynch II syndrome is a notable example of the power of molecular technology. Hereditary non-polyposis colorectal cancer (HNPCC) was classified into two syndromes by Henry Lynch; site-specific hereditary colon cancer (Lynch I syndrome), and families with a predisposition to non-polyposis colorectal cancer in association with other cancers including ovarian and endometrial cancer as well as stomach, pancreas and breast cancer (Lynch II syndrome).[56] Identification of the genes responsible for HNPCC was a result of several developments. First, linkage to a locus on chromosome 2p was demonstrated in affected members of two large HNPCC families.[57,58] Second, it was observed that the tumours from HNPCC patients contained abnormalities of repeating sequences (microsatellites) at numerous loci throughout the genome, suggesting that an abnormality of a DNA mismatch repair gene may be responsible for the pre-disposition.[59,60] Third, it was known that inactivation of bacterial and yeast genes involved in mismatch repair (mutS and mutL) resulted in microsatel-lite instability similiar to that observed in tumour cells.[61] This observation provided the basis for cloning of a human homologue of mutS on chromo-some 2p (hMSH2) and mutL on chromosome 3p (hMLH1), which were found to contain mutations in the germline of HNPCC patients.[62,63] The results indicate that HNPCC is associated with hereditary defects in mis-match repair genes. Available evidence suggests that these genes function as tumour suppressor genes in a manner consistent with Knudson's 'two hit' model. The inherited germline mutation inactivates one copy of the mis-match repair gene, but inactivation of the remaining wild-type (normal) copy by a second somatic mutation is required prior to tumour formation. The basis for the tumour specificity associated with the inherited mutation is unclear, and an interesting issue, because the mismatch repair genes are ubiquitously expressed.

Cervical cancer is a sporadic disease in which viral DNA integration disrupts normal mechanisms of cellular control

The histopathological progression of cervical neoplasia from mild to increas-ingly severe dysplasia and ultimately invasive cervical cancer will be familiar to most readers of this chapter, as will the evidence for an infective aetiology for cervical cancer and the association with human papillomavirus infection. During recent years exciting progress has been made in understanding the mechanism of papillomavirus-induced carcinogenesis and incorporating these findings with the principles of multistep carcinogenesis outlined above. Human papillomaviruses (HPV) are a group of more than 60 viruses, most of which give rise to benign tumours such as wart infections. Risk of cervical neo-plasia is associated with particular HPV types (HPV 16 and 18).[64] The genome of all HPVs have a similiar organization, in that they encode eight major open reading frames comprising early (E1–7) and late (L1–2) viral pro-teins. It is the early proteins E6 and E7 which are responsible for the trans-forming activity of the virus.[65] The E6 and E7 proteins of high-risk HPV types (16 and 18) but not those of low-risk types cause in vitro changes which par-allel the changes in cervical intraepithelial neoplasia (CIN).[66] During a normal viral infection resulting in production and release of new virus the viral genome exists episomally without integration in the nucleus of the infected cell. In tumour cells the viral DNA is integrated with the DNA of the host cell. Although the sites of integration of viral DNA are random in cancer cell lines, and many of the viral genes are lost, the E6 and E7 viral open reading frames are always conserved and are the most abundant viral transcript in such cell lines.[67] Futhermore, integration of E6 and E7 usually occurs in a manner which disrupts the normal viral regulation of expression of these proteins.[68]

These observations suggest that the E6 and E7 proteins have an important role in cervical carcinogenesis; this is supported by recent evidence that these proteins can interact with and inactivate several important cellular proteins. E7 protein binds to the product of the retinoblastoma tumour suppressor gene interfering with normal protein complex formation and disrupting the normal function of Rb protein.[69–71] E6 protein interacts with the protein product of the p53 tumour suppressor gene causing rapid breakdown of the protein and loss of normal p53 function.[72] The overall effect of E6 and E7 expression in the cell is therefore equivalent to loss of the Rb and p53 tumour suppressor genes. This is consistent with the observation that the p53 mutation is uncommon in cervical cancer but is found in HPV 16 and 18 negative cervical cancer cell lines.[73] Clinical and experimental evidence suggests that, in common with other mechanisms of carcinogenesis, HPV infection alone is not sufficient to cause cervical cancer but requires other factors, which may influence local immune responses and/or result in other genetic alterations. First, only a small proportion of women with HPV infection develop cancer and there is a long latent period before this occurs. Second, epidemiological studies suggest that other factors such as smoking and herpes simplex infection may play a role. Third, a number of genetic abnormalities have been identified in cervical cancers. These include amplification or overexpression of c-myc,[74] mutation of c-H-ras[75] and loss of heterozygosity at a number of chromosomal loci.

Sporadic ovarian cancer is associated with abnormalities of oncogenes and tumour suppressor genes

The majority of cases of ovarian cancer are not associated with familial predisposition. There is good evidence from epidemiological studies that the risk of sporadic ovarian cancer is associated with factors which influence the frequency of ovulation (e.g. parity, breast feeding, oral contraceptive use). Ovulation results in disruption of the ovarian epithelium, which is repaired by proliferation of ovarian epithelial cells exposed to growth factors present in follicular fluid. The proliferation of ovarian epithelium at the time of ovulation may provide the opportunity for mutations to occur, resulting in somatic activation of oncogenes and tumour suppressor genes. The genetic abnormalities in ovarian cancer involve genes at each step in the complex pathway of cell regulation (see Fig. 24.1), and include growth factors (M-CSF, TGF-beta), growth factor receptors (fms, EGFR, Her-2/neu), genes involved in signal transduction (ras), genes involved in transcriptional regulation (myc, p53) and loss of heterozygosity at various loci, which occur in a proportion of epithelial ovarian cancers.

Oncogenes in sporadic ovarian cancer

Growth factors. There is good evidence that the response of ovarian cancer cells to growth factors is altered compared with normal ovarian epithelial cells. The proliferative response of ovarian cancer cells in culture to EGF (Epidermal Growth Factor) and TGF-alpha (Transforming Growth Factor alpha) is variable but usually less than normal ovarian epithelium,[76-78] whilst the inhibitory effect of TGF-beta (Transforming Growth Factor beta) is less marked in ovarian cancer cell lines than in normal ovarian epithelium.[79-81] TGF-beta appears to function as an autocrine inhibitory factor in normal ovarian epithelial growth and the loss of this regulatory loop may represent a step in the process of ovarian carcinogenesis. The Macrophage Colony Stimulating Factor (M-CSF) is a ligand for a cell surface receptor (M-CSFr) encoded by the c-fms proto-oncogene. Normal ovarian epithelium does not express M-CSFr whereas the majority of ovarian cancer cells do express this receptor.[82-84] M-CSF is a potent attractant for macrophages and can stimulate the invasiveness of cancer cell lines that express fms.[85] It is possible that M-CSF regulates ovarian cancer cells via an autocrine pathway in cells expressing fms as well as by a paracrine pathway through attraction of macrophages and consequent release of cytokines such as IL-1, IL-6 and TNF.

Growth factor receptors. The growth factor receptors are a family of cell membrane tyrosine kinases, which act as receptors for the growth factors discussed above and are involved in signal transduction via autophosphorylation and phosphorylation of intracellular proteins. The EGF receptor (EGFR also referred to as erbB) and HER-2/neu (also referred to as erbB2) are structurally similiar and both have been shown to be overexpressed in human cancers. EGFR is expressed by most advanced stage ovarian cancers and there is some evidence that EGFR positive tumours have a worse prognosis than tumours not expressing the receptor.[86-87] Her-2/neu is overexpressed in approximately one-third of ovarian cancers[88,89] and overexpression is associated with gene amplification. Berchuck et al[89] and Slamon et al[88] reported a correlation between overexpression of Her-2/neu and poor prognosis for ovarian cancer, but no association with poor outcome was observed in two other studies.[90,91]

Oncogenes involved in signal transduction. Although mutations of the ras oncogene occur in ovarian cancer they are less common than in some other epithelial cancers. Ki-ras mutations in ovarian tumours almost exclusively involve codon 12 and are more frequent in mucinous tumours (48% of borderline and 57% of invasive mucinous tumours) than serous ovarian tumours (27% of borderline and 12% of invasive serous tumours).[92-95]

Nuclear oncogenes. Little is known about the role of most nuclear oncogenes in ovarian cancer. Amplification of c-myc and increased expression of the protein product has been described in approximately one-third of ovarian cancers.[96-98] Tashiro et al[99] found the rate of overexpression of c-myc to be 38% in a series of ovarian tumours.

Tumour suppressor genes in sporadic ovarian cancer

p53. Mutations of the p53 gene are the most common genetic alteration in cancer and occur most frequently in regions of the gene which show the greatest degree of conservation between p53 proteins of different species. Immunohistochemical studies have revealed overexpression of the p53 protein in 50% of advanced stage ovarian cancer.[100] Sequencing of p53 from ovarian cancers overexpressing the p53 protein has in most cases confirmed point mutations in conserved regions of the gene.[100] In most of these tumours loss of heterozygosity studies have revealed that the second copy of the gene is inactivated through deletion of the gene.[101–103] Mutation of p53 is less common in stage I disease than advanced stage disease,[103] and clonal analysis suggests that the occurence of p53 mutation precedes but is temporally associated with metastases.[102,104,105] No clear relationship between p53 mutation and histological grade or prognosis has been established. The location and nature of the p53 mutations in ovarian cancer has now been reported in 149 tumours. A total of 95 different mutations involving 62 different codons have been identified, and most occur in the highly conserved exons 5–8 of the gene.[101–103, 105–110] The codons most frequently involved in p53 mutations are the same as those described in other cancers. The pattern of mutations suggests that most p53 alterations in ovarian cancer arise because of endogenous mutagenic processes rather than exposure to a carcinogen.[106]

Loss of heterozygosity. As tumour suppressor genes inhibit cell proliferation, both copies of the gene must be inactivated for neoplastic effect (i.e. they act recessively at a cellular level). The first 'hit' is frequently a point mutation, whilst the second 'hit', which inactivates the remaining wild-type copy of the gene, is often a larger event involving loss of a portion or the whole of a chromosome. The relatively large losses associated with the second 'hit' are easier to identify than point mutations and have been exploited as a method of mapping the location of tumour suppressor genes by loss of heterozygosity analysis. Studies of loss of heterozygosity in ovarian cancer have revealed a number of regions with high frequencies of loss. The reported frequency of loss of heterozygosity for each chromosome arm is summarized in Fig. 24.7. Losses have been observed on almost all chromosome arms and the background 'random' rate of loss in ovarian cancer is high (15–25%). A high frequency of allelic deletion (>33%) based upon more than 50 tumours in at least three separate studies has been documented for seven chromosome arms: 6p, 6q, 13q, 17p (possibly associated with p53), 17q, 18q and Xp. A number of other chromosome arms have frequencies of loss in the range of 25–33%, which may be above background rates: 4p, 8p, 9p, 9q, 11p, 14q, 16q, 19p and 21q. Further localization of putative tumour suppressor genes in regions with a high rate of LOH requires detailed analysis with a panel of polymorphic markers for the relevant chromosome arm. Available data suggest that a number of as yet unidentified tumour suppressor genes are involved in ovarian carcinogenesis, and recent reports have defined deletion units on chromosome arms with the highest rates of LOH including 6p, 6q, 11p, 13q, 17q and Xp. The high rate of loss of heterozygosity on chromosome 17q was first reported by Eccles et al[111] and Russell et al[112] and is now of particular interest in view of the mapping of BRCA1 to this chromosome

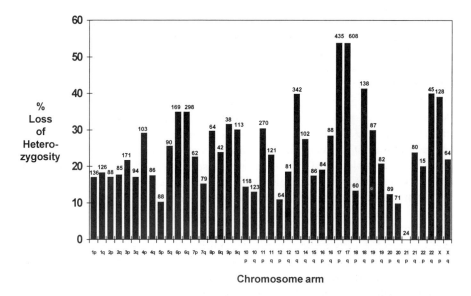

Fig. 24.7 A summary of reports of the frequency of loss of heterozygosity (LOH) at each chromosome arm in ovarian cancer. The data represent the number of tumours with LOH for the chromosome arm/the number of informative tumours for each chromosome arm. The number of tumours studied at each chromosome arm is shown at the top of each bar.[111–135]

arm. The pattern of LOH on chromosome 17 suggests that although BRCA1 may play a role in sporadic disease other, as yet unidentified, tumour suppressor genes on the same chromosome are also of importance.

Some of the genetic events in endometrial carcinogenesis have been identified

A small proportion of endometrial cancers occur as part of the Lynch II syndrome, and it is possible that site-specific hereditary endometrial cancer exists as a distinct entity.[136] The majority of cases of endometrial cancers are, however, sporadic. Although it is known that unopposed oestrogens are important in the aetiology of sporadic endometrial cancer there is limited information about the molecular basis of this disease. Oestrogen and progesterone receptors are frequently expressed by endometrial cancers and loss of expression is correlated with poor prognosis. In contrast to ovarian cancer the majority of endometrial cancers have a diploid DNA content but approximately 25% are aneuploid and this feature is associated with aggressive disease and poor prognosis.[137–139] A number of recent studies have identified mutations of known oncogenes and tumour suppressor genes in endometrial cancer but no genetic alterations specific to this cancer have been documented. Kohler et al[140] reported immunohistochemical evidence of p53 mutations in 21% of a series of 107 endometrial cancers. The results suggested that p53 mutations were more frequent in advanced stage than early stage disease and were associated with non-endometrioid histology, positive peritoneal cytology and metastatic disease. These findings are consistent with other studies of p53 in endometrial cancer; a total of 42/241 endometrial cancers studied (17%) have p53 mutations, usually in conserved regions of the gene with a similiar distribution to p53 mutations in ovarian cancer.[110,141–144] Kohler et al[145] also studied a series of 117 endometrial hyperplasias, none of which were found to have p53 mutations; this suggested that p53 mutation is a relatively late event in endometrial carcinogenesis. A number of studies of ras mutations in endometrial cancer have been reported.[142,146–151] Overall, Ki-ras mutations have been documented in 60/320 (19%) of endometrial cancers analysed. Of the 60 mutations reported all but five were in codon 12 and the remainder in codon 13. The relationship of prognostic factors to Ki-ras mutation is not yet clear. Mizuchi et al[148] found Ki-ras muatations to be an independent indicator of poor prognosis. However, Fujimoto et al[149] found no significant relationship with prognostic factors, and Sasaki et al[147] found Ki-ras mutation to correlate with improved survival rates. In contrast to p53 mutation, Ki-ras mutation appears to be a relatively early event in endometrial carcinogenesis. The frequency of Ki-ras mutation in endometrial hyperplasia is similar to that found in invasive disease.[142,147] Duggan et al[146] found that when Ki-ras mutations were present in areas of invasive endometrial cancer they were present in adjacent areas of atypical hyperplasia but not simple or complex hyperplasia without atypia. Therefore, Ki-ras mutation appears to be involved in progression to atypical hyperplasia. Both overexpression and amplification of the ErbB2 oncogene has been reported to occur in endometrial cancer.[152–154] Small studies also suggest endometrial cancer may be associated with amplification of c-myc and alteration of the retinoblastoma gene.[153–155]

CLINICAL IMPLICATIONS OF MOLECULAR GENETICS IN GYNAECOLOGICAL CANCER

Genetic analysis will allow accurate assessment of familial cancer risk

Epidemiological data, together with a detailed and well documented family history, will identify individuals belonging to cancer syndrome families. However, this information will usually allow only a broad estimate of an individual's risk of malignancy. For familial syndromes such as breast/ovarian cancer, which are not associated with a phenotypic marker (such as polyps in familial adenomatous polyposis), it is not possible to establish precisely which families have a genetic predisposition and which individuals within the family have inherited the predisposition. For example, the available data suggest that in two-thirds of families in which three first degree relatives have breast or ovarian cancer the cause is autosomal dominant inheritance of an abnormality of the BRCA1 gene. Breast or ovarian cancer in the remaining one-third of such families is caused by chance aggregation of these relatively common cancers. For a female first degree relative of an affected family member there is a 2/3 probability that the family history is caused by an inherited abnormality and a 1/2 probability that if this is the case she has inherited the abnormality. As the estimated penetrance for development of either breast or ovarian cancer in female carriers of BRCA1 is 85% and 48%, respectively, by age 70 years[156] she can be told that her risk of developing breast cancer and ovarian cancer by age 70 years is approximately 28% (2/3 $\times$ 1/2 $\times$ 85%) and 16% (2/3 $\times$ 1/2 $\times$ 48%) respectively.

At the present time a more accurate assessment of risk of familial breast/ovarian cancer can only be achieved in large families suitable for linkage analysis. If the relevant DNA samples are available (either from blood or archival pathology material) from several other affected family members it may be possible to establish whether inheritance of the disease is linked to the BRCA1 locus on chromosome 17q and, if so, which individual family members have inherited the disease-linked chromosome. Linkage analysis is not frequently performed in clinical practice. It is costly and time consuming, is only applicable to large families with numerous DNA samples available and can be inaccurate owing to loss of linkage at meiotic crossover. Furthermore, estimation of risk is complicated by the observation that the distribution of breast and ovarian cancer is not homogeneous across all affected families. The pattern of breast and ovarian cancer is best explained by two alleles, one relatively uncommon (11% of mutations) conferring a high lifetime risk of breast and ovarian cancer and another (89% of mutations) conferring a high risk of breast cancer but a relatively lower risk of ovarian cancer.[157] These differences in cancer distribution between families may reflect the effect of different mutations within the BRCA1 gene and will clearly have important implications for counselling and clinical management once the gene is cloned.

It is likely that the BRCA1 gene will be cloned and the spectrum of mutations responsible for familial breast/ovarian cancer identified in the near future. It may then be feasible to screen individuals for mutations and base accurate risk estimates on the precise mutation identified without having to obtain DNA samples from a large number of relatives. The feasibility of such analysis will, however, depend on the size of the gene, the nature and number of different mutations and the effect of different mutations. Furthermore, there are important ethical considerations about the performance of this form of analysis.[158] The information is likely to be valuable to women who have not inherited the mutation as they will not need to undergo preventative or screening procedures. However, for women who are found to be at high risk there are major psychological implications and the possibility of discrimination in obtaining employment, insurance and financial agreements. In

addition, it is far from clear that life expectancy is increased by the identification of genetic risk. The options available to individuals identified as at high
risk for familial ovarian cancer include oophorectomy, screening with tumour
markers or ultrasound and oral contraceptive pill use.[159] A detailed review of
these management options is not possible in this chapter but it should be
noted that none have yet been demonstrated to confer a definite increase in
life expectancy. It is clear that genetic testing for cancer will need to be provided in centres equipped not only to provide accurate genetic analysis but
also psychological support and informed advice concerning preventative and
screening options.

Knowledge of the molecular aetiology of cancer will provide a basis for design of preventative techniques

Genetic approaches may help in the identification of premalignant conditions
amenable to conventional therapy. For example, in contrast to cervical cancer there is no well documented precursor lesion in ovarian carcinogenesis.
The possibility has been raised that ovarian epithelial atypia, inclusion cysts
and benign or borderline ovarian tumours may represent steps in the pathway of ovarian carcinogenesis.[160-163] Genetic studies may establish the relationship between these histopathological features and ovarian cancer and
consequently provide new opportunities for prevention. Where there are
known abnormalities conferring a high risk of cancer it may be possible to
design strategies to correct the abnormality. In familial cancer syndromes it
may ultimately be possible to transfer normal copies of the abnormal gene
(e.g. p53, BRCA1) to the tissue at risk using tissue-specific viral vectors. In
cervical cancer work is in progress to develop a vaccine directed against the
HPV types associated with the disease.[104] It may be possible to generate an
immune response to viral coat particles (L1 and L2) or to viral transforming
proteins (E6 and E7) using either a protein vaccine or presentation of these
antigens in a viral or bacterial vector.

Molecular techniques can be used to detect cancer at an early stage

Knowledge of specific genetic alterations associated with cancer, together
with the high sensitivity of molecular techniques such as the polymerase
chain reaction, may provide new methods for detection of cancer. As direct
sampling of the ovary requires an invasive procedure, any screening test for
ovarian cancer based upon genetic markers will be directed toward identification of a gene product in peripheral blood. The protein product of the M-
CSF gene is detectable at elevated levels in the serum of ovarian cancer
patients. It is possible that the products of other genes coding for secreted
and cell surface proteins produced in abnormal forms or increased amounts
in cancer will be markers for early stage disease. The opportunities may be
even greater for cancers arising from accessible tissues such as the

endometrium. Using techniques such as the polymerase chain or ligase chain reaction it is possible to identify a small proportion of mutated copies of a gene in a background of many thousandfold excess normal copies of the gene. Because it is a relatively simple out-patient procedure to obtain an endometrial sample it may be possible to detect mutation of a gene associated with endometrial cancer at a very early stage of the disease. This approach has been used to detect mutations of p53 and K-ras in urine, sputum and stool specimens in cancers of the bladder, lung and colon.[165-168] Such techniques may be used to identify early stage disease, minimal residual disease and the early stages of recurrent disease.

Genetic markers can be valuable prognostic indicators

The behaviour of a malignancy is a consequence of the complex interaction of all of the genetic alterations which have accumulated during the process of carcinogenesis. As different genetic alterations have different effects, and the set of genetic changes leading to a particular malignancy is not fixed, it is reasonable to infer that genetic analysis will provide important prognostic information. Evidence for this is emerging from studies of ovarian cancer. Although p53 mutation does not appear to correlate with prognosis, there is evidence that erbB2 amplification is associated with decreased survival. Several authors have investigated the relationship between loss of heterozygosity and tumour characteristics. Correlations with frequency of LOH in ovarian cancer have been reported for (i) histological type on chromosomes 6q,13q, 17q and 19q,[113-117] LOH being more frequent in serous than other histological types; (ii) FIGO stage of disease on 17q,[113] with LOH more frequent in advanced stage disease and (iii) tumour grade. Zheng et al[118] found a correlation between tumour grade and frequency of LOH at all loci analysed on nine chromosomes. On the basis of the results it was hypothesized that LOH on chromosomes 3 or 11 results in high-grade malignancy whilst LOH on chromosome 6 is consistent with a well differentiated phenotype. Dodson et al[169] found the average fractional allelic loss in high-grade tumours to be greater than that in low-grade tumours (39.5% versus 16%). Chromosome arms 6p, 17p, 17q and 22q were frequently lost in low and high-grade tumours, whilst LOH on 13q and 15q was more common in high-grade tumours, and LOH on 3p more common in low-grade tumours.[169] These data raise the possibility that pattern of LOH is an independent prognostic indicator for ovarian cancer.

Several strategies for gene therapy are being explored

The increase in understanding of carcinogenesis at a molecular level has raised the possibility that cancer can be treated by selectively targeting cells with specific genetic abnormalities. A broad range of different methods for gene therapy have been suggested and numerous clinical trials are in progress.

Ex vivo approaches to gene therapy

Ex vivo techniques involve removal of cells from the individual, manipulation of the cells in vitro and reinjection of altered cells. One approach is to remove tumour cells from a patient, insert genes in vitro to increase their immunogenicity and reinject them into the patient in order to obtain a systemic immune response that will recognize and destroy tumour cells. Suitable genes for this approach include cytokines, which activate interleukins, and genes for major histocopatibility complex class I antigens. An alternative approach is to transfer a gene that activates a pro-drug to become cytotoxic. For example, transfer of the thymidine kinase gene of the herpes simplex virus results in phosphorylation of the anti-herpes drug gangciclovir, and cell death, owing to inhibition of DNA polymerase. The potential of this approach is enhanced by the observation that adjacent cells which do not have the gene are also affected, presumably because of diffusion of the phosphorylated drug.[170] A trial of intraperitoneal therapy using this strategy is underway in stage III ovarian cancer.[171]

In situ approaches to gene therapy

An exciting possibility is for the correction of specific molecular genetic abnormalities, responsible for carcinogenesis, to be corrected in tumour cells by replacing a normal copy of a tumour suppressor gene, such as p53, or suppressing expression of the product of an oncogene, such as K-ras. There is evidence that insertion of wild-type p53 and antisense K-ras into tumour cells with abnormalities of these genes suppresses tumourigenicity.[172,173] It may also be possible to target genes involved in metastasis. Decreased expression of the nm23 gene is associated with increased metastatic potential in some cancers, and transfection of nm23 into melanoma cells decreases metastatic potential. The technical limitations of corrective gene therapy are currently twofold. First, in order to control a cancer in vivo the gene must be transferred to all tumour cells. The most hopeful method of gene transfer is the use of a recombinant virus, because viral replication and spread may overcome the difficulty of targeting tumour cells with a poor vascular supply which limits other therapeutic approaches such as the use of monoclonal antibodies. Second, the vector used for gene transfer must be targeted to tumour but not normal cells of the individual. It may be possible to construct viral vectors which will bind to cell surface proteins expressed preferentially on tumour cells or which require a transcription factor expressed in tumour cells but not normal cells. Ultimately, a highly sophisticated therapeutic approach may involve a viral vector modified to contain a therapeutic gene, to recognize tumour cell surface antigens and require tumour-specific factors for transcription.

ADDENDUM

This chapter was commissioned and completed in 1994. Since then the BRCA1 and BRCA2 genes have been cloned. Mutations of the BRCA1 gene on chromosome 17q account for the majority of breast/ovarian cancer families and approximately one-third of breast cancer families. Mutations of the BRCA2 gene on chromosome 13q account for a further one-third of breast cancer families and a small proportion of breast/ovarian cancer families. Both of these genes are large and their function is, as yet, unclear. To date, screening for BRCA1 and BRCA2 mutations is largely confined to research studies, due to the size of the genes, the cost of the analysis and the ethical/psychological implications of direct gene testing. As technology for mutation detection improves during the next few years, mutation screening as a clinical service will become available and the complex financial, ethical and psychological implications will need to be addressed.

REFERENCES

1 McCann J, Choi E, Yamasaki E, Ames B N. Detection of carcinogens as mutagens in the Salmonella/microsome test: Assay of 300 chemicals. Proc Natl Acad Sci USA 1975; 84: 4621–4625
2 Ames B N, Durston W E, Yamasaki E, Lee F D. Carcinogens are mutagens: a simple test system combining liver homogenates for activation and bacteria for detection. Proc Natl Acad Sci USA 1973; 70: 2281–2285
3 Fearon E R, Hamilton S R, Vogelstein B. Clonal analysis of human colorectal tumours. Science 1987; 238: 193–197
4 Fialkow P J. Clonal origin of human tumours. Biochim Biophys Acta 1976; 458: 283–321
5 Alberts B, Bray D, Lewis J, Raff M, Robets K, Watson J D. Molecular biology of the cell, 2nd edn. New York: Garland Publishing, 1989
6 Rous P. A sarcoma of the fowl transmissible by an agent separable from the tumour cells. J Exp Med 1911; 13: 396–411
7 Stehelin D, Varmus H E, Bishop J M, Vogt P K. DNA related to the transforming gene(s) of avain sarcoma viruses is present in normal avain DNA. Nature 1976; 260: 170–173
8 Collett M S, Erikson E, Purchio A F, Brugge J S, Erikson R L. A normal cell protein similar in structure and function to the avian sarcoma virus transforming gene product. Proc Natl Acad Sci USA 1979; 3159–3163
9 Oppermann J, Levinson A D, Varmus H E, Levintow L, Bishop J M. Uninfected vertebrate cells contain a protein that is closely related to the product of the avian sarcoma virus transforming gene (src). Proc Natl Acad Sci USA 1979; 76: 1804–1808
10 Parker R C, Varmus H E, Bishop J M. Cellular homologue (c-src) of the transforming gene of Rous sarcoma virus: isolation, mapping and transcriptional analysis of c-src and flanking regions. Proc Natl Acad Sci USA 1981; 78: 5842–5846
11 Krontiris T G, Cooper G M. Transforming activity of human tumour DNAs. Proc Natl Acad Sci USA 1981; 78: 1811–1184
12 Shih C, Padhy L C, Murray M, Weinberg R A. Transforming genes of carcinomas and neuroblastomas introduced into mouse fibroblasts. Nature 1981; 290: 261–264
13 Santos E, Tronick S R, Aaronson S A, Pulciani S, Barbacid M. T24 human bladder carcinoma oncogene is an activated form of the normal human homologue of BALB- and Harvey- MSV transforming genes. Nature 1982; 298: 343–347
14 Parada L F, Tabin C J, Shih C, Weinberg R A. Human EK bladder carcinoma oncogene is homologue of Harvey sarcoma virus ras gene. Nature 1982; 297: 474–478
15 Der C J, Krontiris T G, Cooper G M. Transforming genes of human bladder and lung carcinoma cell lines are homologous to the ra genes of Harvey and Kirsten sarcoma viruses. Proc Natl Acad Sci USA 1982; 79: 3637–3640

16 Birchmeier C, Birnbaum D, Waitches G, Fasano O, Wigler M. Characterisation of an activated human ros gene. Mol Cell Biol 1986; 6: 3109–3116

17 Shimizu K, Yoshimichi N, Sekiguchi M, Hokamura K, Tanaka K. Molecular cloning of an activated human oncogene, homologous to v-raf, from primary stomach cancer. Proc Natl Acad Sci USA 1985; 82: 5641–5645

18 Nowell P C, Hungerford D A. Chromosome studies on normal and leukaemic human leukocytes. J Natl Cancer Inst 1960; 25: 85–109

19 DeKlein A, van Kessel A G, Grosveld G et al. A cellular oncogene is translocated to the Philadelphia chromosome in chronic myelocytic leukemia. Nature 1982; 300: 765–767

20 Harris H, Miller O J, Klein G, Worst P, Tachibana T. Suppression of maligancy by cell fusion. Nature 1969; 223: 363–368

21 Harris H. The analysis of malignancy by cell fusion: the position in 1988. Cancer Res 1988; 48: 3302–3306

22 Stanbridge E J, Flandermeyer R R, Daniels D W, Nelson-Rees W A. Specific chromosome loss associated with the expression of tumorigenicity in human cell hybrids. Somatic Cell Mol Genet 1981; 7: 699–712

23 Knudson A G. Mutation and cancer: statistical study of retinoblastoma. Proc Natl Acad Sci USA 1971; 68: 820–823

24 Knudson A G, Meadows A T, Bichols W W, Hill R. Chromosomal deletion and retinoblastoma. N Engl J Med 1976; 295: 1120–1123

25 Sparkes R S, Murphree A L, Lingua R W, Sparkes M C, Field L L, Funderburk S J, Benedict W F. Gene for hereditary retinoblastoma assigned to human chromosome 13 by linkage to esterase D. Science 1983; 219: 971–973

26 Friend S H, Bernards R, Rogelj S, Weinberg R A, Rapaport J M, Albert D M, Dryja T P. A human DNA segment with properties of the gene that predisposes to retinoblastoma and osteosarcoma. Nature 1986; 323: 643–646

27 Lee W-H, Bookstein R, Hong F, Young L-J, Shew J-Y, Lee E Y-H P. Human retinoblastoma susceptibility gene: cloning, identification and sequence. Science 1987; 235: 1394–1399

28 Fung Y-K T, Murphree A L, T'Ang A, Qian J, Hinrichs S H, Benedict W F. Structural evidence for the authenticity of the human retinoblastoma gene. Science 1987; 236: 1657–1661

29 Cavanee W K, Dryja T P, Phillips R A et al. Expression of recessive alleles by chromosomal mechanisms in retinoblastoma. Nature 1983; 305: 779–784

30 Dryja T P, Rapaport J M, Joyce J M, Petersen R A. Molecular detection of deletions involving band q14 of chromosome 13 in retinoblastomas. Proc Natl Acad Sci USA 1986; 83: 7391–7394

31 Baker S J, Fearon E R, Nigro J M et al. Chromosome 17 deletions and p53 gene mutations in colorectal carcinomas. Science 1989; 244: 217–221

32 Groden J, Thliveris A, Samovitz W et al. Identification and characterisation of the familial adenomatous polyposis coli gene. Cell 1991; 66: 589–600

33 Kinzler K W, Nilbert M C, Su L-K et al. Identification of FAP locus genes from chromosome 5q21. Science 1991; 253: 661–665

34 Fearon E R, Cho K R, Nigro J M et al. Identification of a chromosome 18q gene that is altered in colorectal cancers. Science 1990; 247: 49–56

35 Cairns J. Mutation selection, and the natural history of cancer. Nature 1975; 255: 197–200

36 Armitage P, Doll R. The age distribution of cancer and a multi-stage theory of carcinogenesis. Br J Cancer 1954; 8: 1–12

37 Land H, Parada L F, Weiberg R A. Tumorigenic conversion of primary embryo fibroblasts requires at least two cooperating oncogenes. Nature 1983; 304: 596–602

38 Sinn E, Muller W, Pattengale P, Tepler I, Wallace R, Leder P. Coexpression of MMTV/v-Ha-ra and MMTV/c-myc genes in transgenic mice: synergistic action of oncogenes in vivo. Cell 1987; 49: 465–475

39 Fearon E R, Cho K R, Nigro J M et al. Identification of a chromosome 18q gene that is altered in colorectal cancers. Science 1990; 247: 49–56

40 Standbridge E J. Identifying tumour suppressor genes in human colorectal cancer. Science 1990; 247: 12–13

41 Vogelstein B, Kinzler K W. The multistep nature of cancer. Trends Genet 1993; 9(4): 138–141

42 Hollstein M, Sidransky D, Vogelstein B, Barris C. p53 mutations in human cancer. Science 1991; 253: 49–53

43 Malkin D, Li F P, Strong L C et al. Germ line p53 mutations in a familial syndrome of breast cancer, sarcomas, and other neoplasms. Science 1990; 250: 1233–1238

44 Miyoshi Y, Nagase H, Ando H et al. Somatic mutations in the APC gene in colorectal tumours: mutation cluster region in the APC gene. Hum Mol Genet 1992; 1: 229–233

45 Powell S M, Zilz N, Beazer-Barclay Y et al. APC mutations occur early during colorectal tumorigenesis. Nature 1992; 359: 235–237

46 Bewtra C, Watson P, Conway T, Read-Hippee C, Lynch H T. Hereditary ovarian cancer: a clinicopathological study. Int J Gynecologic Pathol 1992; 11(3): 180

47 Hall J M, Lee M K, Newman B et al. Linkage of early-onset familial breast cancer to chromosome 17q21. Science 1990; 250: 1684–1689

48 Narod S A, Feunteun J, Lynch H T et al. Familial breast-ovarian cancer locus on chromosome 17q12-q23 (see comments). Lancet 1991; 338(8759): 82

49 Easton D F, Bishop D T, Ford D, Crockford G P. Genetic linkage analysis in familial breast and ovarian cancer: results from 214 families. The breast cancer linkage consortium. Am J Hum Genet 1993; 52(4): 678

50 Simard J, Feunteun J, Lenoir G et al. Genetic mapping of the breast-ovarian cancer syndrome to a small interval on chromosome 17q12–21: exclusion of candidate genes EDH17B2 and RARA. Hum Mol Genet 1993; 2: 1193–1199

51 Goldgar D E, Cannon-Albright L A, Oliphant A et al. Chromosome 17q linkage studies of 18 Utah breast cancer kindreds. Am J Hum Genet 1993; 52(4): 743

52 Bowcock A M, Anderson L A, Friedman L S et al. THRA1 and D17S183 flank an interval of: 4 cM for the breast-ovarian cancer gene (BRCA1) on chromosome 17q21. Am J Hum Genet 1993; 52(4): 718

53 Chamberlain J S, Boehnke M, Frank T S et al. BRCA1 maps proximal to D17S579 on chromosome 17q21 by genetic analysis. Am J Hum Genet 1993; 52(4): 792

54 Kelsell D P, Black D M, Bishop D T, Spurr N K. Genetic analysis of the BRCA1 region in a large breast/ovarian family: refinement of the minimal region containing BRCA1. Hum Mol Genet 1993; 2: 1823–1828

55 Smith S A, Easton D F, Evans D G, Ponder B A. Allele losses in the region 17q12–21 in familial breast and ovarian cancer involve the wild-type chromosome. Nature Genet 1992; 2(2): 128

56 Lynch H T et al. Hereditary nonpolyposis colorectal cancer (Lynch syndromes I and II). Cancer 1985; 15: 938

57 Pättomäki P et al. Genetic mapping of a locus predisposing to human colorectal cancer. Science 1993; 260: 810–812

58 Aaltonen L A et al. Clues to the pathogenesis of familial colorectal cancer. Science 1993; 260: 812–816

59 Ionov Y, Peinado M A, Miakhosyan S, Shibata D, Penucho M. Ubiquitous somatic mutations in simple repeated sequences reveal a new mechanism for colonic carcinogenesis. Nature 1993; 363: 558–561

60 Thibodeau S N, Bren G, Schaid D. Microsatellite instability in cancer of the proximal colon. Science 1993; 260: 816–819

61 Strand M, Prolla T A, Liskey R M, Petes T D. Nature 1993; 365: 274

62 Leach F S, Nicolaides N C, Papadopoulos N et al. Mutations of a mutS homolog in hereditary nonpolyposis colorectal cancer. Cell 1993; 75: 1215–1225

63 Fishel R, Lascoe M K, Rao M R S et al. The human mutator gene homolog MSH2 and its association with hereditary nonpolyposis colon cancer. Cell 1993; 75: 1027–1038

64 Vousden K H. Human papillomaviruses and cervical cancer. Cancer Cells 1989; 1: 43–49

65 Vousden K H. Human papillomavirus transforming genes. Semin Virol 1991; 2: 307–317

66 Hudson J B, Bedell M A, McCance D J, Laimins L A. Immortalisation and altered differentiation of human keratinocytes in vitro by the E6 and E7 open reading frames of human papillomavirus type 18. J Virol 1990; 64: 519–526

67 Shirashawa J, Tomita Y, Sekiya S, Takamizawa H, Simizu B. Integration and transcription of human papillomavirus type 16 and 18 sequences in cell lines derived from cervical carcinomas. Journal of General Virology 1987; 68: 583–591.

68 Durst M, Kleinheinz A, Hotz M. The physical state of human papillomavirus type 16 DNA in benign and malignant genital tumours. J Gen Virol 1985; 66: 1515–1522

69 Vousden K H. Interactions of human papillomavirus transforming proteins with the products of tumour suppressor genes. FASEB J 1993; 7: 872–879

70 Chellappan S, Kraus V, Kroger B, Munger K, Howley P M, Phelps W C, Nevins J R.

Adenovirus E1A simian virus 40 tumour antigen, and human papillomavirus E7 protein share the capacity to disrupt the interaction between transcription factor E2F and the retinoblastoma gene product. Proc Natl Acad Sci USA 1992; 89: 4549–4553

71 Dyson N, Howley P M, Münger K, Harlow E. The human papilloma virus-16 E7 oncoprotein is able to bind the retinoblastoma gene product. Science 1989; 243: 934–937

72 Scheffner M, Werness B A, Huibregtse J M, Levine A J, Howley P M. The E6 oncoprotein encoded by human papillomavirus types 16 and 18 promotes the degradation of p52. Cell 1990; 63: 1129–1136

73 Crook T, Wrede D, Tidy J A, Mason W P, Evans D J, Vousden K H. Clonal p53 mutation in primary cervical cancer: association with human-papillomavirus-negative tumours. Lancet 1992; 339: 1070–1073

74 Riou G, Barrois M, Dutronquay V, Orth G. In: Howley P, Broker T, eds. Papillomaviruses: Molecular and clinical aspects. New York: A R Liss, 1985: pp 47–57

75 Riou G, Barrois M, Zong-Mei Sheng, Lhomme C. Somatic deletions and mutations of c-Ha-ras gene in human cervical cancer. Oncogene 1988; 3: 329–333

76 Berchuck A, Rodriguez G, Kamel A, Soper J T, Clarke-Pearson D L, Bast R Jr. Expression of epidermal growth factor receptor and HER-2/neu in normal and neoplastic cervix, vulva, and vagina. Obstet Gynecol 1990; 76(3): 381

77 Rodriguez G C, Berchuck A, Whitaker R S, Schlossman D, Clarke-Pearson D L, Bast R Jr. Epidermal growth factor receptor expression in normal ovarian epithelium and ovarian cancer. II. Relationship between receptor expression and response to epidermal growth factor. Am J Obstet Gynecol 1991; 164(3): 745

78 Mills G B, Hashimoto S, Hurteau J et al. Regulation of growth of human ovarian cancer cells. In: Sharp F, Mason W P, Creasman W, eds. Ovarian cancer II, biology, diagnosis and management. London: Chapman and Hall Medical, 1992: pp 127–148

79 Berchuck A, Rodriguez G, Olt G et al. Regulation of growth of normal ovarian epithelial cells and ovarian cancer cell lines by transforming growth factor-beta. Am J Obstet Gynecol 1992; 166(2): 676

80 Bartlett J M, Rabiasz G J, Scott W N, Langdon S P, Smyth J F, Miller W R. Transforming growth factor-beta mRNA expression and growth control of human ovarian carcinoma cells. Br J Cancer 1992; 65(5): 655

81 Jozan S, Guerrin M, Mazars P et al. Transforming growth factor beta 1 (TGF-beta 1) inhibits growth of a human ovarian carcinoma cell line (OVCCR1) and is expressed in human ovarian tumors. Int J Cancer 1992; 52(5): 766

82 Kacinski B M, Carter D, Mittal K et al. Ovarian adenocarcinomas express fms-complementary transcripts and fms antigen, often with coexpression of CSF-1. Am J Pathol 1990; 137(1): 135

83 Baiocchi G, Kavanagh J J, Talpaz M, Wharton J T, Gutterman J U, Kurzrock R. Expression of the macrophage colony-stimulating factor and its receptor in gynecologic malignancies. Cancer 1991; 67(4): 990

84 Bast R C, Rodriguez G C, Wu S et al. Factors regulating the growth of normal and malignant ovarian epithelium. In: Sharp F, Mason W P, Creasman W, eds. Ovarian cancer II, biology, diagnosis and management. London: Chapman and Hall Medical, 1992: pp 61–65

85 Kacinski B M, Carter D, Mittal K et al. High level expression of fms proto-oncogene mRNA is observed in clinically aggressive human endometrial adenocarcinomas. Int J Rad Oncol Biol Phys 1988; 15: 823–829

86 Berchuck A, Rodriguez G C, Kamel A et al. Epidermal growth factor receptor expression in normal ovarian epithelium and ovarian cancer. I. Correlation of receptor expression with prognostic factors in patients with ovarian cancer. Am J Obstet Gynecol 1991; 164(2): 669

87 Foekens J A, van Putten W L, Portengen H et al. Prognostic value of pS2 protein and receptors for epidermal growth factor (EGF-R), insulin-like growth factor-1 (IGF-1-R) and somatostatin (SS-R) in patients with breast and ovarian cancer. J Steroid Biochem Mol Biol 1990; 37(6): 815

88 Slamon D J, Godolphin W, Jones L A et al. Studies of the HER-2/neu proto-oncogene in human breast and ovarian cancer. Science 1989; 244(4905): 707

89 Berchuck A, Kamel A, Whitaker R et al. Overexpression of HER-2/neu is associated with poor survival in advanced epithelial ovarian cancer. Cancer Res 1990; 50(13): 4087

90 Haldane J S, Hird V, Hughes C M, Gullick W J. c-erbB-2 oncogene expression in ovarian cancer. J Pathol 1990; 162(3): 231

91 Kacinski B M, Mayer A G, King B L, Carter D, Chambers S K. NEU protein

overexpression in benign, borderline, and malignant ovarian neoplasms. Gynecol Oncol 1992; 44(3): 245

92 Mok S C, Bell D A, Knapp R C et al. Mutation of K-ras protooncogene in human ovarian epithelial tumors of borderline malignancy. Cancer Res 1993; 53(7): 1489

93 Teneriello M G, Ebina M, Linnoila R I et al. p53 and Ki-ras gene mutations in epithelial ovarian neoplasms. Cancer Res 1993; 53(13): 3103

94 Enomoto T, Weghorst C M, Inoue M, Tanizawa O, Rice J M. K-ras activation occurs frequently in mucinous adenocarcinomas and rarely in other common epithelial tumors of the human ovary. Am J Pathol 1991; 139(4): 777

95 Ichikawa Y, Nishida M, Suzuki H et al. Mutation of K-ras protooncogene is associated with histological subtypes in human mucinous ovarian tumors. Cancer Res 1994; 54(1): 33

96 Kohler M, Janz I, Wintzer H O, Wagner E, Bauknecht T. The expression of EGF receptors, EGF-like factors and c-myc in ovarian and cervical carcinomas and their potential clinical significance. Anticancer Res 1989; 9(6): 1537

97 Baker V V, Borst M P, Dixon D, Hatch K D, Shingleton H M, Miller D. c-myc amplification in ovarian cancer. Gynecol Oncol 1990; 38(3): 340

98 Schreiber G, Dubeau L. C-myc proto-oncogene amplification detected by polymerase chain reaction in archival human ovarian carcinomas. Am J Pathol 1990; 137(3): 653

99 Tashiro H, Miyazaki K, Okamura H, Iwai A, Fukumoto M. c-myc over-expression in human primary ovarian tumours: its relevance to tumour progression. Int J Cancer 1992; 50(5): 828

100 Marks J R, Davidoff A M, Kerns B J et al. Overexpression and mutation of p53 in epithelial ovarian cancer. Cancer Res 1991; 51(11): 2979

101 Okamoto A, Sameshima Y, Yokoyama S et al. Frequent allelic losses and mutations of the p53 gene in human ovarian cancer. Cancer Res 1991; 51(19): 5171

102 Mazars R, Pujol P, Maudelonde T, Jeanteur P, Theillet C. p53 mutations in ovarian cancer: a late event? Oncogene 1991; 6(9): 1685

103 Kohler M F, Kerns B J, Humphrey P A, Marks J R, Bast R Jr, Berchuck A. Mutation and overexpression of p53 in early-stage epithelial ovarian cancer. Obstet Gynecol 1993; 81(5): 643

104 Jacobs I J, Kohler M F, Wiseman R W et al. Clonal origin of epithelial ovarian carcinoma: analysis by loss of heterozygosity, p53 mutation, and X-chromosome inactivation. J Natl Cancer Inst 1992; 84(23): 1793

105 Mok C H, Tsao S W, Knapp R C, Fishbaugh P M, Lau C C. Unifocal origin of advanced human epithelial ovarian cancers. Cancer Res 1992; 52(18): 5119

106 Kohler M F, Marks J R, Wiseman R W et al. Spectrum of mutation and frequency of allelic deletion of the p53 gene in ovarian cancer. J Natl Cancer Inst 1993; 85(18): 1513

107 Milner B J, Allan L A, Eccles D M et al. p53 mutation is a common genetic event in ovarian carcinoma. Cancer Res 1993; 53(9): 2128

108 Kihana T, Tsuda H, Teshima S, Okada S, Matsuura S, Hirohashi S. High incidence of p53 gene mutation in human ovarian cancer and its association with nuclear accumulation of p53 protein and tumor DNA aneuploidy. Jap J Cancer Res 1992; 83(9): 978

109 Kupryjanczyk J, Thor A D, Beauchamp R et al. p53 gene mutations and protein accumulation in human ovarian cancer. Proc Natl Acad Sci USA 1993; 90(11): 4961

110 Naito M, Satake M, Sakai E et al. Detection of p53 gene mutations in human ovarian and endometrial cancers by polymerase chain reaction-single strand conformation polymorphism analysis. Jap J Cancer Res 1992; 83(10): 1030

111 Eccles D M, Cranston G, Steel C M, Nakamura Y, Leonard R C. Allele losses on chromosome 17 in human epithelial ovarian carcinoma. Oncogene 1990; 5(10): 1599

112 Russell S E, Hickey G I, Lowry W S, White P, Atkinson R J. Allele loss from chromosome 17 in ovarian cancer. Oncogene 1990; 5(10): 1581

113 Jacobs I J, Smith S A, Wiseman R W et al. A deletion unit on chromosome 17q in epithelial ovarian tumors distal to the familial breast/ovarian cancer locus. Cancer Res 1993; 53(6): 1218

114 Sato T, Saito H, Morita R, Koi S, Lee J H, Nakamura Y. Allelotype of human ovarian cancer. Cancer Res 1991; 51(19): 5118

115 Saito H, Inazawa J, Saito S et al. Detailed deletion mapping of chromosome 17q in ovarian and breast cancers: 2-cM region on 17q21.3 often and commonly deleted in tumors. Cancer Res 1993; 53(14): 3382

116 Foulkes W D, Ragoussis J, Stamp G W, Allan G J, Trowsdale J. Frequent loss of hetero-zygosity on chromosome 6 in human ovarian carcinoma. Br J Cancer 1993; 67(3): 551

117 Saito S, Saito H, Koi S et al. Fine-scale deletion mapping of the distal long arm of chromosome 6 in 70 human ovarian cancers. Cancer Res 1992; 52(20): 5815

118 Zheng J P, Robinson W R, Ehlen T, Yu M C, Dubeau L. Distinction of low grade from high grade human ovarian carcinomas on the basis of losses of heterozygosity on chromosomes 3, 6, and 11 and HER-2/neu gene amplification. Cancer Res 1991; 51(15): 4045

119 Foulkes W D, Campbell I G, Stamp G W, Trowsdale J. Loss of heterozygosity and amplification on chromosome 11q in human ovarian cancer. Br J Cancer 1993; 67(2): 268

120 Foulkes W D, Black D M, Stamp G W, Solomon E, Trowsdale J. Very frequent loss of heterozygosity throughout chromosome 17 in sporadic ovarian carcinoma. Int J Cancer 1993; 54(2): 220

121 Lee J H, Kavanagh J J, Wildrick D M, Wharton J T, Blick M. Frequent loss of heterozygosity on chromosomes 6q, 11, and 17 in human ovarian carcinomas. Cancer Res 1990; 50(9): 2724

122 Li S B, Schwartz P E, Lee W H, Yang-Feng T L. Allele loss at the retinoblastoma locus in human ovarian cancer. J Natl Cancer Inst 1991; 83(9): 637

123 Yang-Feng T L, Li S, Han H, Schwartz P E. Frequent loss of heterozygosity on chromosomes Xp and 13q in human ovarian cancer. Int J Cancer 1992; 52(4): 575

124 Yang-Feng T L, Han H, Chen K C et al. Allelic loss in ovarian cancer. Int J Cancer 1993; 54(4): 546

125 Eccles D M, Gruber L, Stewart M, Steel C M, Leonard R C. Allele loss on chromosome 11p is associated with poor survival in ovarian cancer. Dis Mark 1992; 10(2): 95

126 Eccles D M, Russell S E, Haites N E et al. Early loss of heterozygosity on 17q in ovarian cancer. The Abe ovarian cancer genetics group. Oncogene 1992; 7(10): 2069

127 Eccles D M, Brett L, Lessells A et al. Overexpression of the p53 protein and allele loss at 17p13 in ovarian carcinoma. Br J Cancer 1992; 65(1): 40

128 Vandamme B, Lissens W, Amfo K et al. Deletion of chromosome 11p13–11p15.5 sequences in invasive human ovarian cancer is a subclonal progression factor. Cancer Res 1992; 52(23): 6646

129 Viel A, Giannini F, Tumiotto L, Sopracordevole F, Visentin M C, Boiocchi M. Chromosomal localisation of two putative 11p oncosuppressor genes involved in human ovarian tumours. Br J Cancer 1992; 66(6): 1030

130 Cliby W, Ritland S, Hartmann L et al. Human epithelial ovarian cancer allelotype. Cancer Res 1993; 53(suppl 10): 2393

131 Ehlen T, Dubeau L. Loss of heterozygosity on chromosomal segments 3p, 6q and 11p in human ovarian carcinomas. Oncogene 1990; 5(2): 219

132 Chenevix-Trench G, Leary J, Kerr J et al. Frequent loss of heterozygosity on chromosome 18 in ovarian adenocarcinoma which does not always include the DCC locus. Oncogene 1992; 7(6): 1059

133 Phillips N, Ziegler M, Saha B, Xynos F. Allelic loss on chromosome 17 in human ovarian cancer. Int J Cancer 1993; 54(1): 85

134 Tavassoli M, Ruhrberg C, Beaumount V et al. Whole chromosome 17 loss in ovarian cancer. Genes Chromosom Cancer 1993; 8: 195–198

135 Osborne R J, Leech V. Polymerase chain reaction allelotyping of human ovarian cancer. Br J Cancer 1994; 69: 429–438

136 Sandles L G, Shulman L P, Elias S et al. Endometrial adenocarcinoma: genetic analysis suggesting heritable site-specific uterine cancer. Gynecol Oncol 1992; 47(2): 167

137 Lukes A S, Kohler M F, Pieper C F et al. Multivariable analysis of DNA ploidy, p53, and HER-2/neu as prognostic factors in endometrial cancer. Cancer 1994; 73(9): 2380

138 Ikeda M, Watanabe Y, Nanjoh T, Noda K. Evaluation of DNA ploidy in endometrial cancer. Gynecol Oncol 1993; 50(1): 25

139 Melchiorri C, Chieco P, Lisignoli G, Marabini A, Orlandi C. Ploidy disturbances as an early indicator of intrinsic malignancy in endometrial carcinoma. Cancer 1993; 72(1): 165

140 Kohler M F, Berchuck A, Davidoff A M et al. Overexpression and mutation of p53 in endometrial carcinoma. Cancer Res 1992; 52(6): 1622

141 Honda T, Kato H, Imamura T et al. Involvement of p53 gene mutations in human endometrial carcinomas. Int J Cancer 1993; 53(6): 963

142 Enomoto T, Fujita M, Inoue M et al. Alterations of the p53 tumor suppressor gene and its association with activation of the c-K-ras-2 protooncogene in premalignant and malignant lesions of the human uterine endometrium. Cancer Res 1993; 53(8): 1883

143 Okamoto A, Sameshima Y, Yamada Y et al. Allelic loss on chromosome 17p and p53 mutations in human endometrial carcinoma of the uterus. Cancer Res 1991; 51(20): 5632

144 Risinger J I, Dent G A, Ignar-Trowbridge D et al. p53 gene mutations in human endometrial carcinoma. Mol Carcin 1992; 5(4): 250

145 Kohler M F, Nishii H, Humphrey P A et al. Mutation of the p53 tumor-suppressor gene is not a feature of endometrial hyperplasias. Am J Obstet Gynecol 1993; 169(3): 690

146 Duggan B D, Felix J C, Muderspach L I, Tsao J L, Shibata D K. Early mutational activation of the c-Ki-ras oncogene in endometrial carcinoma. Cancer Res 1994; 54(6): 1604

147 Sasaki H, Nishii H, Takahashi H et al. Mutation of the Ki-ras protooncogene in human endometrial hyperplasia and carcinoma. Cancer Res 1993; 53(8): 1906

148 Mizuuchi H, Nasim S, Kudo R, Silverberg S G, Greenhouse S, Garrett C T. Clinical implications of K-ras mutations in malignant epithelial tumors of the endometrium. Cancer Res 1992; 52(10): 2777

149 Fujimoto I, Shimizu Y, Hirai Y et al. Studies on ras oncogene activation in endometrial carcinoma. Gynecol Oncol 1993; 48(2): 196

150 Ignar-Trowbridge D, Risinger J I, Dent G A et al. Mutations of the Ki-ras oncogene in endometrial carcinoma. Am J Obstet Gynecol 1992; 167(1): 227

151 Enomoto T, Inoue M, Perantoni A O et al. K-ras activation in premalignant and malignant epithelial lesions of the human uterus. Cancer Res 1991; 51(19): 5308

152 Hetzel D J, Wilson T O, Keeney G L, Roche P C, Cha S S, Podratz K C. HER-2/neu expression: a major prognostic factor in endometrial cancer. Gynecol Oncol 1992; 47(2): 179

153 Borst M P, Baker V V, Dixon D, Hatch K D, Shingleton H M, Miller D M. Oncogene alterations in endometrial carcinoma. Gynecol Oncol 1990; 38(3): 364

154 Berchuck A, Rodriguez G, Kinney R B et al. Overexpression of HER-2/neu in endometrial cancer is associated with advanced stage disease. Am J Obstet Gynecol 1991; 164(1): 15

155 Enomoto T, Fujita M, Inoue M et al. Alterations of the Rb gene and its association with Ki-ras activation and p53 inactivation in endometrial adenocarcinoma. Mol Carcin 1993; 8: 132–137

156 Ford D, Easton D F, Bishop D T, Narod S A, Breast Cancer Linkage Consortium. The risks of cancer in BRCA1 mutation carriers. Am J Hum Genet 1993; 53: A298

157 Easton D, Ford D, Peto J. Inherited susceptibility to breast cancer. In: Fentiman I S, Taylor-Papadimitrious J, eds. Breast Cancer. Cold Spring Harbor New York: Cold Spring Harbor Laboratory Press,

158 Nowak R. Genetic testing set for takeoff. Nature 1994; 265: 464–467

159 Jacobs I J, Ponder B A J. The genetics of ovarian cancer. In: Studd J, Jardine Brown C, eds. The Yearbook of The Royal College of Obstetricians and Gynaecologists. London: RCOG Press, 1993: pp 169–183

160 Plaxe S C, Deligdisch L, Dottino P R, Cohen C J. Ovarian intraepithelial neoplasia demonstrated in patients with stage I ovarian carcinoma. Gynecol Oncol 1990; 38(3): 367

161 Mittal K R, Zeleniuch-Jacquotte A, Cooper J L, Demopoulos R I. Contralateral ovary in unilateral ovarian carcinoma: a search for preneoplastic lesions. Int J Gynecol Pathol 1993; 12(1): 59

162 Resta L, Russo S, Colucci G A, Prat J. Morphologic precursors of ovarian epithelial tumors. Obstet Gynecol 1993; 82(2): 181

163 Puls L E, Powell D E, DePriest P D et al. Transition from benign to malignant epithelium in mucinous and serous ovarian cystadenocarcinoma. Gynecol Oncol 1992; 47(1): 53

164 Crawford L. Prospects for cervical cancer vaccines. In: Lemoine N R, Wright N A, eds. The molecular pathology of cancer. Cold Spring Harbor, New York: Cold Spring Harbor Laboratory Press, 1993: pp 215–229

165 Caldas C, Hahn S A, Hruban R H et al. Detection of K-ras mutations in stool of patients with pancreatic adenocarcinoma and pancreatic duct hyperplasia. Cancer Res 1994; 54: 3568–3573

166 Mao L, Hruban R H, Boyle J O, Tockman M, Sidransky D. Detection of oncogene mutations in sputum precedes diagnosis of lung cancer. Cancer Res 1994; 54: 1634–1637

167 Sidransky D, Von Eschenbach A, Tsai Y et al. Identification of p53 mutations in bladder cancers and urine samples. Science 1991; 252: 706–709

168 Sidransky D, Tokino T, Hamilton S R et al. Identification of ras oncogene mutations in the stool of patients with curable colorectal tumours. Cancer 1992; 256: 102–104

169 Dodson M K, Hartmann L C, Cliby W A et al. Comparison of loss of heterozygosity patterns in invasive low-grade and high-grade epithelial ovarian carcinomas. Cancer Res 1993; 53: 4456–4460
170 Culver K W et al. In vivo gene transfer with retroviral vector-producer cells for treatment of experimental brain tumours. Science 1992; 256: 1550–1552
171 Freeman S M et al. The 'bystander effect': tumour regression when a fraction of the tumour mass is genetically modified. Cancer Res 1993; 53: 5274–5283
172 Harris C C, Hollstein M. Clinical implications of the p53 tumor-suppressor gene. N Engl J Med 1993; 329: 1318–1327
173 Zhang Y et al. Retroviral vector-mediated transduction of K-ras antisense RNA into human lung cancer cells inhibits expression of the malignant phenotype. Hum Gene Ther 1993; 4: 451–460

Index

PROGRESS IN OBSTETRICS AND GYNAECOLOGY
Edited by John Studd

All backlist volumes are available.
You can place your order by contacting your local medical bookseller or the Sales Promotion Department,
Robert Stevenson House, 1-3 Baxter's Place, Leith Walk, Edinburgh EH1 3AF, UK
Tel: (0131) 556 2424

PROGRESS IN OBSTETRICS AND GYNAECOLOGY

Contents of Volume 3

Contents of Volume 4

PROGRESS IN OBSTETRICS AND GYNAECOLOGY

PROGRESS IN OBSTETRICS AND GYNAECOLOGY

PROGRESS IN OBSTETRICS AND GYNAECOLOGY

PROGRESS IN OBSTETRICS AND GYNAECOLOGY

Contents of Volume 11

ISBN 0443 05059 7